28 Update in Intensive Care and Emergency Medicine

Edited by J.-L. Vincent

Springer

Berlin
Heidelberg
New York
Barcelona
Budapest
Hong Kong
London
Milan
Paris
Santa Clara
Singapore
Tokyo

M. R. Pinsky (Ed.)

Applied Cardiovascular Physiology

With 72 Figures and 24 Tables

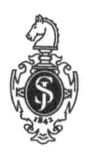

Springer

Series Editor

Prof. Dr. Jean-Louis Vincent
Clinical Director, Department of Intensive Care
Erasme University Hospital
Route de Lennik 808, B-1070 Brussels, Belgium

Volume Editor

Prof. Dr. Michael R. Pinsky
University of Pittsburgh, Dept. of Anesthesiology
and Critical Care Medicine
604 Scaife Hall, Pittsburgh, PA 15261, USA

ISBN-13:978-3-642-64512-9

Library of Congress Cataloging-in-Publication Data applied for

Die Deutsche Bibliothek – CIP-Einheitsaufnahme
Applied cardiovascular physiology / M. R. Pinsky (ed.). – Berlin ; Heidelberg ; New York ;
Barcelona ; Budapest ; Hong Kong ; London ; Milan ; Paris ; Santa Clara ; Singapore ; Tokyo :
Springer, 1997
  (Update in intensive care and emergency medicine ; 28)
  ISBN-13:978-3-642-64512-9   e-ISBN-13:978-3-642-60696-0
  DOI: 10.1007/978-3-642-60696-0

NE: Pinsky, Michael R. [Hrsg.]; GT

Typesetting and printing: Zechnersche Buchdruckerei, Speyer
Bookbinding: J. Schäffer, Grünstadt
SPIN: 10565476   19/3133-5 4 3 2 1 0 – Printed on acid-free paper

Preface

This book represents the collective efforts of several excellent clinician-scientists who have devoted many years of their lives and many hours in each day to the application of physiological principles to the bedside care of critically ill patients. The universal challenge of cardiovascular instability confronts all health care providers who treat patients in an acute care setting. Whether that be in the field or Emergency Department, general ward, operating suite or intensive care unit, all patients carry a common theme of potential life-taking processes which must to identified and treated in a timely fashion or severe morbidity and death rapidly follow.

Since the cardiovascular system subserves the body in maintaining metabolic stability through global and regional blood flow at an adequate pressure to insure appropriate autoregulation of blood flow distribution, it would be difficult to describe the mechanisms of cardiovascular instability their diagnosis and treatment without placing them within the context of overall metabolism and tissue viability. Accordingly, this book has been grouped into four arbitrary subsets. First, we address issues of basic cardiovascular physiology. Classic developments of ventricular pump function and arterial resistance are balanced with newer applications of ventriculo-arterial coupling, right ventricular function, and tissue oxygen delivery. Next, new and established aspects of hemodynamic monitoring are presented with in a clinical-physiologic context. This section is unique in critical care textbooks because it presents issues of applications and limitations in a highly focused fashion, beginning with the rationale for hemodynamic monitoring and progressing through exciting aspects of analogues of hemodynamic variables to echocardiography, the latest and very powerful imaging technique used at the bedside. The third section tackles the important issue; now that you have the patient's data, what are you going to do? Goals of resuscitation have been developed and tested in many large clinical trials. Although some controversies exist, and one.can ever define in exact terms the proper end-points of resuscitation for all patients certain important guide posts have been validated in the recent past which should aid the care giver on focusing cardiovascular support in a rational fashion. Finally, to aid in the management of specific disease process, the final section was developed to focus attention on four important aspects of cardiovascular support: hemorrhagic shock, cardiogenic shock, septic shock, and the use of extracorporeal support systems in the management of patients with severe lung injury.

Our goal in this textbook is to comprehensively address the entire area of cardiovascular instability from a pragmatic stand point allowing the clinician at the bedside to deliver care more efficiently and effectively based on recent published data and a firm understanding of cardiovascular pathophysiology.

Pittsburgh, USA, February 1997   *Michael R. Pinsky*

Table of Contents

Goals of Resuscitation

Cardiovascular Support by Hemodynamic Subsets

List of Contributors

Jan Bakker, MD
Department of Intensive Care,
ZcA Lukas Hospital,
PO Box 90 14,
7300 DS Apeldoorn, The Netherlands

S. Beloucif, MD
Department of Anesthesiology,
Hopital Lariboisiere,
2 rue Ambroise Pare,
75475 Paris cx 10, France

Giorgio Berlot, MD
Via dell'Eremo 106/I,
I-34100 Trieste, Italy

Timothy R. Billiar, MD
Department of Surgery,
University of Pittsburgh,
A1O11 PUH,
Pittsburgh PA 15213, USA

Arthur Boujoukos, MD
Division of Critical Care Medicine,
University of Pittsburgh,
612B Scaife Hall,
Pittsburgh PA 15261, USA

Charles Buffington, MD
Department of Anesthesiology,
910 Lilianne Kaufmann Building,
3471 Fifth Avenue,
Pittsburgh PA 15213, USA

Paul Christensen, MD
Department of Intensive Care,
Glostrup University Hospital,
2600 Glostrup, Denmark

Bernard Cholley, MD
Departement d'Anesthesiologie,
Hopital Lariboisiere,
2 rue Ambroise Pare,
75475 Paris Cx 10, France

Jean-Francois Dhainaut, MD PhD
Service de Reanimation Polyvalénte,
Groupe Hospitalier Cochin,
27 rue du Fg. St. Jacques,
F-75674 Paris cedex 14, France

John Gorcsan III, MD
Department of Cardiology,
University of Pittsburgh,
548 Scaife Hall,
Pittsburgh PA 15261, USA

Johan B. J. Groenveld, MD
ICU, Free University Hospital,
De Boelelaan 1117,
NL-1081 HV Amsterdam,
The Netherlands

John A. Kellum, MD
Division of Critical Care Medicine,
University of Pittsburgh,
640B Scaife Hall,
Pittsburgh PA 15261, USA

Sheldon Magder, MD
Department of Cardiology,
McGill University,
Royal Victoria Hospital,
687 Pine Avenue W,
Montreal Quebec H3A 1A1, Canada

A. Meier-Hellmann, MD
Klinik für Anästhesiologie und
Intensivtherapie, Klinikum der
Friedrich-Schiller-Universität Jena,
Bachstr. 18, 07740 Jena, Germany

Laurel A. Omert, MD
Department of Surgery,
University of Pittsburgh,
A 1 O 11 PUH,
Pittsburgh PA 15213, USA

X   List of Contributors

Didier Payen, MD
Departement d'Anesthesiologie,
Hopital Lariboisiere,
2 rue Ambroise Pare,
75475 Paris Cx 10, France

Azriel Perel, MD
Department of Anesthesiology and
Intensive Care Medicine,
Sheba Medical Center,
Tel Hashomer, Israel 52621

Antonio Pesenti, MD
Institute of Anesthesia,
Ospedale San Gerardo,
Via Donzetti 106,
20052 Monza, Italy

Michael R. Pinsky, MD
Division of Critical Care Medicine,
University of Pittsburgh,
604 Scaife Hall,
Pittsburgh PA 15261, USA

Konrad Reinhart, MD
Klinik für Anästhesiologie und
Intensivtherapie, Klinikum der
Friedrich-Schiller-Universität Jena,
Bachstr. 18, 07740 Jena, Germany

Paul Rogers, MD
Department of Anesthesia,
Veterans Affairs Medical Center,
University Drive C,
Pittsburgh PA 15240, USA

Kenneth P. Rothfield, MD
Department of Anesthesiology,
University of Pittsburgh,
604 Scaife Hall,
Pittsburgh PA 15261, USA

Jukka Takala, MD
Department of Intensive Care,
Kuopio University Hospital,
PO Box 1777, SF-70211 Kuopio,
Finland

B. Vallet, MD
Laboratoire de Pharmacologie,
Centre Hospitalier Regional
Universitaire,
1 Place de verdun,
Lille 59065 Cedex, France

Jean-Louis Vincent, MD PhD
Department of Intensive Care,
Erasme University Hospital,
Route de Lennik 808,
B-1070 Brussels, Belgium

Basic Cardiovascular Physiology

Left Ventricular Pump Function

C. W. Buffington

Introduction

The heart is a cleverly designed organ that propells blood around the body. Satisfactory performance depends on competent cardiac valves and powerful contraction of cardiac muscle. The heart's performance is often compared to that of a hydraulic pump where efficiency is computed as the ratio of work performed to oxygen consumed. Any understanding of the factors governing left ventricular performance must begin with the events of the cardiac cycle.

Events of the Cardiac Cycle

The events of the cardiac cycle are shown in Fig. 1 in a format initiated by Carl Wiggers. Ventricular volume during diastole is enhanced by atrial contraction. Ventricular pressure increases during isovolumic systole until it exceeds aortic pressure. Then the aortic valve opens, and blood is ejected into the aorta. The active tension generated by the fibers in the ventricular wall is proportional to LV pressure and volume and inversely proportional to wall thickness as modelled by Laplace's law. Contraction of the papillary muscles during systole helps maintain apposition of the mitral valve leaflets. Active tension reaches a maximum early in systole when the ventricle is large, even though maximum aortic pressure occurs later. Ejection is followed by isovolumic relaxation which starts when the aortic valve closes and lasts until the mitral valve opens. Vigorous contractions deform elastic elements in the ventricular wall; early in diastole, the relaxation of these elements creates a suction effect that helps move blood into the ventricular cavity from the left atrium. The ventricle fills almost completely early in diastole. Tachycardia can limit late filling. End-diastolic pressure is relatively easily measured in clinical practice and often used as a substitute for end-diastolic volume. There may not be a predictable relation between these two variables.

LV Pressure-Volume Relations

The events of the cardiac cycle can be thought of as loops in the pressure volume plane (Fig. 2). Each loop is bounded by the diastolic relation between pressure

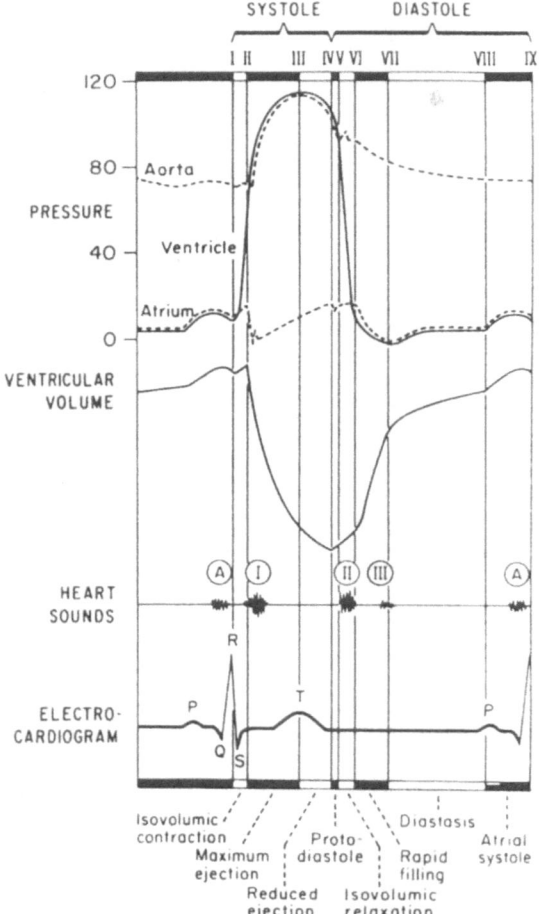

Fig. 1. Events of the cardiac cycle in the format of Dr. Carl Wiggers. [From Katz (1992) with permission]

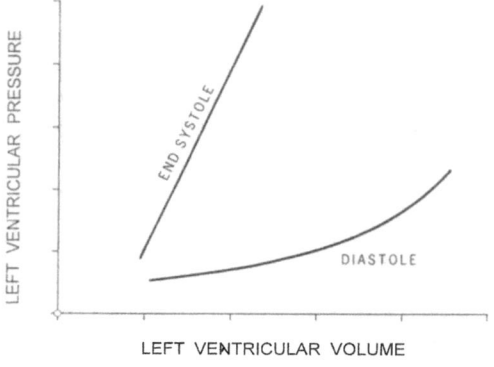

Fig. 2. The left ventricular pressure-volume plane. Each contraction begins on the diastolic relation and finishes on the end-systolic line. These "boundaries" change depending on the diastolic compliance and contractile state of the ventricle

and volume (an indication of ventricular compliance) and the end-systolic relation (a measure on ventricular contractility). Each heart beat starts on the diastolic relation and ends somewhere on the end-systolic relation depending on the afterload imposed on the ventricle (Fig. 3). Stroke volume is the horizontal distance between these points, and ejection fraction is the ratio of stroke volume to end-diastolic volume. The processes that determine these interactions are described below.

Preload

A fundamental property of the heart is that increases in myofibril length during diastole produces a more vigorous contraction during the subsequent systole. If the ventricle is not allowed to empty, this enhancement translates into increased pressure generation. If ejection occurs, then stroke work is increased (Fig. 4). The traditional 2-dimensional description of this phenomenon is the Frank-Starling relation in which initial length (or some co-variant) is plotted against stroke volume. This description is adequate in the normal heart because stroke volume is

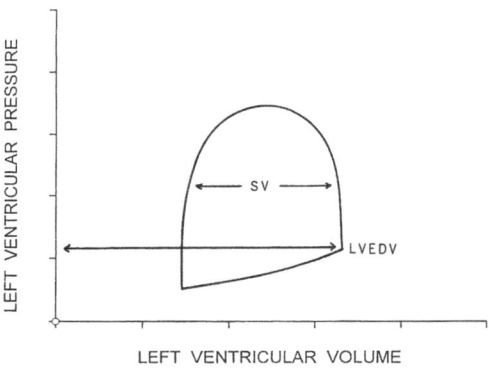

Fig. 3. A single heart beat forms a loop in the pressure-volume plane. The horizontal distance from the left ventricular end-diastolic volume (LVEDV) to the end-systolic line (not shown) is the stroke volume (SV). The area inside the loop is the stroke work. The quotient of SV and LVEDV is the ejection fraction

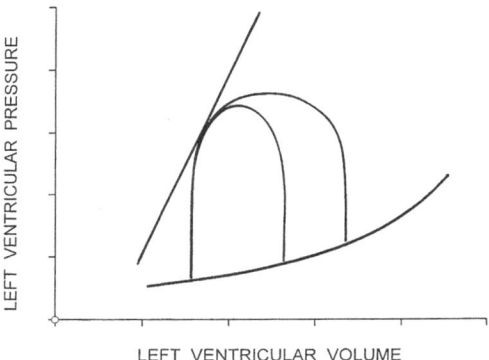

Fig. 4. Increases in end-diastolic volume increase stroke volume when afterload and contractility stay constant

not much affected by afterload (see below); however, in the failing heart, pump function is better described by the relation between preload and stroke work (the product of stroke volume and the average ventricular pressure during ejection). This refinement was suggested by Sarnoff.

Basis of Starling's Law

Individual sarcomeres generate force that is directly proportional to their initial length over the range of 1.6 to 2.4 µM. Experiments in "skinned" myocytes devoid of their cell membrane allow careful control of intercellular calcium and reveal that the force generated by a given intracellular Ca^{++} concentration is increased at longer sarcomere lengths (Fig. 5). This is evidence that the sensitivity of Troponin C to Ca^{++} is altered by the physical change in sarcomere length. The exis-

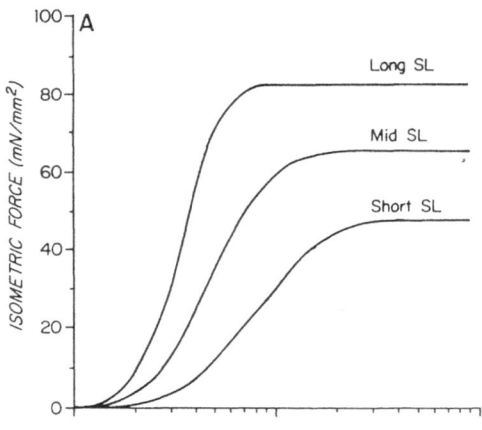

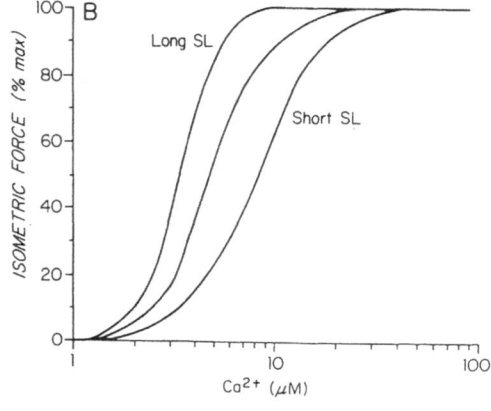

Fig. 5. Isometric force generated by an isolated strip of cardiac muscle is greater at a given intracellular Ca^{++} level when the strip is stretched to a longer segment length (SL) before contraction. This is the basis of the Frank-Starling relation in the heart. [From Huntsman and Feigl (1989) with permission]

tence of length-dependent variations in calcium sensitivity of the contractile proteins has blurred the distinction between two types of regulation: control by changing initial muscle length, and control by changing myocardial contractility. Both can now be explained by variations in excitation-contraction coupling. The connective tissue within the heart muscle combined with the pericardium limits the length of sarcomeres to around 2.5 µM. A decrease in active tension generation beyond this length (the "descending limb" of the Frank-Starling relation) probably results from tissue disruption in isolated muscle preparations and from subendocardial ischemia in intact models.

Afterload

Afterload is estimated by the aortic diastolic pressure that the ventricle must overcome to eject blood. Total peripheral resistance (MAP/CO) provides another way to estimate afterload and is a better reflection of the load faced by the ventricle than systemic vascular resistance ((MAP-CVP)/CO). The active force necessary for ejection is greater in a large ventricle than a small one because, by Laplace's Law, fiber tension increases as volume increases. The normal ventricle's ejection is not influenced much by afterload over a normal range of arterial pressures (Fig. 6). In contrast, a failing ventricle's output may be dramatically decreased if afterload increases (Fig. 7).

Contractility

The vigor of cardiac contraction depends not only on preload, but also on a strange and mystical concept called cardiac contractility. Everyone has an intuitive concept of contractility, and it is easy to see the effects of calcium, norepinephrine (which increase contractility) or failure (which decreases it). However, it is difficult to sort out whether contractility has changed with an intervention, because ventricular performance is influenced strongly by both preload and

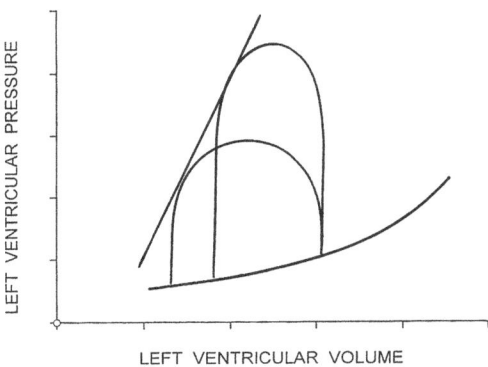

Fig. 6. Increases in afterload change the shape of the pressure-volume loop but do not alter stroke volume much in a heart with normal contractility

LEFT VENTRICULAR VOLUME

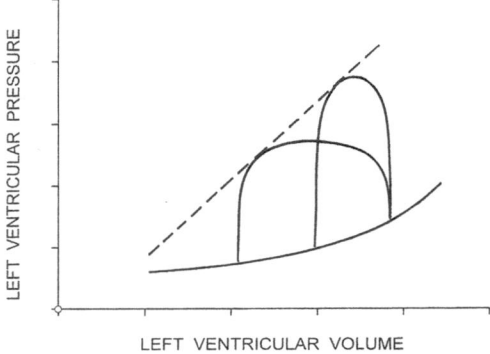

Fig. 7. Increases in afterload dramatically reduce stroke volume when contractility is depressed, such as in cases of heart failure. The decrease in contractility is reflected in the reduced slope of the end-systolic pressure-volume relation (*dashed line*)

afterload, cardiovascular variables that are difficult to control in the clinical setting. One approach to access contractility that was popularized by Sarnoff is to plot LV stroke work against end-diastolic pressure (Fig. 8). Thus preload (x-axis) and afterload are included in the analysis. Clear changes can be seen in such plots when a positive (or negative) inotropic agent is given. On the other hand, the curvalinearity of these plots complicates analysis of treatment effects. The use of end-diastolic volume instead of pressure as the x-axis variable linearizes the plots (Fig. 9) because of the exponential relation between LV diastolic pressure and volume (Fig. 10). This approach yields an updated Sarnoff curve called the "preload recruitable stroke work (PRSW) relation". The linearity of the relations simplifies statistical analysis of treatment effects. Technically, these approaches should be called "load inclusive" rather than "load independent" indexes of contractility.

An approach to defining contractility popularized by Suga and Sagawa uses the relation of ventricular pressure to ventricular volume at end systole (ESPVR). This relation is obtained from sequential heart beats in which preload (or afterload) is progressively varied. The slope of the ESPVR is termed "end-systolic elastance" (Ees) and increases with increasing contractility. "Elastance" is a term

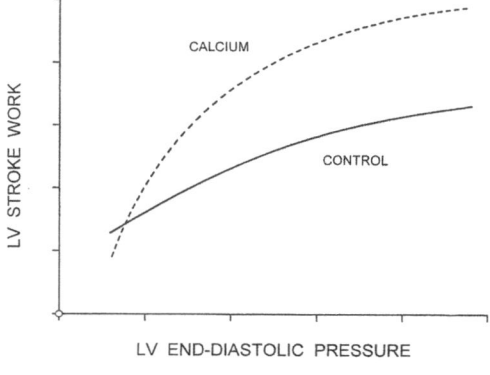

Fig. 8. Stroke work is plotted as a function of left ventricular end-diastolic pressure (LVEDP), an approach to quantifying myocardial contractility popularized by Sarnoff. Administration of calcium increases the stroke work obtained at a given LVEDP by increasing contractility (*dashed line*)

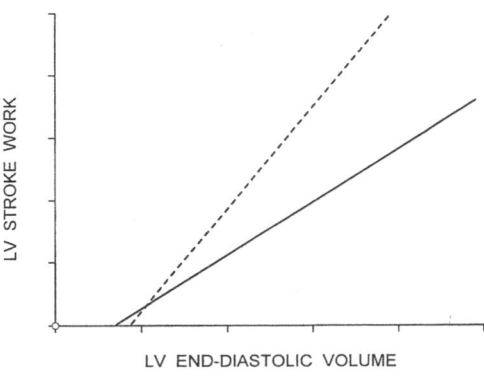

Fig. 9. Plotting stroke work against end-diastolic volume instead of pressure results in linear relations for control data (*solid line*) as well as those with calcium (*dashed line*). The new plot is called "preload recruitable stroke work" (PRSW). The data are the same as in Fig. 8

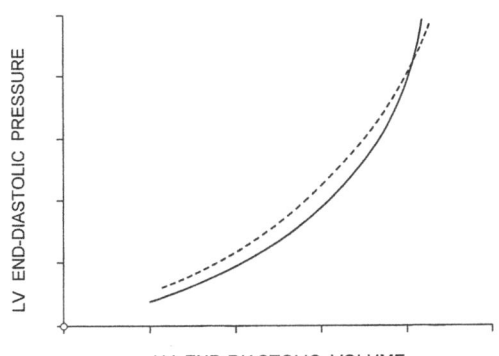

Fig. 10. The PRSW data are linear because volume is used as the independent variable instead of pressure

from engineering that is synonymous with "stiffness". Engineers like to imagine that the heart muscle stiffens in a progressive way that imparts energy to the blood in the LV cavity during systole and ultimately propells some of it out of the heart. The ratio of instantaneous ventricular volume to pressure (elastance) can be plotted over time to further characterize the process of contraction and relaxation. This approach avoids the problem of defining the precise end of systole that is necessary for an accurate measurement of "end-systolic elastance" and thus provides more reliable information about the level of contractility. However, none of these approaches is readily used in the routine care of patients because of the difficulty of measuring LV volume.

Oxygen Consumption

The amount of oxygen consumed by the myocardium per unit time is a good measure of ATP produced by oxidative metabolism. Even though oxidation of a gram of fat produces twice the ATP produced by oxidation of the same amount of carbohydrate or protein, it also requires twice the amount of oxygen. The efficiency of LV contraction can be estimated as the ratio of work produced to oxygen consumed. Several problems beset this analysis, however. For example, even a non-beating ventricle consumes a basal amount of oxygen for protein synthesis. A beating ventricle that is empty and does no external work has an additional component of oxygen consumption related to excitation-contraction coupling and the pumping of calcium. Changes in contractility affect this component by altering the amount of calcium released from the sarcoplasmic reticulum with each heart beat that subsequently must be actively pumped back in. Even when these components are taken into account, the relation between external work and oxygen consumption is not regular because the ventricle stretches internal elastic components during contraction and, hence, wastes energy on internal work. Suga has provided a useful conceptual approach to the problem (Fig. 11) based on experiments in which oxygen consumption was found to be related to the pressure-volume area (PVA), a sum of the area accounted for by external work and that related to internal work or "potential energy" (Fig. 12). This approach clarifies the concept that "pressure work" is more expensive (in terms of oxygen consumption) that "volume work" (Figs. 13, 14). Even if the product of stroke volume and ejection pressure is constant for the two conditions, the internal work

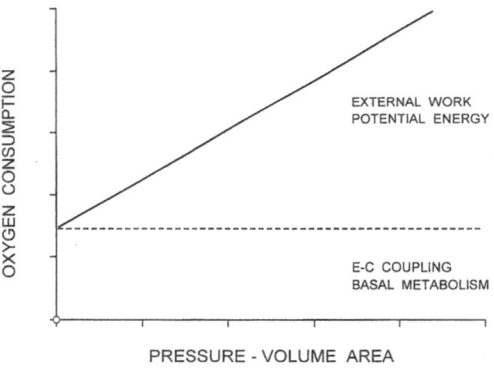

Fig. 11. Suga's approach to partitioning the components of myocardial oxygen consumption. The dashed line represents the amount of oxygen consumed by excitation-contraction (EC) coupling and basal metabolism, a value influenced by temperature and contractile state. The solid line represents an additional component due to internal and external work

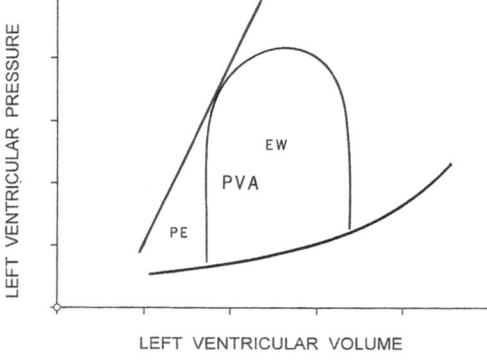

Fig. 12. The Pressure-Volume Area (PVA) is defined as the sum of external work (EW) and the small triangular area labeled PE for "potential energy", a value related to "internal work"

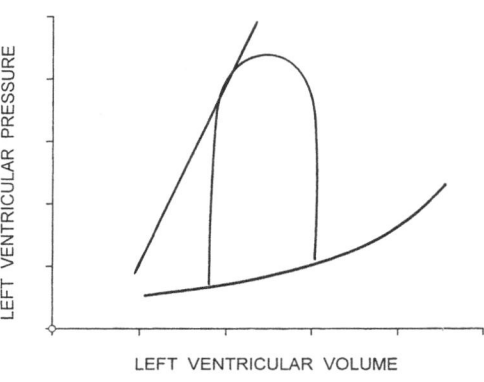

Fig. 13. Increased afterload results in increased oxygen use related to internal work, reflected in a larger PE area. Hence the concept that "pressure work is expensive" in terms of oxygen consumption

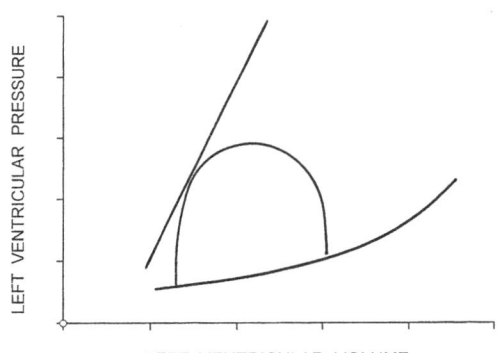

Fig. 14. In contrast to Fig. 13, reduced afterload reduces the size of the PE area. Hence the concept that "volume work is less expensive than pressure work". The stroke work areas of Figures 13 and 14 are drawn to be equivalent

contributing to the potential energy term is much greater when pressure is elevated than when stroke volume is increased.

Pathophysiology

Ischemia rapidly reduces myocardial contractile force generation, a potential disaster if the entire ventricle is affected. Fortunately, however, only a segment related to one coronary artery is usually involved, producing a region of akinesis or dyskinesis. The remainder of the ventricle compensates for this reduced function, although cardiogenic shock may occur in severe cases. The ischemic region often bulges during systole, absorbing energy that would normally go into ejection. When ventricular pressure falls at the start of diastole, the ischemic region may manifest a weak, late contraction (Fig. 15). This heterogeneity confounds interpretation of regional contraction during systole by "unloading" the active elements. It also confounds interpretation of various pressure-based indices of relaxation because the late, weak contraction supports ventricular pressure. If infarction results, the scar tissue is not only non-contractile, but also stiff, reducing ventricular filling.

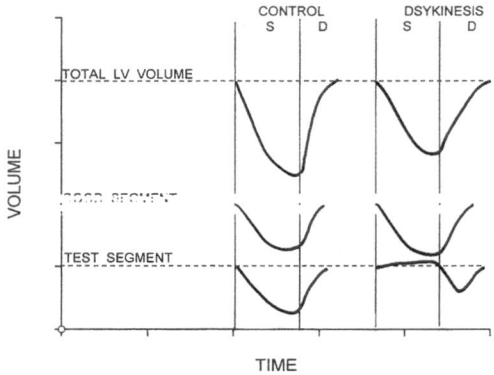

Fig. 15. Dyskinesis of a segment of myocardium reduces stroke volume of the entire left ventricle and complicates pressure-based analysis of LV relaxation. S = systole, D = diastole

If ischemia is of limited duration, then myocardial "stunning" occurs. Contraction is reduced from normal in post-ischemic myocardium. Ischemia and reperfusion cause widespread damage to the cell, mediated in part by free-radicals generated at the time of re-oxygenation. Damage to the myofibrils results in decreased calcium sensitivity and less force generation. Stunned myocardium displays creep, meaning that end-diastolic segment length will be increased at any given diastolic pressure. Paradoxically, the muscle is less stretchy when creep sets in, so the ventricle appears less distensible rather than more. Stunned myocardium resembles failing myocardium in that it displays a reduced response to increased preload. Response to afterload is normal, however. Stunned myocardium is less "efficient" (in the strict sense of oxygen consumed per unit of external work produced) than normal myocardium, as a result of increased oxygen cost to handle raised intracellular calcium levels, an effect that is reflected in the E–C coupling component of Suga's framework (Fig. 11). Stunned myocardium responds to inotropic stimulation with increased contraction, although the dose-response curve is shifted to the right. Inotropic stimulation does not produce ischemia in stunned myocardium.

Conclusion

The interplay of preload, afterload, and contractility determine the pump performance of the left ventricle. These concepts are easily understood on an intuitive basis even though precise characterization is difficult. The use of the pressure-volume paradigm provides a useful framework for the concepts.

References

Glower DD, Spratt JA, Snow ND, Kabas JS, Davis JW, Olsen CO, Tyson GS, Sabiston DC, Rankin JS (1985) Linearity of the Frank-Starling relationship in the intact heart: the concept of preload recruitable stroke work. Circulation 71:994–1009

Huntsman LL, Feigl EO (1989) Cardiac Mechanics. In: Patton HD, Fuchs AF, Hille B, Scher AM, Steiner R (eds) Textbook of Physiology. 21st ed, W. B. Saunders, Philadelphia, Chapter 39

Kass DA, Maughan WL, Guso ZM, Kono A, Sunagawa K, Sagawa K (1987) Comparative influence of load versus inotropic states on indexes of ventricular contractility: experimental and theoretical analysis based on pressure-volume relationships. Circulation 76 : 1422–1436

Katz AM (1992) Physiology of the Heart. 2nd Edition, Raven Press, New York

Kentish JC, ter Keurs HEDJ, Ricciardi L, Bucx JJJ, Nobel MIM (1986) Comparison between the sarcomere length-force relations of intact and skinned trabeculae from rat right ventricle. Circ Res 58 : 755–768

Ohgoshi Y, Gotto Y, Futaki S, Yaku H, Kawaguchi O, Suga H (1991) Increased oxygen cost of contractility in stunned myocardium of dog. Circ Res 69 : 975–988

Left Ventricular Afterload and Ventriculo-Arterial Coupling

B. Cholley and D. Payen

Ventriculo-Arterial Coupling

The study of the left ventricle and the arterial circulation as a "coupled" system is an engineering concept rather than a medical one. It means the study of the energy transfer between a source and the load attached to it, receiving a part of that energy [1]. The ideal coupling is achieved when the maximum of energy is transferred by the source to the load, with minimal waste in friction and heat. In the case of the heart and the systemic circulation, this supposes that a maximum of the energy produced by the left ventricle is converted into forward flow to perfuse the body organs. The best matching between the source and the load, allowing optimal energy transfer, is governed by the mechanical properties of the two units. For example, a battery connected to an electrical circuit as a load will achieve maximum output power when its internal impedance equals the input impedance of the load [1]. In the cardiovascular system, some insight on ventriculo-arterial coupling and arterial load properties can be obtained by a detailed analysis of instantaneous pressure-flow relationships [2–4]. Such an analysis allows one to describe the arterial load with the aortic input impedance spectrum, to quantify the hydraulic power "thrown" by the left ventricle into the systemic circulation and the efficiency of the arterial tree in converting these bursts of energy into forward flow to perfuse the body organs. Two examples (treatment of hypertension and septic shock) are presented to illustrate how alterations in arterial mechanical properties influence ventriculo-arterial coupling. An other approach to ventriculo-arterial coupling has been derived from the left ventricular and arterial pressure-volume relationships. This approach translates in a very simple graphic representation based on the pressure-volume diagrams and provides a rationale for the physiological values of left ventricular ejection fraction.

Aortic Input Impedance

The most exhaustive representation of arterial load is given by the aortic input impedance spectrum [5, 6]. This approach provides information on the relation between pressure and flow at any frequency of these pulsatile signals. To obtain the impedance spectrum, one needs to decompose pressure and flow into a sum

of elementary sinusoids called harmonics using Fourier transform [7]. Each harmonic is characterized by three elements:
1) *frequency* (always an integer multiple of heart rate, the first harmonic),
2) *magnitude*,
3) *phase* delay or advance relatively to the first harmonic.

Impedance magnitude at each frequency is obtained as the ratio of pressure to flow magnitudes and quantifies the opposition to the corresponding flow harmonic. The impedance magnitude at 0 Hz is the ratio of the steady components of pressure and flow, that is to say mean pressure and mean flow, and is equal to total peripheral resistance (TPR). Impedance phase at each frequency is obtained as the difference between pressure and flow phases. A negative difference is usually observed at low frequencies and indicates a capacitive phenomenon because volume (or flow) leads pressure. Instead, at higher frequencies a positive difference is noted, suggesting a resistive effect at these frequencies. As can be seen in the example of impedance spectrum shown in Fig. 1, impedance magnitude is high for steady flow (Harmonic zero of impedance, or TPR) and falls rapidly as frequency increases. Such a pattern attests for the perfect design of the normal arterial circulation that ensures maintenance of adequate mean blood pressure for organ perfusion together with minimal opposition to pulsatile ejection. These properties are related to arterial geometric and viscoelastic characteristics as well as wave propagation and reflection phenomena [8].

Peripheral Resistance:
An Oversimplification of Arterial Mechanical Properties

Peripheral resistance is the only parameter used by clinicians to characterize the arterial circulation. This simple number, reflecting the level of vasoconstriction or vasodilation, has proved useful for guiding vasoactive therapy in critically ill patients and to correlate with outcome [9]. Total peripheral resistance (TPR) rep-

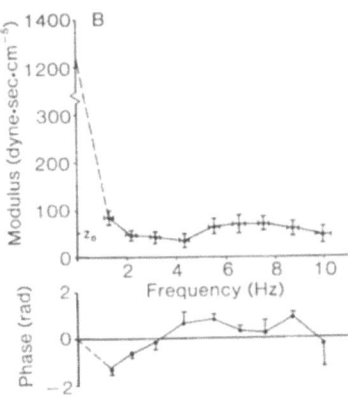

Fig. 1. Averaged impedance spectra obtained from 5 normal human subjects. Note the high value for the magnitude (=modulus) at 0 Hz (=TPR) as opposed to the low values for the different frequencies. (From Nichols et al. [6].)

resents the opposition to mean, continuous flow as it exists at the level of very small vessels, therefore, it is a quantification of arteriolar smooth muscle tone. However, the accuracy of a single resistance model to describe the arterial tree is questionable [10]. According to Poiseuille's Law, TPR is calculated as the ratio of mean pressure to mean flow [11].

$$TPR = \frac{\bar{P}}{\bar{Q}}$$

This method of calculation is analogous to Ohm's Law for a single resistance and direct current. Obviously, the transposition to the arterial tree and pulsatile flow is a gross simplification. The physiological irrelevance of this trivial model of the arterial circulation can be emphasized by the following computerized simulation (Fig. 2) [12]. Using a real aortic flow wave as an input, a single resistance (R) model of the circulation (model 1) would generate a pressure waveform that is morphologically identical to the flow wave, differing only in magnitude by a factor of R. As a consequence, the predicted pressure waveform differs from the measured one by outrageously high systolic values and zero diastolic pressure! Since arterial pressure and flow are pulsatile, additional parameters should be considered to describe arterial load more accurately. When a capacitive element representing compliance (C) is incorporated in the model (Fig. 2, model 2), the predicted pressure waveform begins to exhibit many of the morphological characteristics of its measured counterpart. And if a third element representing characteristic impedance (Z) is introduced (Fig. 2, model 3), the morphologies of the predicted and measured pressure waveforms become very similar. These two additional elements take into account arterial geometric and viscoelastic properties as well as wave propagation-reflection phenomena. These physical properties and phenomena are distributed over the entire vasculature and are represented in our simplified models of the circulation as lumped parameters. For example, arterial compliance incorporates arterial elasticity and geometry as well as wave propagation and reflection phenomena [13]. Characteristic impedance of the aorta, on the other hand, is a function of local aortic material and geometric properties [5, 14]. When instantaneous pressure-flow relationships are to be described accurately, it is very important to include arterial compliance and characteristic impedance in the arterial model [12].

Energy Dissipation in the Arteries

Instantaneous analysis of pressure-flow relationships provides information about energy dissipation within the systemic circulation [8]. The product of pressure by flow has dimensions of power:

$$(mmHg) \times (cm^3 \times s^{-1}) \Leftrightarrow (1333 \text{ dynes} \times cm^{-2}) \times (cm^3 \times s^{-1})$$
$$\Leftrightarrow (1333 \times 10^{-7} \text{ J} \times cm^{-3}) \times (cm^3 \times s^{-1}) \Leftrightarrow 1333 \times 10^{-7} \text{ Watts}$$

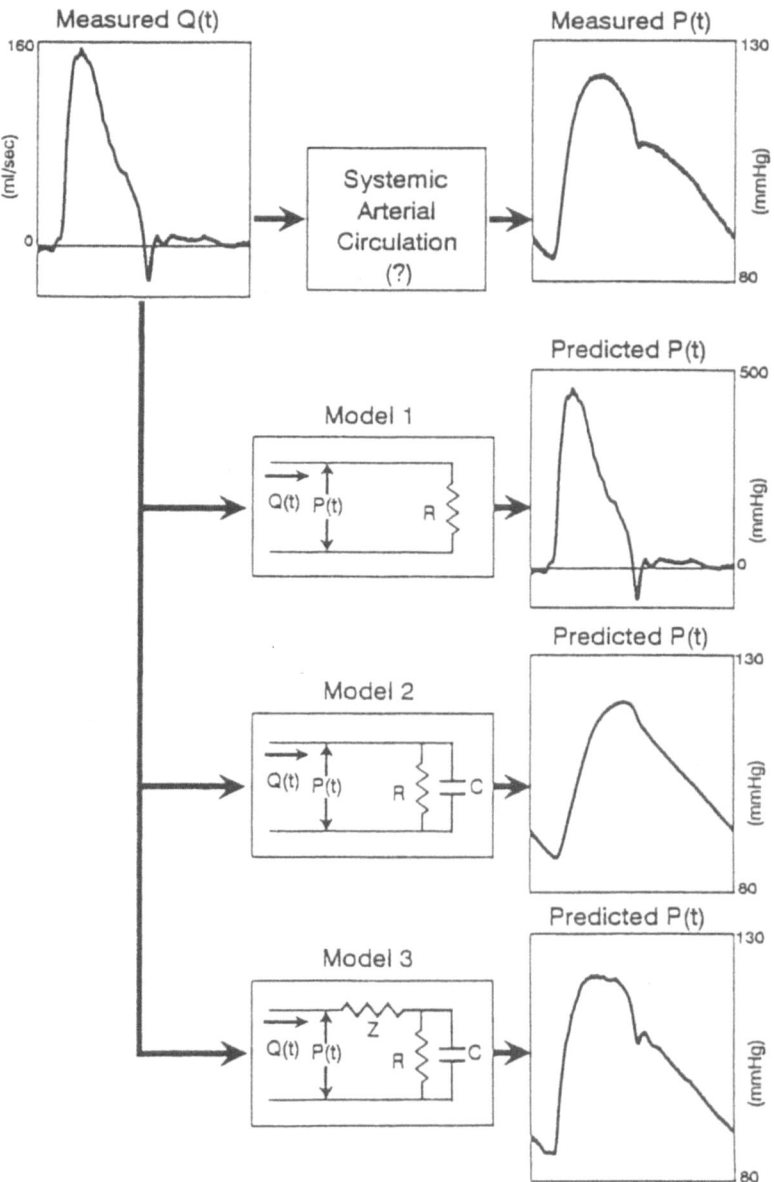

Fig. 2. Conceptual diagram depicting the importance of various components of arterial load in describing instantaneous pressure-flow relations. See text for details. (From Cholley et al. [12].)

The instantaneous product of pressure by flow represents the total hydraulic power, or total energy transferred from the left ventricle to the systemic circulation:

$$\dot{W}_{tot} = \frac{1}{T} \int_0^T P(t)\, Q(t)\, dt$$

The product of mean pressure by mean flow, or steady power, corresponds to the part of that energy that is converted into forward flow, useful for organ perfusion:

$$\dot{W}_{std} = \bar{P} \times \bar{Q}$$

Conversely, the difference between total power and steady power represents the energy that is "wasted" in pulsatile phenomena and is called oscillatory power:

$$\dot{W}_{osc} = \dot{W}_{tot} - \dot{W}_{std}$$

The fraction of energy wasted or percent oscillatory power quantifies the efficiency of energy dissipation in the systemic circulation, and is therefore an index of coupling:

$$\% \, \dot{W}_{osc} = \frac{\dot{W}_{osc}}{\dot{W}_{tot}} \times 100$$

The value for percent oscillatory power is usually close to 10% in normal subjects, attesting for the minor fraction of energy used for purposes other than producing forward flow.

Alterations in Arterial Mechanical Properties and Efficiency of Energy Dissipation

Alterations in arterial mechanical properties occur with aging [15, 16], hypertension [17–19], and certain disease states such as Marfan syndrome [20] or septic shock [21]. How these processes affect cardiac ejection from a mechanical and energetic point of view is an important issue. We will describe here two situations where arterial loading conditions were modified and evaluate the consequences in terms of ventriculo-arterial coupling.

Treatment of Systemic Hypertension

Among the complex alterations in arterial properties that occur during systemic hypertension are elevated peripheral resistance and characteristic impedance, reduced arterial compliance, and abnormal propagation/reflection of pressure and flow waves [17–19]. Despite the high prevalence of hypertension, few data are available regarding how the different antihypertensive drugs affect these parameters [19, 22]. Using Doppler and calibrated subclavian pulse tracings we were able to acquire the instantaneous pressure and flow required for the computation of pulsatile load characteristics (Fig. 3) [23]. In addition, by combining echocardiographic measurements of left ventricular geometry with calibrated subclavian pulse tracings, it is possible to obtain indexes of left ventricular energetics noninvasively [24]. An ACE inhibitor (ramipril), a calcium channel blocker (nifedipine), and a beta-blocker (atenolol) can achieve similar reductions in diastolic pressure, one of the "official" criteria to define hypertension [25], and still have very different effects on arterial properties. In a double blind, placebo-controlled, cross-over study comparing these three drugs in a group of hypertensive African American patients, we found differential responses in heart rate, arterial load characteristics, and left ventricular energetics [12]. Results concerning arterial hemodynamics are presented in Table 1. Both, the steady and pulsatile components of arterial load as well as the integrals of wall stress during ventricular ejection (index of myocardial oxygen consumption, data not shown) decreased with ramipril and nifedipine, but not with atenolol. None of the antihypertensive

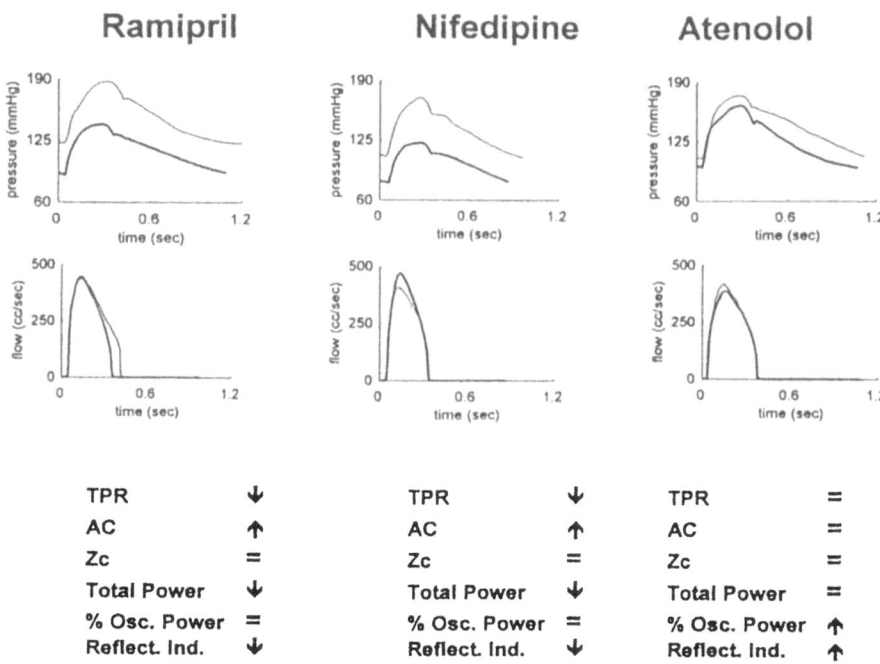

Fig. 3. Representative example of the changes in pressure and flow waveforms observed in a patient before and after 6-week of treatment with ramipril, nifedipine, and atenolol. Qualitative changes in calculated parameters between predrug control (*light line*) and after treatment (*heavy line*) are indicated as ↑ for increase, ↓ for decrease, and = for no change. *TPR* indicates total peripheral resistance; *AC*, arterial compliance; *Zc*, characteristic impedance; *% Osc. Power*, fraction of oscillatory power; *Reflect. Ind.*, reflection index. (From Cholley et al. [12].)

Table 1. Arterial load characteristics, reflection indexes and mechanical power data

	Pre-ramipril	Ramipril	Pre-nifedipine	Nifedipine	Pre-atenolol	Atenolol
TPR	1740 ± 292	1437 ± 290[a]	1744 ± 398	1290 ± 215[a]	1756 ± 451	1722 ± 321[c,d]
AC_L	1.214 ± 0.19	1.569 ± 0.424[a]	1.234 ± 0.253	1.776 ± 0.415[a,b]	1.291 ± 0.278	1.478 ± 0.353[c]
Z_c	107 ± 49	98 ± 31	106 ± 28	92 ± 41	117 ± 46	96 ± 27
Z_1	212 ± 55	167 ± 42[a]	196 ± 42	137 ± 32[a,b]	199 ± 54	204 ± 59[c,d]
Z_2	134 ± 50	101 ± 20[a]	125 ± 33	91 ± 25[a]	130 ± 39	121 ± 29[c,d]
RI_1	0.67 ± 0.08	0.61 ± 0.12	0.65 ± 0.1	0.57 ± 0.15	0.61 ± 0.1	0.64 ± 0.07
RI_2	0.62 ± 0.12	0.55 ± 0.13	0.60 ± 0.1	0.52 ± 0.18	0.57 ± 0.15	0.60 ± 0.07
$\dot{W}_{tot}$	1.99 ± 0.42	1.92 ± 0.49	2.03 ± 0.491	1.88 ± 0.41	2.08 ± 0.42	1.74 ± 0.36
$\dot{W}_{std}$	1.73 ± 0.39	1.65 ± 0.42	1.67 ± 0.4	1.62 ± 0.34	1.8 ± 0.379	1.47 ± 0.29
$\dot{W}_{osc}$	0.26 ± 0.09	0.27 ± 0.08	0.28 ± 0.11	0.25 ± 0.1	0.28 ± 0.11	0.27 ± 0.09
% $\dot{W}_{osc}$	13.4 ± 3.9	14.0 ± 2.1	13.3 ± 3.2	13.2 ± 3.9	13.4 ± 3.9	15.4 ± 2.9

Values are mean ± standard deviation (n = 16). TPR: total peripheral resistance (dyn-sec/cm⁵); AC_L: arterial compliance derived from a linear model (ml/mmHg); Zc: characteristic impedance (dyn-s/cm⁵); Z_1, Z_2: first and second harmonics of aortic input impedance (dyn-sec/cm⁵); RI_1 and RI_2: wave reflection indexes; $\dot{W}_{tot}$, $\dot{W}_{std}$, $\dot{W}_{osc}$: left ventricular total, steady and oscillatory power (Watts); % $\dot{W}_{osc}$: percent of oscillatory power.
[a] p < 0.05, drug vs. pre-drug; [b] p < 0.05, nifedipine vs. ramipril; [c] p < 0.05, atenolol vs. nifedipine; [d] p < 0.05, atenolol vs. ramipril

treatment used in this study resulted in a significant decrease in total hydraulic power. For ramipril and nifedipine, this was the result of a slight increase in cardiac output that counterbalanced the decrease in pressure. For atenolol, the pressure and flow decrements were not sufficient to significantly reduce $\dot{W}_{tot}$. The fraction of the total energy dissipated in pulsation was small ($< 15\%$ of $\dot{W}_{tot}$) and was not further reduced by any antihypertensive treatment. Conflicting results have been published on whether blood pressure reduction in hypertensive patients decreases % $\dot{W}_{osc}$, thereby indicating an improvement in efficiency of power dissipation in the arterial system [6, 19, 22]. Recent theoretical findings however indicate that there are multiple determinants of oscillatory power (e.g. TPR, pulse wave velocity, arterial compliance, heart rate). Thus, offsetting effects of simultaneous changes in these determinants might account for the lack of change observed in % $\dot{W}_{osc}$ after ramipril and nifedipine. In terms of ventriculo-arterial coupling, unaltered total vascular mechanical power at a time myocardial oxygen consumption was reduced indicates an improvement in the efficiency of the cardiovascular system after treatment with ramipril in this group of patients. Similar improvements in efficiency were observed with nifedipine in the subgroup of patients in whom heart rate remained unchanged with this agent.

Septic Shock with and without Fluid Resuscitation

Septic shock is characterized by profound alterations of the cardiovascular system, including low blood pressure, high cardiac output (CO), low TPR and impaired vascular responsiveness to vasoconstrictive agents [26, 27]. Studies that have addressed the effects of septic shock on arterial mechanical properties have mainly characterized arteriolar tone in terms of peripheral resistance. As a result, little information is available during septic shock regarding the pulsatile component of left ventricular vascular load and the way it is affected by fluid resuscitation. Because pulsatile load plays a major role in shaping pressure and flow waveform, alterations in large vessel properties and characteristics of wave propagation/reflection can potentially impair the coupling between the left ventricle and the peripheral circulation. This hypothesis was tested in a rabbit septic shock model induced by endotoxin (EDTX) administration [21]. Animals were studied during three hours following EDTX injection, with (EDTX + fluids) or without (EDTX-alone) fluid resuscitation. Instantaneous pressure and flow were recorded using micromanometers (Millar) and ultrasonic flowmeters (Transonic) located at the aortic root. At 3 hours of EDTX shock, EDTX-alone rabbits had elevated total peripheral resistance ($+30\%$, $p < 0.05$), reduced cardiac output (-40%, $p < 0.05$), and increased aortic characteristic impedance ($+78\%$, $p < 0.05$). In contrast, the EDTX + fluids group responded with decreased TPR (-30%, $p < 0.05$), a tendency to increase CO ($+23\%$), and elevated characteristic impedance ($+46\%$, $p < 0.05$). Input impedance spectra at baseline (control 1) and 3 hours following EDTX injection are presented in Figure 4. The unresuscitated group had an increase in impedance magnitude for all frequencies (Fig. 4, A and B). In contrast, the fluid resuscitated group had a differential response with re-

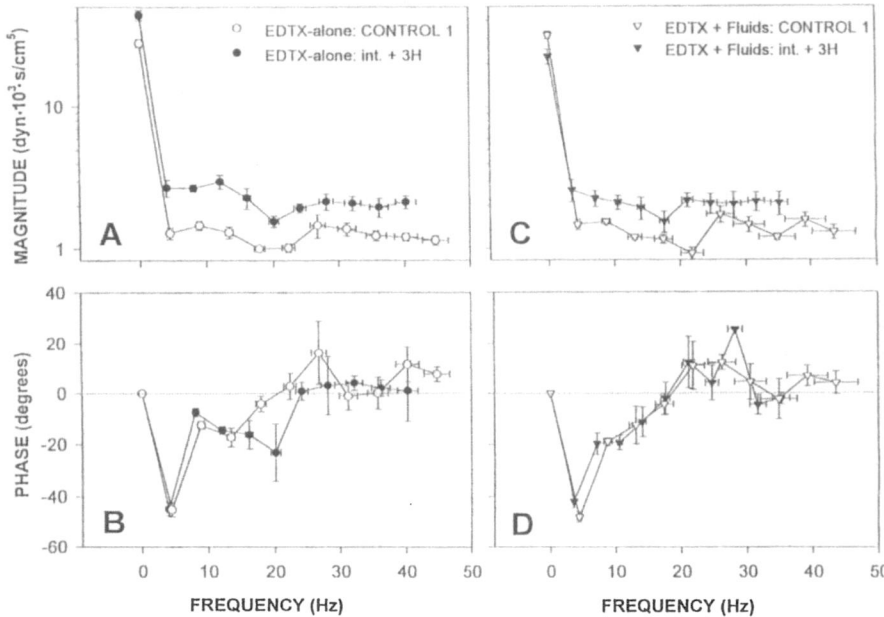

Fig. 4. Aortic impedance spectra (mean ± SE) of unresuscitated (**A** and **B**) and fluid resuscitated (**C** and **D**) rabbits before and 3 hours after EDTX administration. Magnitude spectra are presented with a logarithmic scale. Note that the opposition to pulsatile components of the flow is increased after 3 hours of septic shock in both groups whereas opposition to steady flow (0 Hz component, or TPR) is reduced in the EDTX + fluids group and increased in the EDTX-alone group. (From Cholley et al. [21].)

duced opposition to steady flow (i.e.: 0 Hz) and increased opposition to pulsatile flow (Fig. 4, C and D). This indicates that the mechanical properties of large and small arteries were affected differently during fluid resuscitation. One factor that might contribute to the persistent elevation in characteristic impedance (Zc) is the presence of aortic wall edema during septic shock. Additionally, because smooth muscle tone is a major determinant of both Zc and TPR, the differential response to fluid resuscitation suggested a difference between the responses of aortic and arteriolar smooth muscle tone to increased flow during endotoxemia. EDTX-induced impairment of endothelium dependent vasodilation has been demonstrated in rabbit aorta [28] and in large canine arteries [29]. Thus reflex vasoconstriction may not have been counterbalanced by local flow-induced vasodilatory stimulus, resulting in persistent elevation of large vessel tone. In contrast, Cryer et al. have shown that the dilation ability of third- and fourth-order arterioles of rat cremaster muscle (resistance vessels) is preserved during hyperdynamic endotoxemia [30]. These experiments together with our data corroborate the hypothesis of a differential response between small and large vessels to increased flow during endotoxemia. Vascular mechanical power data obtained at baseline and 3 hours following endotoxin injection are presented in Table 2. The

Table 2. Vascular mechanical power data

		Control 1	Injection + 3H
$\dot{W}_{tot}$	EDTX alone:	57 ± 6	23 ± 4*
	SHAM:	52 ± 4	44 ± 6*
	EDTX + Fluid	46 ± 8	43 ± 9
$\dot{W}_{std}$	EDTX alone:	53 ± 5	20 ± 3*
	SHAM:	48 ± 4	38 ± 5*
	EDTX + Fluid	44 ± 8	39 ± 9
$\dot{W}_{osc}$	EDTX alone:	4 ± 1	3 ± 1
	SHAM:	3 ± 1	4 ± 1
	EDTX + Fluid	3 ± 1	6 ± 1
% $\dot{W}_{osc}$	EDTX alone:	7 ± 1	12 ± 1*
	SHAM:	7 ± 1	10 ± 1
	EDTX + Fluid	7 ± 1	14 ± 3*

Total, steady, and oscillatory powers ($\dot{W}_{tot}$, $\dot{W}_{std}$, and $\dot{W}_{osc}$, respectively; mW) and percent oscillatory power (% $\dot{W}_{osc}$) values (mean ± SEM) obtained at baseline (control 1) and 3 hours after endotoxin administration are presented for all three groups: (1) endotoxin shock without fluid resuscitation (EDTX alone), (2) endotoxin shock with fluid resuscitation (EDTX + Fluids), and (3) Sham-operated animals (SHAM). * $p < 0.05$, vs. control 1.

reduced total power in the EDTX group was a result of reduced arterial pressure and flow. However, the proportion of energy wasted in pulsation (% $\dot{W}_{osc}$) increased. In the EDTX + fluids group, although total power returned to the control value, the percent oscillatory power remained significantly elevated. This marked increase in percent oscillatory power following fluid resuscitation is consistent with the notion that it is directly related to Zc and inversely related to TPR and heart rate [31, 32]. Thus septic shock, both with or without fluid resuscitation, resulted in a reduction in the efficiency of hydraulic power transfer from the left ventricle to the peripheral circulation. Similar effects of increased Zc on ventriculo-arterial coupling have been observed in other pathophysiological conditions [1]. Increased pressure pulsation may also be detrimental from the point of myocardial oxygen consumption. For example, Kelly et al. [33] have shown that for a given stroke volume and mean blood pressure, increased pressure pulsation is associated with increased myocardial oxygen consumption.

Pressure-Volume Relationship and Ventriculo-Arterial Coupling

To analyze the coupling between the heart and the arterial circulation, the mechanical properties of each unit can also be described in terms of pressure-volume relationship. The left ventricular contractility can be characterized by the slope of the end-systolic pressure-volume relation called end-systolic elastance (Ees) [34, 35]. The slope of the vascular end-systolic pressure-volume relationship represents the "effective elastance" of the arterial system (Ea) [36]. By analogy to the coupling between cardiac output and venous return curves, a given hemodynamic situation may be seen as the result of the interaction between ventricular and arterial mechanical characteristics (i.e.: Ees and Ea, respectively). Sunagawa et al. have presented a conceptual framework that illustrates this concept [36]. Arterial elastance (Ea) can be included in the ventricular end-systolic, pressure-volume diagram, so that its origin on the volume axis lies at end-diastolic volume. The intersection of Ea and Ees yields a unique pair of values for stroke volume and Pes, corresponding to that given hemodynamic situation (Fig. 5).

The pressure-volume diagram of the left ventricle also contains information about ventricular energetics [37]. The area contained within the loop itself has the dimensions of work and represents the external work (SW) of the left ventricle. According to basic geometrical rules, the SW area will be maximized when Ees equals Ea, meaning that the mechanical output of the cardiovascular system is optimum in that specific situation [38, 39] (Fig. 5). The area between the end-systolic and end-diastolic P-V relation curves on the origin side of the P-V loop represents the elastic potential energy (PE) of the left ventricle (Fig. 5). The sum of SW and PE is denominated systolic pressure-volume area (PVA) and represents the total mechanical energy generated by the contraction [37]. The PVA has been shown to correlate tightly with myocardial oxygen consumption [40–42]. Therefore, the metabolic efficiency of myocardial contraction may be evaluated as the ratio of SW to PVA [37, 38]. Regarding this issue, the geometrical rules tell us that metabolic efficiency is maximized when the value of Ea is half of that of Ees [38, 39].

Ejection fraction (EF) can be expressed as a function of Ea and Ees [39, 43] such that:

$$EF = \frac{Ees}{Ea + Ees}$$

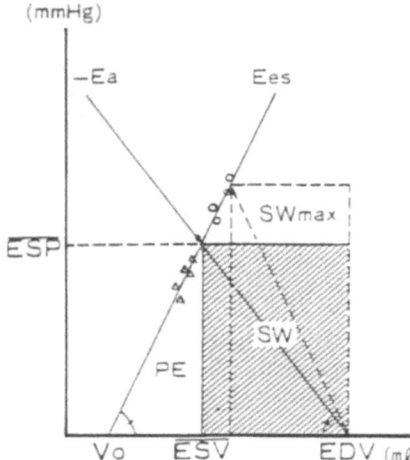

Fig. 5. Schematic representation of ventriculo-arterial coupling on the pressure-volume diagram. The shaded area represents the stroke work (SW) and the triangular area shows end-systolic potential energy (PE). Maximum stroke work (SW max) for a given end-diastolic volume can be determined when the slope of the end-systolic pressure-volume relation (Ees) is assumed to be equal to that of arterial elastance (Ea). (From Asanoi et al. [38].)

From this it results that optimal mechanical efficiency occurs for an ejection fraction of 0.5 and optimal metabolic efficiency is obtained when EF equals 0.67. Most of the "normal" ejection fractions are close to 0.6 suggesting that a normal cardiovascular system is optimizing metabolic efficiency rather than maximizing external work [38, 39, 43]. A low ejection fraction reflects the inability of the cardio-vascular system to match the mechanical properties of the two units in order to work at the lowest energetic cost. This is one of the reasons why an abnormal EF does appear as a potent predictor of cardiovascular mortality [44, 45].

Conclusion

Even though the heart itself has received much more attention than its vascular load, the latter plays a major role in determining the performance of the coupled ventriculo-arterial system. New noninvasive methods provide access to instantaneous pressure and flow measurements in humans. The detailed study of their relationships allows a better understanding of the physiopathologic changes affecting the cardiovascular system. This approach may offer a tool to guide the therapeutic strategy aimed at improving ventriculo-arterial coupling.

The ventricular and arterial end-systolic pressure-volume relationships are also a powerful tool to characterize ventriculo-arterial coupling. The normal cardiovascular system keeps arterial and ventricular mechanical properties such that metabolic efficiency of the circulatory function is optimized. This translates into a normal value for left ventricular ejection fraction close to 0.6. Ejection fraction reflects the adequacy of the ventriculo-arterial coupling rather than the myocardial function.

References

1. Yin F (1987) Ventricular/vascular coupling. Clinical, physiological and engineering aspects. Springer, New York
2. Chiu Y, Arand P, Caroll J (1992) Power-afterload relation in the failing human ventricle. Circ Res 70:530–535
3. Binkley P, Van Fossen D, Nunziata E, Unverferth D, Leier C (1990) Influence of positive inotropic therapy on pulsatile hydraulic load and ventricular-vascular coupling in congestive heart failure. J Am Coll Cardiol 15:1127–1135
4. O'Rourke MF, Avolio AP, Nichols WW (1987) Left ventricular-systemic arterial coupling in humans and strategies to improve coupling in disease states. In: Yin FCP (ed) Ventricular-arterial coupling. Springer, Berlin Heidelberg New York, pp 1–19
5. Milnor WR (1975) Arterial impedance as ventricular afterload. Circ Res 36:565–570
6. Nichols W, Conti R, Walker W, Milnor W (1977) Input impedance of the systemic circulation in man. Circ Res 40:451–458
7. Nichols WW, O'Rourke MF (1990) Measuring principles of arterial waves (ed) Mac Donald's blood flow in arteries. Edward Arnold, pp 143–195
8. Milnor W (1989) Hemodynamics. Williams & Wilkins, Baltimore
9. Groenveld ABJ, Nauta JPP, Thijs LG (1988) Peripheral vascular resistances in septic shock: its relation to outcome. Intens Care Med 14:141–147

10. Lang R, Borrow K, Neuman A, Janzen D (1986) Systemic vascular resistance: an unreliable index of left ventricular afterload. Circulation 74:1114–1123
11. Poiseuille J (1840) Recherches experimentales sur le mouvement des liquides dans les tubes de très petits diamètres. Comptes Rendus Acad Sci 11:1041–1048
12. Cholley B, Shroff S, Sandelski J, Korcarz C, Balasia B, Shelly J, Berger D, Murphy M, Marcus R, Lang R (1995) Differential effects of chronic oral antihypertensive therapies on systemic arterial circulation and ventricular energetics in African-American patients. Circulation 91:1052–1062
13. Berger D, Robinson K, Shroff S (1996) Wave propagation in coupled left ventricle-arterial system. Implications for aortic pressure. Hypertension 27:1079–1089
14. Dujardin J, Stone D, Paul L, Pieper H (1980) Response of systemic arterial input impedance in volume expansion and hemorrhage. Am J Physiol 238:H902–H908
15. Learoyd B, Taylor M (1966) Alteration with age in the viscoelastic properties of human arterial walls. Circ Res 18:278–292
16. Lang R, Cholley B, Korcarz C, Marcus R, Shroff S (1994) Measurements of regional elastic properties of the human aorta: a new application of transesophageal echocardiography with automated border detection and calibrated subclavian pulse tracings. Circulation 90:1875–1882
17. O'Rourke M (1990) Arterial stiffness, systolic blood pressure, and logical treatment for arterial hypertension. Hypertension 15:339–347
18. Liu Z, Ting C-T, Zhu S, Yin FCP (1989) Aortic Compliance in Human Hypertension. Hypertension 129–136
19. Ting C, Brin K, Lin S, Wang S, Chang M, Chiang B, Yin F (1986) Arterial hemodynamics in human hypertension. J Clin Invest 78:1462–1471
20. Yin F, Brin K, Ting C, Pyeritz R (1989) Arterial hemodynamic indexes in Marfan's syndrome. Circulation 79:854–862
21. Cholley B, Lang R, Berger D, Korcarz C, Payen D, Shroff S (1995) Alterations in systemic arterial mechanical properties during septic shock: role of fluid resuscitation. Am J Physiol 269:H375–H384
22. Merillon JP, Fontenier GJ, Lerallut JF, Jaffrin MY, Motte GA, Genain CP, Gourgon RR (1982) Aortic Input Impedance in Normal Man and Arterial Hypertension: its modification during changes in aortic pressure. Cardiovasc Res 646–656
23. Marcus R, Korcarz C, McGray G, Neuman A, Murphy M, Borrow K, Weinert L, Bednarz J, Gretler D, Spencer K, Sarelli P, Lang R (1994) Noninvasive method for determination of arterial compliance using Doppler Echocardiography and subclavian pulse tracings: validation and clinical application of a physiological model of the circulation. Circulation 89:2688–2699
24. Borrow K, Neuman A, Lang R (1986) Milrinone versus dobutamine: contribution of altered myocardial mechanics and augmented inotropic state to improved left ventricular performance. Circulation 73 (suppl III):III-153–III-161
25. Materson B, Reda D, Cushman W, Massie B, et al (1993) Single-drug therapy for hypertension in men: a comparison of six antihypertensive agents with placebo. N Engl J Med 328:914–921
26. Parker MM, Shelhamer JH, Bacharach SL, Green MV, Natanson C, Frederick TM, Damske BA, Parillo JE (1984) Profund but reversible myocardial depression in patients with septic shock. Ann Intern Med 100:483–490
27. Parillo JE, Parker MM, Natanson C, et al (1990) Septic Shock in Humans: Advances in the understanding of pathogenesis, cardiovascular dysfunction, and therapy. Ann Intern Med 113:227–242
28. Umans J, Wylam M, Samsel R, Edwards J, Schumacker P (1993) Effects of endotoxin in vivo on endothelial and smooth muscle function in rabbit and rat aorta. Am Rev Respir Dis 148:1638–1645
29. Wylam M, Samsel R, Umans J, RW M, Leff A, Schumacker P (1990) Endotoxin in vivo impairs endothelium-dependant relaxation of canine arteries in vitro. Am Rev Respir Dis 142:1263–1267
30. Cryer H, Garrison R, Harris P (1988) Role of microvasculature during hyperdynamic and hypodynamic phases of endotoxin shock in decerebrated rats. J Trauma 28:312–318

31. Cox R (1974) Determinants ofsystemic hydraulic power in unanesthetized dogs. Am J Physiol 226:579–587
32. O'Rourke MF (1967) Steady and pulsatile energy losses in the systemic circulation under normal conditions and in simulated arterial disease. Cardiovasc Res 1:313–326
33. Kelly RP, Tunin R, Kaas DA (1992) Effect of reduced aortic compliance on cardiac efficiency and contractile function of in situ canine left ventricle. Circ Res 71:490–502
34. Suga H, Sagawa K, Shoukas A (1973) Load independance of instantaneous pressure-volume ratio of the canine left ventricle and effects of epinephrine and heart rate on the ratio. Circ Res 32:314–322
35. Suga H, Sagawa K (1974) Instantaneous pressure-volume relationships and their ratio in the excised, supported canine left ventricle. Circ Res 35:117–126
36. Sunagawa K, Maughan W, Burkhoff D, Sagawa K (1983) Left ventricular interaction with arterial load studied in isolated canine ventricle. Am J Physiol 245:H773–H780
37. Suga H (1990) Ventricular energetics. Physiol Rev 70:247–277
38. Asanoi H, Sasayama S, Kameyama T (1989) Ventriculo-arterial coupling in normal and failing hearts in humans. Circ Res 65:483–493
39. Hayashida K, Sunagawa K, Noma M, Sugimachi M, Ando H, Nakamura M (1992) Mechanical matching of the left ventricle with the arterial system in exercising dogs. Circ Res 71:481–489
40. Suga H, Hayashi T, Shirahata M (1981) Ventricular systolic pressure-volume area as predictor of cardiac oxygen consumption. Am J Physiol 240:H39–H44
41. Suga H, Hayashi T, Suehiro S, Hisano R (1981) Regression of cardiac oxygen consumption on ventricular pressure-volume area in dog. Am J Physiol 240:H320–H325
42. Nozawa T, Yasumura Y, Futaki S, Nobuaki T, Igarashi Y, Goto Y, Suga H (1987) Relation between oxygen consumption and pressure-volume area of in situ dog heart. Am J Physiol 253:H31–H40
43. Robotham JL, Takata M, Berman M, Harasawa Y (1991) Ejection fraction revisited. Anesthesiology 74:172–183
44. Mock M, Ringqvist I, Fisher L, Davis K, Chaitman B, Kouchoukos N, Kaiser G, Alderman E, Ryan T, Russel RJ, Mullin S, Fray D, Killip TI (1982) Survival of medically treated patients in the Coronary Artery Surgery Study (CASS) registry. Circulation 66:562–568
45. Nelson G, Cohn P, Gorlin R (1975) Prognosis in medically-treated coronary artery disease. Circulation 52:408–412

The Cardiovascular Management of the Critically Ill Patient

S. Magder

Volume management is a major activity in the intensive care unit, because of the importance of blood volume as a determinant of venous return and cardiac output. The basic principles that I will discuss in this chapter can be summarized as *there needs to be "enough but not too much"* and *"quantity must be differentiated from quality"*. Cardiac output is dependent upon the interaction of two functions: *circuit function (or venous return) and cardiac function* [1, 2]. I will begin by reviewing the basics for venous return.

Determinants of Venous Return

A common misconception is that arterial blood pressure is an important determinant of the total cardiac output [3]. Arterial pressure determines flow to individual regions, such as cerebral flow, coronary flow and renal flow, but does not determine the total amount of blood flowing around the body. The reason for this, is that there is a large compliant region in the veins which effectively dampens out the effects of arterial pressure. A useful analogy is that of water flowing out of a bathtub. The flow of water out of a bathtub is determined by the height of the water above the opening at the bottom of the tub, the resistance in the drain leaving the tub and any downstream pressures in the drain. The height of water in the tub is determined by the surface area of the tub and the volume of water filling the tub. If the tub has a large surface area, this is the equivalent of a large compliance and a small surface area is the equivalent of a small compliance. If the plug is removed from the bottom of the tub, and the tap is turned off, there will be very little change in the height of the water in the tub for the first minute or so (depending on how functional the drain is!). Water flows out of the tub at a relatively constant rate during this time period and is little affected by whether the tap is on or not. If one tries this with a sink instead of a bathtub, the water level will fall much faster because of its smaller surface area. Similarly, the veins in the body act as a large bathtub, for 70 percent of the total blood volume is present in small veins and venules [2]. Drainage from the venous compartment is then determined by the pressure in the venous compartment, the resistance draining them, and the downstream pressure. Although the resistance in the vessels draining the compliant region is only 10–15 percent of the total resistance from the aorta to the right atria, it is an absolutely crucial resistance, for it determines the drainage of blood flow from the veins. Mathematically, venous drainage can then be given by [2]:

$$\text{venous return} = (\text{MCFP} - \text{Pra})\,\text{Rv}$$

where MCFP is the mean circulatory filling pressure which in turn is determined by the volume in the veins and their compliance, Pra is the right pressure or the downstream pressure for the venous drainage and Rv is the resistance between the two. When venous return is zero, the right atrial pressure is equal to MCFP. Since venous volume is so large relative to the volume in the rest of the body, the pressure in this region remains relatively constant during changing flow conditions. With increasing cardiac output, the arterial pressure rises and the right atrial pressure falls, but MCFP remains essentially constant. What the heart essentially does to produce a cardiac output is to lower right atrial pressure. Arthur Guyton used this principle to develop his very useful venous return curves [2, 4]. Since the major function of the heart is to lower right atrial pressure, Guyton made right atrial pressure the independent variable on his graph and plotted venous return against right atrial pressure. When the venous return is zero, right atrial pressure equals MCFP. When right atrial pressure is lowered, there is linear increase in venous return (Fig. 1).

A very interesting and important phenomena occurs when the right atrial pressure reaches zero, or atmospheric pressure. Further decreases in right atrial pressure produce no further increase in flow. This is because the pressure inside the veins becomes less than the pressure outside the vein as they enter the thorax and the thin-walled veins collapse to produce a Starling resistor or vascular waterfall [5]. Further increases in right atrial pressure then do not have any further effect on the venous return. This brings up the ironic point that maximum venous return occurs when the heart is removed and the heart only appears to produce a blockage to venous return! Unfortunately, it is also true that if the heart is removed, none of the blood will recirculate and maximum venous return would only occur for a brief glorious instant!

Effect of Increasing Volume

How then does volume affect cardiac output? Increasing vascular volume increases MCFP. An increase in vascular volume shifts the venous return curve in parallel to the right and produces two important consequences. The venous return is higher at any right atrial pressure and, importantly, the maximum venous return is increased. This is because the veins collapse at a higher venous return value (Fig. 1). This has very important clinical implications. As noted above, the major role of the heart is to control right atrial pressure. Thus, improving cardiac function can only increase venous return by lowering right atrial pressure. When right atrial pressure is low, as in hypovolemic shock, venous return and thus cardiac output are improved by giving volume which shifts the venous return curve to the right and raises the plateau of the venous return curve. This is also dramat-

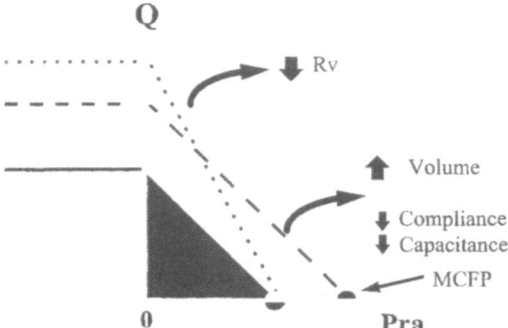

Fig. 1. Venous return curves. The abscissa is right atrial pressure and the ordinate is flow. An increase in volume, decrease in venous compliance or decrease in capacitance produce a parallel shift to the venous return curve to the right. This results in a higher flow for any right atrial pressure and a higher maximum venous return. A decrease in venous resistance (Rv) rotates the venous return curve and also produces a higher maximum venous return. MCFP refers to the mean systemic filling pressure and it is equal to right atrial pressure at zero flow

ically seen when one uses a device such a left ventricular assist device. The pump technician will report that the tubing is fluttering when the limits of the circuit are reached, and the pump can only put out more when the patient is given more volume.

Venous return can also be increased by a decrease in the resistance to venous return (Fig. 1). This shifts the venous return curve upward but does not change MCFP. This occurs during exercise and perhaps with drugs such as dobutamine. On the other hand, alpha-agonists and inhibitors of nitric oxide production increase the resistance [6].

Quantity versus Quality

In the model described above, the opening of the bathtub was at the bottom, as is the usual case. If the opening was on the side of the tub instead, relationships of total volume to output are different. Once the water in the tub reaches the lower part of the opening, no further water can leave the tub. The volume that is left will remain trapped, and only the volume above the opening creates the pressure which pushes the water out of the tub. The volume above the opening is called stressed volume, for it produces the pressure head to push the volume out, and the volume below this is called the unstressed volume [7]. The unstressed volume is essential to get to the opening but does not itself contribute to the flow out of the tub. Similarly, vessels have a stressed and unstressed volume. The unstressed volume is required to give the round shape to the vessels, but it is only the stressed volume that stretches vascular walls and creates the pressure which is responsible for MCFP. Under normal resting conditions, approximately 25 percent of blood volume is stressed and 75 percent is unstressed [7]. This means that there are very large reserves of unstressed volume that can be recruited through neurohumeral mechanisms to maintain stressed volume. Normally stressed and unstressed volume cannot be distinguished in an intact person [8]. However, we were able to measure stressed vascular volume in patients undergoing surgery on the aorta. These patients underwent hypothermic circulatory arrest for their surgery. This was achieved by putting them on a heart-lung bypass circuit and then cooling them to a cerebral temperature of 19 °C. The bypass was then turned off and the patients' blood was allowed to passively drain into the reservoir of the circuit. We simply measured the blood volume that came out and it was approximately 30% of their predicted total volume.

It is important to appreciate that only stressed volume determines MCFP and thus affects hemodynamics, and there is no clinical method to detect the reserves in unstressed volume. The pressure-volume relationship is graphically represented in Figure 2. An increase in sympathetic activity [9, 10] or vasoactive agents, such as norepinephrine [11], can produce a leftward shift of the pressure-volume relationship without changing the slope of the relationship which is elastance or 1/venous compliance. This results in a higher MCFP for any given total volume. A shift to the left of the pressure-volume relationship of the vasculature is called a decrease in capacitance, for capacitance represents the pressure for the total volume of the system which includes stressed and unstressed volume. Of importance, agents such as nitroglycerine [12] and morphine [13] can shift the pressure-volume relationship to the right which means that a greater volume is needed to maintain the same MCFP. If a patient's catecholamine levels are high, whether due to high sympathetic activity or exogenous catecholamine infusions, then vascular capacitance is reduced. If there is then a loss of volume, there may not be any vascular reserves remaining to compensate with a further shift to the

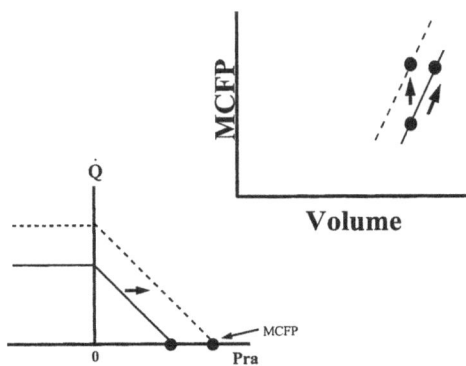

Fig. 2. The right upper corner shows the relationship of mean circulatory filling pressure (MCFP) and total blood volume. The slope of this line is 1/venous compliance. An increase in blood volume results in a rise in MCFP along the same compliance line. A decrease in capacitance results in a shift to the left of the total pressure-volume relationship. The effect of this is shown on the venous return curve in the lower left corner. Both an increase in total volume and a decrease in capacitance result in a parallel shift to the right of the venous return curve

left of the pressure-volume curve. The loss of volume then will result in a direct decrease in MCFP and a fall in cardiac output and, importantly, in maximum cardiac output. Furthermore, a decrease in vascular tone from a vasodilating agent may result in a very precipitous fall in cardiac output by decreasing MCFP. An important clinical and research point is that the response of cardiac output to various physical agents such as ventilation, external pumps or drugs will vary considerably depending on the available reserves in unstressed volume, for this determines the potential for volume compensation.

Cardiac Function

Venous return (or circuit function) interacts with cardiac function to produce the final cardiac output. The Starling relationship plots the cardiac output versus the preload of the heart. Preload relates to the pressure which distends the cardiac muscle prior to contraction, although, in fact, it is the sarcomere length and thus cardiac volume which is the crucial factor determining cardiac output. However, since preload is a force term, it should refer to the pressure rather than the volume. The compliance of the heart determines what pressure is needed to produce a given volume and a given stretch of the sarcomeres. It is obvious that whatever the right heart puts out, the left heart must also put out in the steady state. Guyton thus evaluated total cardiac function by looking at the preload of the right heart which is Pra, and the output of the whole heart which is cardiac output [2]. He could then plot cardiac function on the same graph as venous return, for the abscissa was right atrial pressure and the ordinate, flow. However, it is necessary to have the cardiac function curve start from a slightly negative right atrial pressure rather than zero. This is because the pressure surrounding the heart is pleural pressure which, at end-expiration, is negative relative to atmosphere. The intersection of the cardiac function curve and venous return curve gives the cardiac output (Fig. 3). The actual cardiac output can thus be changed by changing the cardiac function curve or changing the venous return curve, although under most physiological conditions, changes occur in both these relationships. However, one can still talk about a dominant cardiac effect or a domi-

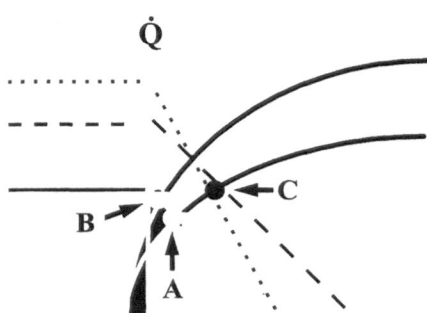

Fig. 3. Interaction of venous return curve and cardiac function curve. An increase in cardiac function will increase cardiac output from A to B with a fall in right atrial pressure. An increase in circuit function will increase cardiac output from A to C with a rise in right atrial pressure

nant venous return or circuit effect. If the cardiac output rises with a fall in right atrial pressure, then the dominant effect was improvement in cardiac function. If the cardiac output rises with a rise in right pressure, then the dominant effect was an improvement in the circuit function [1] as would occur for example with an infusion of volume.

Plateau of the Cardiac Function Curve

A very important point is that the cardiac function curve has a plateau. For the right heart under normal conditions, this occurs at around 6–12 mmHg, which is much lower than the plateau for the left heart. However, the left heart can only put out what the right heart gives it. The plateau of the cardiac function curve is, under normal conditions, due to the pericardium, although even when the pericardium is removed, the cytoskeleton of the heart limits distention of the heart and there is still a plateau in the cardiac function curve. It is very important to appreciate that when the plateau of the cardiac function curve is reached [14], further increases in right atrial pressure will not result in a further increase in cardiac output. This increase in right atrial pressure then becomes "wasted" preload. It is also important to appreciate that it is the right atrial pressure which determines the total cardiac output and not the pulmonary capillary wedge pressure or left atrial pressure. The wedge pressure gives the clinician an indication of the function of the left heart and the status of the pulmonary capillaries, but it does not give an indication of what is happening to cardiac output in relationship to the circuit and thus how the output of the heart compares to its input. When a patient's right atrial pressure is on the flat part of the cardiac function curve, cardiac output can only be increased by improving cardiac function. Further increases in volume will not have any beneficial effect and will, in fact, have negative effects. This is because the increased pressure in the heart from the excess volume can then compromise myocardial blood flow and potentially produce myocardial ischemia. Distention of the right ventricle will also compress the left ventricle and decrease its compliance. Furthermore, the increase in right atrial pressure will be transmitted to the left heart without actually distending the heart and improving its output. This rise in left-sided pressures will increase pulmonary artery pressures and add to the load on the right heart. Finally, the increased central venous pressures will increase systemic capillary pressures and increase the patient's edema. It is thus very important for the clinician to recognize when the limits of cardiac filling have been reached and not continue to infuse volume.

Volume limitation in a patient can be determined by giving a volume challenge. I usually give sufficient volume to raise the right atrial pressure by an observable amount. I usually choose about 2 mmHg. I then quickly measure the cardiac output. If cardiac output does not increase with an increase in Pra, then the patient is on the flat part of the cardiac function curve, and further volume loading will not be of help. This is even true when the wedge pressure is low. For example, a fairly common scenario after cardiac surgery is to observe a patient with a central venous pressure of approximately 12 mmHg, a wedge pressure of 8 mmHg and a cardiac index of $1.9 \ l/m^2$. If this patient's right heart is on the flat part of the function curve, even though the wedge pressure is low, a volume infusion will not increase this patient's cardiac output, because the output cannot get from the right heart to the left heart to alter the filling of the left heart and improve output. An inotrope must be used.

We presented another test that can be useful to assess volume status in patients who have spontaneous breaths [15]. Normally, an inspiratory effort produces a fall in pleural pressure which is transmitted to the right atrium and presents as a fall in right atrial pressure. If the right heart is maximally filled, it is then on the steep part of its compliance curve and the change in pleural pressure is not transmitted to the heart and there is no inspiratory fall in right atrial pressure. Thus, patients who have no inspiratory fall in right atrial pressure will not respond to a fluid challenge.

Changes in intrathoracic pressure change the position of the cardiac function curve relative to the venous return curve. Positive pleural pressure shifts the cardiac function curve to the right, and negative pleural pressure shifts the cardiac function curve to the left. Of importance, positive pleural pressure also changes the collapse point of the veins as they enter the thorax, for with positive pleural pressure, the collapse occurs at a positive Pra rather than zero Pra or atmospheric pressure. This has very important implications for cardiac output, for the higher collapse pressure reduces the maximum potential cardiac output [16, 17]. Cardiac output can then only be restored by having an increase in the MCFP which can come about by an increase in sympathetic activity, assuming that adequate vascular reserves still remain, or further volume is given [17–19]. On the other hand, if the patient's right atrial pressure is on the flat part of the cardiac function curve, then the application of positive pressure will not affect cardiac output until the cardiac function curve is shifted enough to the right that the venous return curve intersects with the ascending part of the cardiac function curve. This means that the effect of positive pleural pressure on cardiac function is variable and highly dependent upon the initial volume status of the patient. This extra volume must also be considered when the positive intrathoracic pressure is removed. If the patient's cardiac function is limited, the large increase in venous return that occurs with the removal of positive pressure could result in acute distention of the heart, a marked rise in filling pressures and pulmonary edema. In such patients it is important to gradually reduce the positive pressure to allow the appropriate volume redistributions to occur [20]. It also must be appreciated that removing vascular tone from a patient on a ventilator, whether by sedation or by the use of vasodilating agents, potentially removes a very important compensatory mechanism and can result in a marked fall in cardiac output and blood pressure.

In summary, volume is a very important determinant of venous return and thus cardiac output. The clinician must be careful to make sure that the patient has enough volume, but not too much, and to consider the potential reservoirs of unstressed volume, for it is not only the quantity of volume that it important, but also the quality, for only stressed volume determines venous return.

References

1. Magder S (1992) Shock Physiology. In: Pinsky MR, Dhainault JF (eds) Physiological Foundations of Critical Care Medicine. Williams and Wilkins, Philadelphia, pp 140–160
2. Guyton AC, Jones CE, Coleman TG (1973) Circulatory physiology: cardiac output and its regulation. In: Guyton AC (ed), W. B. Saunders Co.
3. Berne RM, Levy MN (1983) The cardiovascular system. In: Berne RM, Levy MN (eds) Physiology. Mosby, St. Louis, pp 439–638
4. Guyton AC (1955) Determination of cardiac output by equating venous return curves with cardiac response curves. Physiol Rev 35:123–129 (Abstract)
5. Permutt S, Riley S (1963) Hemodynamics of collapsible vessels with tone: the vascular waterfall. J Appl Physiol 18 (5):924–932
6. Vanelli G, Magder S (1996) Circuit factors in the high cardiac output of sepsis. J Crit Care (in press)
7. Rothe CF (1983) Reflex control of veins and vascular capacitance. Physiol Rev 63 (4):1281–1295
8. Magder S, De Varennes B, Ralley F (1994) Clinical death and the measurement of stressed vascular volume in humans. Am Rev Respir Dis 149:A1064 (Abstract)
9. Deschamps A, Magder S (1992) Baroreflex control of regional capacitance and blood flow distribution with or without alpha adrenergic blockade. J Appl Physiol 263:H1755–H1763
10. Shoukas AA, Sagawa K (1973) Control of total systemic vascular capacity by the carotid sinus baroreceptor reflex. Circ Res 33:22–33
11. Appleton C, Olajos M, Morkin E, Goldman S (1985) Alpha-1 adrenergic control of the venous circulation in intact dogs. J Pharmacol Exp Ther 233:729–734
12. Manyari DE, Wang Z, Cohen J, Tyberg JV (1993) Assessment of human splanchnic venous volume-pressure relation using radionuclide plethysmography. Circulation 87:1142–1151
13. Green JF, Jackman AP, Parsons G (1978) The effects of morphine on the mechanical properties of the systemic circulation in the dog. Circ Res 42 (4):474–478
14. Bishop VS, Stone HL, Guyton AC (1964) Cardiac function curves in conscious dogs. Am J Physiol 207 (3):677–682
15. Magder SA, Georgiadis G, Tuck C (1992) Respiratory variations in right atrial pressure predict response to fluid challenge. J Crit Care 7:76–85
16. Wilson CR, Vanelli G, Magder S, Hussain SNA (1991) The effect of phrenic afferent stimulation by bradykinin on the distribution of ventilatory drive. Clin and Invest Med 14 (4):A112 (Abstract)
17. Fessler HE, Brower RG, Wise RA, Permutt S (1992) Effects of positive end-expiratory pressure on the gradient for venous return. Am Rev Respir Dis 146:4–10
18. Fessler HE, Brower RG, Wise RA, Permutt S (1991) Effects of positive end-expiratory pressure on the gradient for venous return. Am Rev Respir Dis 143:19–24
19. Nanas S, Magder S (1992) Adaptations of the peripheral circulation to PEEP. Am Rev Respir Dis 146:688–693
20. Lemaire F, Teboul J-L, Cinotti L, et al (1988) Acute left ventricular dysfunction during unsuccessful weaning from mechanical ventilation. Anesthesiology 69:171–179

Right Ventricular Function

J.-F. Dhainaut

Thirty years ago, the right ventricle (RV) was considered to be little more than a conduit for blood flow between the peripheral venous circulation and the pulmonary arterial tree. The physiologic role of the RV systole has been revisited, especially because of the observations of acute cor pulmonale and RV infarction where the RV failure may be responsible for a circulatory shock (Laver et al. 1979).

Right Ventricular Function: Physiology

Anatomic Background

Low resistance is the main physical characteristic of the normal pulmonary circulation. The RV wall is normally thinner than the left ventricular (LV) wall. This highlights the inability for the RV to face an acute increase in pulmonary resistance such as may occur in pulmonary embolism. However, the adaptation to chronic pulmonary hypertension may induce a thickness that may nearly equal that of the LV. The RV chamber is anatomically composed of three walls: anterior, inferior, and postero-lateral, i.e. the ventricular septum that bulges into the RV cavity under normal conditions. The ventricular septum normal contraction contributes essentially to decrease LV diameter. Nevertheless, the septum position is responsive to the transseptal gradient throughout the cardiac cycle. Then, marked displacement may occur depending on the respective left and right intra-chamber pressure. In any case of increased RV intra-chamber pressure, a leftward septal displacement is expected that further reduces the apparent LV compliance and accounts for possible decrease in LV stroke output. Such a displacement is of less magnitude is systole than in diastole due to the different myocardial stiffness.

Role of the RV in Overall Hemodynamics

The RV and LV are mechanically coupled (Pinsky 1989). Experimental studies performed by cauterizing electively the RV free wall, demonstrated that both the right atrial and pulmonary arterial pressures did not change, illustrating that this function is not significantly impaired by elective RV free wall destruction. By virtue of the anatomic continuity, tension developed during contraction of the intact

LV is transmitted to the damaged RV wall, thus preserving the RV pump function. In contrast, it has been shown, in a hemodynamic model of exclusion of the RV, that this acute elimination of RV function leads to a marked fall in cardiac output. When the fluid volume was increased sufficiently, cardiac output was restored to the control level, but central venous pressure markedly increased. The normal role of the RV seems to maintain a low systemic venous pressure.

RV Systole

The RV is crescent shaped with an angle of 60°, divided into sinus (inflow) and conus (outflow) regions. During systole, the greatest relative motion occurs in the tricuspid valve, suggesting a sphincter-like action. Even in absence of tricuspid annulus dilatation, a slight tricuspid regurgitation may be detected in half of the normal subjects by doppler echocardiography. RV contraction proceeds sequentially from the sinus to the conus. During the sinus contraction, the conus dilates concomitantly with the initial part of the pulmonary artery, acting as a reservoir. Rather than a booster, the RV contraction has been compare to a peristaltic movement, initiated by the atrial systole (Pouleur et al. 1980). When the RV ejection is impeded by acute pulmonary hypertension the functional difference between inflow and outflow tract persists. We can speculate that this sinus-conus asynchronism is adequate to protect the sensitive pulmonary arteries from high peaks of pressure and to promote a continuous blood flow in the pulmonary vessels for optimal hematosis.

Since the RV ejects against a low resistance circuit, the blood ejection continues after peak pressure is developed within the RV. Consequently the shape of the global RV pressure-volume loop differs from those of the LV. The more triangular shape makes end-systole more difficult to point out. However, it has been demonstrated that the end-systolic pressure-volume relation defined by maximal elastance (max P/V-V0) is a more reliable index to assess RV function.

RV Diastole

These considerations also account for particular feature of the RV diastole. Diastole begins at the end of systole. Then, up to one third of the stroke volume may be ejected during the active relaxation phase. This explains the very short isovolumic relaxation period. The passive part of diastole is associated with ventricle filling. It is now accepted that filling is favored by a ventricular suction that may approximate -5 mmHg. The RV is highly compliant during filling, allowing low systemic venous pressure that favors tissue perfusion, and preventing acute pulmonary edema in the settings associated with LV dysfunction. The passive pressure-volume relationship of the normal RV is quite horizontal and linear inside its usual limits (Weber et al. 1983). Consequently, the measurement of RV end-diastolic volume appears to be critical, and the complex geometry of the RV explain the difficulties to model volume calculations from one or several measured dimensions. Moreover, since the RV is functioning below its unstressed volume, changes in volume do not result in measurable changes in pressure, but only changes in ventricular geometry. Therefore, since the RV distending pressure changes little during filling, it is clear that muscle length and tension must also not change greatly, i.e. under normal conditions, RV preload may be poorly related to end-diastolic volume.

Finally, even the filling pressure could be an acceptable evaluation of the RV preload when positioned on the ascending limb of the pressure-volume relationship, the heart fills, not as a function of absolute intra-chamber pressure, but according to transmural pressure (intra-chamber pressure minus juxta-cardiac pressure). Changes in juxta-cardiac pressure are dependent of pericardial capacity, changes in regional lung volume and chest wall compliance. The pericardial stress-strain relationship is "J" shape. In most clinical circumstances, the pericardial cavity is unstressed and pericardectomy is followed by no hemodynamic consequences. However, in important volume dilatation, both ventricles compete in the inextensible pericardial space amplifying the ventricular interdependence. In addition, the lungs may directly compress the heart and induce an anterior heart rotation. In practice, measuring juxta-cardiac pressure is complex and often underestimated when evaluated by esophageal or pleural pressure.

Right Ventricular Function: Pathophysiology

In isolated contracting intact heart preparations, the effects of changes in preload on RV performance may be studied independent of changes in afterload, heart rate and contractile state. In contrast, in the clinical setting, abnormalities in RV loading conditions and function often coexist and interact in the same patient. Despite this feature, we analyze the RV responses to volume- and pressure-overload respectively, to simply the understanding of this issue.

RV Response to Volume-Overload

Acute and chronic volume-overload alter the architecture of the RV wall and cavity, as well as the pattern of systolic motion (Feneley et al. 1986). In patients with RV volume-overload, the interventricular septum is flattened at end-diastole, resulting in inequality of the LV minor axes. Theoretically, in pure volume overloaded RV, the flattened end-diastolic septum must reassure its normal concave leftward configuration at end-systole since the normal trans-septal systolic pressure gradient is conserved. Depending of the degree of diastolic leftward septal shift (and of frequent associated pressure overloaded) RV proto-systolic motion may be paradoxic. This motion pattern should be additionally distinguished from one in which septal contractile function is decreased which is characterized by a depressed septal systolic thickening.

The acute effect of increased end-diastolic volume on ventricular systolic function may be expressed by the Starling relation when RV stressed volume is reached. Accordingly, the volume overload of the RV results in a marked increase in stroke volume but may not be fully explain by an increased segment length. The more spheric RV end-diastolic shape could induce a better mechanical effect of the contractile force. A quicker relaxation when diastolic fiber length is enlarged may contribute to a better RV filling. The existence of a true descending limb of the Starling curve in clinical setting associated with excessive preload remains debated. An apparent descending limb may result from functional tricuspid regurgitation.

Experimental chronic RV volume-overload, in contrast to the LV, has not been found to exhibit significant alteration of contractile function and energetics (Cooper et al. 1973). However, patients with left-to-right shunt that provides acceptable models for RV volume-overload, RV rarely fails in the absence of significant pulmonary vascular obstructive disease. With surgical repair, RV ejection fraction often falls, thus revealing systolic dysfunction which had been masked through the Starling mechanism. In addition, the return to normal pattern of septal motion is in part related to the duration of the volume overload prior to repair and often needs long period of time to appear. These findings should be interpreted cautiously, since cardiac surgery is followed by the appearance of paradoxical septal motion presumably related to an alteration in the geometry of the entire heart rather than altered RV load.

RV Response to Pressure-Overload

Specific configurational changes in the presence of RV pressure-overload are less well described, because of the constant coexistence of pressure and volume-overload in such circumstances. The RV pressure increases and may compete with the LV pressure to position the interventricular septum. The systolic leftward septal shift optimizes the mechanical effect of the RV contraction. Changes in both ventricles configuration have been observed during acute RV pressure loading in dogs (Smith et al. 1985). Following acute pulmonary artery constriction, the LV septal-free wall dimension and shortening are reduced as well as its contribution to global LV systolic function, whereas in chronic RV pressure-overload, the LV septal-free wall dimension and shortening are maintained.

This leftward shift of the ventricular septum has at least two mechanisms:
1) competition between both ventricle inside an inextensive pericardial cavity, and
2) series interactions with a decreased LV filling due to a decreased RV stroke volume.

To what degree the contractile state of RV myocardium is altered by chronic pressure overload remains uncertain. Indeed, since the ventricular response to chronic pressure overload has been extensively studies in animals, the results of these investigations differ somewhat, and special attention must be given to the species utilized, the magnitude of hypertrophy produced, and the duration of pressure load produced. Usually, RV and LV hypertrophy was produced by constriction of the pulmonary artery and aorta, respectively. In the former, ventricle/body weight ratios increased 44–90%, while in reports of LV pressure overload, the hypertrophy was more modest (30–40%). In most studies, the maximum active tension developed by hypertrophied papillary muscles, the time derivative of tension development, Vmax and the maximum measured velocity of shortening were observed to be reduced. Time to peak tension, a measure of the duration of active state was found to be normal or most frequently prolonged. The rate at which the pressure load is applied to the ventricle does not appear to influence these mechanical abnormalities since the same findings are observed in models where the pressure load is gradual as when it is abrupt.

The long-term effects of chronic pressure overload on ejection phase indice of contractile function were rapidly depressed but returned to baseline values after several weeks (Williams and Potter 1974). Interestingly, ejection phase indices of systolic performance in the intact RV correlated poorly with the findings in isolated papillary muscles, suggesting that compensatory mechanisms in intact animal mask the intrinsic functional abnormalities of hypertrophied heart muscle. In clinical studies of chronic RV pressure overload, decreased ejection fraction is frequently present essentially due to the systolic load present at the time of study, but abnormalities in RV contractility are generally absent.

Finally, the early response to pressure overload of the RV is a reduction in the intrinsic velocity of the contractile apparatus, associated with a compensatory prolonged duration of force development. In the intact organism, these defects may be masked by neurohumoral effects and are not easily detected by clinical indices of systolic pump function. With sustained pressure overload, there is good evidence that these mechanical abnormalities may revert towards normal. However, further depression of contractile function during prolonged and severe pressure-overload is demonstrated in isolated heart muscle.

Response of Right Coronary Circulation to RV Overload

The RV is mainly perfused by the right coronary artery. It has been shown than the volume work needs less energy than the pressure work. Relatively to the myocardial mass, the sub-endocardial coronary vasculature of the RV is less developed than in the LV. However, the RV coronary perfusion is maintained during both systole and diastole since the driving pressure (intracoronary pressure – right myocardial tissue pressure) remains always positive. As for LV, the RV myocardial oxygen extraction is quite maximum, and consequently an increase in RV oxygen requirement must be mainly met by an increased coronary blood flow, mostly obtained by a vasodilatation.

For the LV, it has been shown a close relation between myocardial oxygen consumption and the total pressure volume area determined by both systolic and diastolic pressure volume lines and the portion of the pressure volume loop from end-diastole to end-systole. Thus increased afterload increases LV oxygen consumption. Since RV oxygen consumption is difficult to measure, no clinical data are available for the RV. However Calvin and Quinn (1989) argue, from experimental studies, for the hypothesis of an increased RV myocardium oxygen demand in acute pressure overload. In many other pathologic circumstances, a RV ischemia has been hypothesized, even in absence of significant coronary disease, when the systolic coronary perfusion driving pressure decreased. This is likely to occur and consequently to induce a decreased contractility when an acute pulmonary hypertension coexists with a reduced systemic pressure. Furthermore, it has been shown an increased RV performance when increasing aortic pressure in canine studies where two models of pulmonary hypertension have been performed. The precise mechanism was not fully demonstrated, a global decreased RV ischemia was not founded, but the authors have speculated an increased perfusion of the deeper layers of the RV myocardium. However, the last study shows that RV ischemia is not necessary for RV failure to occur in acute pulmonary hypertension. Therefore, in patients without coronary disease, a decreased in contractility due to a RV ischemia may be only advocated in extreme situations.

Hypertrophied hearts may have a particular sensitivity to hypoxia that could be clinically relevant. If the coronary blood flow per unit weight of muscle is normal in hypertrophied hearts, coronary vascular resistance is higher in hypertrophied than in normal myocardium, and a greater proportion of the total vasodilation reserve is used to maintain resting flow in hypertrophy. An important expression of this defect has been the finding of a disproportionate decrease in the endocardial/epicardial flow ratio in hypertrophy during the stress of pacing and during exercise. While most of these studies have involved models of LV hypertrophy, reduced vasodilatator response has been observed in dogs with RV hypertrophy and in the RV of patients with atrial septal defects and pulmonary hypertension.

RV Response to Decreased Contractile State

There are few available data to investigate the specific RV response to elective contractile impairment. The reason is the lack of valid model. When studying global cardiomyopathy or inferior LV-associated RV infarction, the RV response account for both ventricular interdependence and post-capillary RV pressure overload. The RV free wall infarction may be considered as a better model, but several associated factors as modifyied ventricular coupling, geometric consequences of infarction or post-ischemic particular relaxation impairment may have important additional, but non valuable effects. Furthermore, the constraining effect of the pericardium seems to be a major contributor to hemodynamic consequences of impaired RV contractility.

With the pericardium intact, Goldstein et al. (1982) showed that the experimental RV free wall infarction was followed by a fall in cardiac output, an increase in both RV filling pressure and size and a decrease in LV end-diastolic dimension and pressure leading to the classic diastolic pressures equalization. However, in accordance with other studies in open chest models, when the pericardium is open, right and left dimensions increase as do cardiac output and both right and left stroke work indices. RV pressure decreased and diastolic equalization resolved. Therefore, when face to a decreased contractile state at least three factors may preserve ejection and cardiac output: ventricular coupling, RV dilation-related increase in the contractile force via a Starling effect, and a slower RV relaxation that may favor ejection. In such circumstances, the pericardium decreases the apparent ventricle compliance, promotes ventricular interference and acts as a limiting factor for both RV dilatation and ejection force (Dhainaut et al. 1989).

In summary, to maintain RV stroke volume (hence, end-systolic pressure remains constant) a decreased Emax should be balanced by an increased RV end-diastolic volume in the same proportion. Therefore, the respective levels of
1) maximum diastolic volume (according to extra-mural: pleural, pericardial, right atrial and LV constrains),
2) pulmonary resistance and
3) minimum forward stroke volume to maintain adequate cardiac output are the determinants of a given decreased contactility-induced RV failure.

Since natural life implies exercises and various situations of increased oxygen demand (i.e. increased pulmonary resistance and increased needed cardiac output), RV performance may become an important limiting factor to cardiac output and may be of great prognostic value in global cardiomyopathy with comparable LV performance.

Right Heart as an Endocrine Organ

Right atrium contains granules of an immunoreactive peptide, the atrial natriuretic factor. To date, vasodilatation, diuresis, natriuresis, inhibition of angiotensin II, release of aldosterone, relaxe of smooth muscles, negative inotrope power on the myocardium have been shown.

Both experimental and clinical studies have evidenced that the release of atrial natriuretic factor is dependent of atrial stretching as it may occur during RV acute failure (Raine et al. 1986). During RV infarction, a significant increase in the atrial natriuretic factor has been shown, and the biological effects of atrial natriuretic factor may participate to the specific hemodynamic pattern of the RV infarction syndrome.

References

Calvin JE, Quinn B (1989) Right ventricular pressure overload during acute lung injury: Cardiac mechanics and the pathophysiology of right systolic dysfunction. J Crit Care 4:251–265
Cooper G, Tomanek RJ, Ehrhardt JC, Marcus ML (1981) Chronic progressive pressure overload of the cat right ventricle. Circ Res 48:488–497

Dhainaut JF, Ghannad E, Brunet F, Villemand D, Devaux JY, Shremmer B, Squara P, Weber S, Monsallier JF (1989) The role of tricuspid regurgitation and left ventricular damage in the treatment of right ventricular infarction-induced cardiogenic shock. Am J Cardiol 66:289–295

Feneley MP, Gavaghan T (1986) Paradoxical and pseudoparadoxical interventricular septal motion in patients with right ventricular volume overload. Circulation 74:230–238

Goldstein JA, Vlahakes GJ, Verrier ED, Schiller NB, et al (1982) The role of right ventricle systolic dysfunction and elevated intra-pericardial pressure in the genesis of low output in experimental right ventricle infarction. Circulation 65:513–522

Laver MB, Strauss HW, Pohost GM (1979) Right and left ventricular geometry: adjustments during acute respiratory failure. Crit Care Med 7:509–519

Pinsky MR (1989) Assessment of the right ventricle in the critically ill: facts, fancy, and perspectives. In: Update in intensive care and emergency medicine. JL Vincent (ed). Springer Verlag, Berlin, pp 518–523

Pouleur H, Lefevre J, Van Mechelem H, Charlier AA (1980) Free wall shortening and relaxation during ejection of the canine right ventricle. Am J Physiol 239:H601

Raine AE, Erne P, Burgisser E, et al (1986) Atrial natriuretic peptide and atrial pressure in patients with congestive heart failure. N Engl J Med 315:533–537

Smith ER, Kingma I, Smiseth OA, et al (1985) Ventricular response to acute constriction of the pulmonary artery in conscious dogs. Am Rev Respir Dis 131:A57

Weber KT, Janicki JS, Shroff SG, et al (1983) The right ventricle: Physiologic and pathophysiologic considerations. Crit Care Med 11:323–328

Williams JF, Potter RD (1974) Normal contractile state of hypertrophied myocardium after pulmonary artery constriction in the cat. J Clin Invest 54:1266–1272

Pharmacologic Support of Critically Ill Patients

K. P. Rothfield

Introduction

Cardiovascular collapse is a devastating clinical entity frequently observed in both medical and surgical intensive care unit patients. Despite the gravity of this condition, advances in cardiovascular physiology, molecular biology, and pharmacology, now allow physicians to offer rational therapeutic interventions to such patients. This chapter will review the basic pathophysiology of cardiac failure, identify cellular targets for pharmacologic intervention, and discuss the actions and uses of some of the newer inotropic agents.

Heart Failure

Heart failure may be defined as either inadequate pump function to meet tissue metabolic demands, or adequate pump function with abnormally elevated filling pressures. Heart failure can be further subdivided into *systolic failure* (inadequate cardiac output or inotropy) or *diastolic failure* (inadequate ventricular relaxation or filling). Although the distinction between systolic and diastolic failure may be subtle in individual patients, it is important to recognize that a combination of the two frequently exists.

Typical causes of systolic failure include dilated cardiomyopathy, myocardial ischemia or infarction, and myocardial stunning. A common cause of heart failure which is sometimes overlooked is right ventricular failure secondary to acute pulmonary embolus. The sudden pressure overload of the right ventricle leads to chamber dilatation and a low-flow state which may mimic decompensation of the left ventricle (LV).

Diastolic failure may result from hypertrophic cardiomyopathy, subendocardial fibrosis, and pericardial disease. Cardiac tamponade is the most frequent cause of acute diastolic failure seen in cardiac surgical patients. Mediastinal blood and clots compress the heart and limit its filling, producing a life-threatening low-flow state. Although aggressive fluid and inotropic therapy may be used as temporizing measures, surgical decompression is the mainstay of therapy.

Cardiac Physiology and the Goals of Pharmacologic Therapy

Pathological processes may affect cardiac performance by altering preload, afterload, heart rate, contractility (inotropy), and distensibility (lusitropy). Accordingly, the goals of ideal pharmacologic therapy may include preload reduction, afterload reduction, heart rate optimization, increased inotropy, improved lusitropy, and patient survival. Notable exceptions to these goals include the avoidance of preload reduction in relatively hypovolemic patients, and the use of *negative* inotropes in patients with hypertrophic cardiomyopathy, in which inotropic stimulation frequently worsens LV outflow obstruction.

Importantly, acute and chronic therapy for heart failure are not one and the same. Although treatment with positive inotropic agents may be lifesaving in acutely ill hospitalized patients, chronic outpatient management with high doses of such drugs, as discussed later in this chapter, has been associated with increased cardiac mortality. Surprisingly, negative inotropic modulation is sometimes helpful in prolonging survival in such patients.

Cellular Anatomy of Myocardial Contraction

An understanding of myocardial function at the cellular level is necessary in order to identify and target specific cellular events for pharmacologic intervention (Fig. 1).

Myocyte contraction begins with stimulation of the β-receptor, which activates adenyl cyclase through modulation of the G protein. Adenyl cyclase is the enzyme which catalyzes the conversion of adenosine triphosphate (ATP) to the so-called "second messenger" cyclic adenosine monophosphate (cAMP). cAMP, which is degraded by phophodiesterases (PDE), serves to stimulate protein kinases, which in turn phosphorylate phospholambin, leading to release of calcium from the sarcoplasmic reticulum. This increase in cytosolic calcium concentrations leads to increased actin-myosin cross-linkage [1]. cAMP also serves to regulate myocardial relaxation by activating phospholambin and Troponin I, which play a role in sequestering cytosolic calcium and decreasing the affinity of troponin C for this ion.

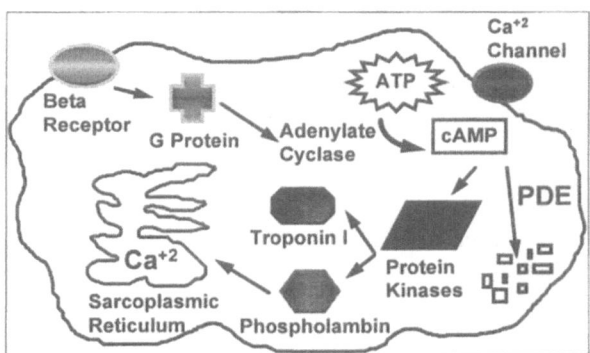

Fig. 1. Cellular events during myocyte contraction

Because of the multitude of individual steps involved in this cellular mechanism, as well as the dual roles of cAMP, there exists many potential opportunities for the therapeutic alteration of cardiac function.

β-Adrenergic Therapy

β-receptors may be subdivided into two groups. The effector organ of β_1-receptors is the heart, where stimulation leads to increased chronotropy, inotropy, automaticity, and impulse conduction (dromotropy). β_2-stimulation causes bronchodilatation and arterial vasodilatation, as well hypokalemia, increased glucagon secretion, and decreased secretion of insulin. Vasoconstriction is mediated by α_1-receptors. Presynaptic α receptors inhibit norepinephrine release, whereas postsynaptic α-receptors constrict venous capacitance vessels [2]. Most β-adrenergic agonists exert a combination of β_1-, β_2-, and α-effects (Table 1). Dopamine is unique in that its spectrum of receptor affinities is dose dependent; at low doses (1–5 mcg/kg/min), dopaminergic receptor stimulation causes renovascular dilatation. At moderate infusions (5–15 mcg/kg/min), β-adrenergic stimulation is most prominent, while intense α effects are noted at higher doses.

Disadvantages of Catecholamines

Despite their efficacy, catecholamines possess several additional properties which limit their usefulness in individual patients. The most important of these is increased myocardial oxygen demand (MVO_2), which becomes critically important in the setting of myocardial ischemia. Furthermore, β-adrenergic receptors may be decreased in number and density in the hearts of patients with chronic congestive failure [3]. This down-regulation of β-receptors causes impaired responsivity to conventional doses of β-agonist drugs. Furthermore, because cAMP levels may also be depressed in patients with heart failure [4], β-adrenergic therapy may be ineffective. Catecholamines predispose to tachydysrhythmias, and may cause peripheral shunting due to β_2-stimulation. Prolonged administration, even in patients without a history of chronic congestive heart

Table 1. Comparison of relative alpha- and beta-adrenergic receptor affinities of commonly used catecholamines

	β-1	β-2	α-1
Isoproterenol	+ + +	+ + +	0
Norepinephrine	+ +	0	+ + +
Epinephrine	+ +	+ +	+
Dopamine	+ +	+	variable
Dobutamine	+ + +	+	+

failure, frequently results in receptor down-regulation, thus limiting the utility of catecholamine therapy in subacute and chronic management.

Newer Catecholamines

Dopexamine is a synthetic analogue of dopamine with many similarities to its parent molecule. It acts primarily at both subsets of dopamine receptors as well as at β_2-receptors. There is moderate affinity for the β_1-receptor, but only minimal α activity. Like dopamine, its actions include inotropy, chronotropy, and renovascular dilatation [5]. Unlike dopamine, however dopexamine produces systemic vasodilatation, which may improve hemodynamics by increasing myocardial contractility while also unloading the left ventricle. Augmentation of cardiac function is comparable or even greater than that produced by dobutamine [6, 7]. Dopexamine appears to be less disrhythmogenic than other catecholamines, and does not significantly increase MVO_2 at lower doses. β_1-downregulation is not profound. Furthermore, hepatosplanchnic perfusion may be augmented by dopexamine infusion [8]. As with all other catecholamines, however, therapy with dopexmine is limited by adverse properties which include tachycardia and systemic hypotension, as well as nausea and vomiting.

For several years, some investigators have postulated that providing supranormal oxygen delivery may improve outcome in high risk patients [9]. Dopexamine, titrated to provide oxygen delivery of 600 ml/m^2 was recently compared to standard perioperative care in 107 high risk surgical patients [10]. The investigators concluded that patients in the dopexamine group experienced significantly less morbidity and mortality during the 28 day postoperative follow-up period.

Phosphodiesterase Inhibitors

A relatively recent addition to the pharmacologic armamentarium available to intensivists is the class of inotropic agents whose action derives from inhibition of the phosphodiesterase enzyme (Fig. 2). These so-called "inodilators" take advantage of the fact that cAMP modulates the energy requiring cellular mechanisms that control both ventricular contraction and relaxation. By preventing the breakdown of cAMP, phosphodiesterase inhibitors amplify the effects of beta-adrenergic stimulation. The inodilators, which include amrinone, milrinone, enox-

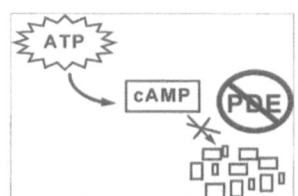

Fig. 2. Mechanism of action of the inodilators. Inhibition of phosphodiesterase prevents breakdown of cAMP

imone, and piroximone, all cause increased inotropy, vasodilatation, and venodilatation, usually without significant effects on heart rate or rhythm. Amrinone and milrinone are currently available in the United States, the most significant difference being a 20-fold increase in potency of the latter drug. Therapy with phosphodiesterase inhibitors may unload the ventricle to the point that decreases in LV wall stress overshadow increases in contractile function, such that net MVO$_2$ is reduced. cAMP accumulation may also augment diastolic function by promoting the activity of troponin 1 (Fig. 3). Evidence to support these lusitropic effects includes increases in peak negative dP/dt and the rate of peak LV diastolic filling, as well as decreases in the time constant of ventricular relaxation.

Because of their unique hemodynamic effects, the phosphodiesterase inhibitors may be useful in several clinical settings, including post cardiotomy shock, right ventricular dysfunction with pulmonary hypertension, as well as a pharmacologic bridge to cardiac transplantation. Because inotropic effects do not rely on beta-adrenergic stimulation, they are particularly useful in patients with pre-existing LV dysfunction who may have significant β-receptor down regulation as well as cAMP depletion.

Unfortunately, phosphodiesterase inhibitors may increase AV nodal conduction and predispose to supraventricular tachycardia and rapid atrial fibrillation. Excessive preload and afterload reduction may cause significant systemic hypotension. This becomes especially problematic in pulmonary hypertension, in which decreases in coronary perfusion pressure may lead to ischemia of the hypertrophied right ventricle. Thrombocytopenia and impaired platelet aggregation, although less of a problem with milrinone than amrinone, remain a disadvantage.

The fact that milrinone may be administered orally prompted its evaluation as a chronic medication in patients with heart failure. The Prospective Randomized Milrinone Survival Evaluation (PROMISE) study [11], initiated in 1991, compared milrinone to combined therapy with digoxin, diuretic, and angiotensin converting enzyme inhibitors in 1100 patients with heart failure. A 28% increase in cardiac mortality in the milrinone group prompted early termination of the study. Furthermore, milrinone did not appear to offer any clinical benefits to patients when compared to standard therapy. This study underscores the notion that treatment with potent positive inotropes is best carried out in the acute setting.

Recently, however, it has become apparent that lower doses of inotropic agents may be beneficial for prolonging survival in chronic heart failure patients, even in the absence of dramatic hemodynamic improvement [12–14]. For example,

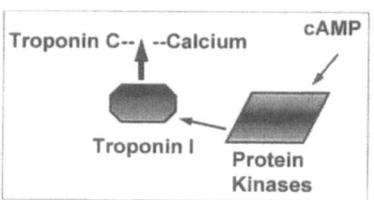

Fig. 3. Effect of phosphodiesterase inhibition on ventricular relaxation. Increased cAMP levels increase activity of troponin 1, which serves to decrease the affinity of calcium and tropinin C

low doses of vesnarinone, an orally active mild phosphodiesterase inhibitor, improves quality of life and prolongs survival in patients with congestive heart failure [15]. However, higher doses increase mortality, underscoring the narrow therapeutic range of this and probably other potentially useful agents.

Triiodothyronine in Heart Failure and Cardiac Surgery

The use of hormonal therapy in acute cardiac decompensation represents a novel approach based on clinical observations of the hemodynamic manifestations of severe hypothyroidism, in which bradycardia, decreased stroke volume, and increased arterial tone are typically present. The cornerstone of therapy in this setting is hormonal replacement. In contrast, the "euthyroid sick syndrome (ESS)" signifies an imbalance of the active and inactive forms of thyroid hormone. Diagnosis is based on the measurement of decreased free T_3 levels in combination with increased reverse T_3 levels. ESS may be observed in patients with surgical stress, sepsis, hepatic dysfunction, burns, and chronic congestive heart failure [16]. Unlike frank hypothyroidism, therapy is directed at the underlying cause. Recently, however, investigators have postulated that ESS may play a role in the hemodynamic derangements seen in brain-dead organ donors as well as in patients undergoing procedures in which cardiopulmonary bypass (CPB) is used [17, 18]. Acute administration of T_3 has been shown to be of benefit in improving hemodynamic status in potential organ donors [19] as well as separation from cardiopulmonary bypass [20].

The mechanism of action of T_3, however, remains unclear. Although the effects of thyroid hormone in most tissues are typically mediated by activities within the cell nucleus, mechanisms in cardiac muscle are probably more diverse [21], and defy simplistic explanations. For example, improvement in left ventricular function was documented in an animal model of ischemia and reperfusion [22], in which enhanced contractile performance and subcellular preservation could not be explained by increased availability of high-energy phosphates, since ATP levels were similarly diminished in both control and experimental animals.

Although T_3 holds promise as a novel inotropic agent, further investigations are necessary before its role in acute hemodynamic management can be fully defined.

Summary

Recent advancements in pharmacology have enabled clinicians to more precisely target therapy for cardiovascular dysfunction, particularly with regard to novel synthetic catecholamines and inodilators. The next challenge for investigators is to more precisely define the cardiovascular actions of these agents, as well as improve technology for bedside diagnosis of hemodynamic instability. Such advancements should bring clinicians closer to the goal of improving patient outcomes through rational application of pharmacologic support.

References

1. Shore-Lesserson L, Konstadt S (1994) Recent advances in cardiac pharmacology. Anesth Clin North Am 12:133–168
2. Lindeborg DM, Pearl RG (1993) Inotropic therapy in the critically ill patient. Int Anes Clin 31:49–71
3. Bristow MR, Ginsburg R, Minobe W, Cubicciotti RS, Sageman WS, Lurie K, Billingham ME, Harrison DC, Stinson EB (1982) Decreased catecholamine sensitivity and beta-adrenergic-receptor density in failing human hearts. N Engl J Med 307:205–211
4. Feldman MD, Copelas L, Gwathmey JK, Phillips SP, Warren SE, Schoen FJ, Grossman W, Morgan JP (1987) Deficient production of cyclic AMP: pharmacologic evidence of an important cause of contractile dysfunction in patients with end-stage heart failure. Circulation 75:331–339
5. Magrini F, Foulds R, Macchi G, Mondadori C, Zanchetti A (1987) Human renovascular effects of dopexamine hydrochloride: a novel agonist of peripheral dopamine and beta 2-adreno-receptors. Eur J Clin Pharmacol 32:1–4
6. MacGregor DA, Butterworth JF 4th, Zaloga CP, Prielipp RC, James R, Royster RL (1994) Hemodynamic and renal effects of dopexamine and dobutamine in patients with reduced cardiac output following coronary artery bypass grafting. Chest 106:835–841
7. Boyd O, Lamb G, Mackey CJ, Grounds RM, Bennett ED (1995) A comparison of the efficacy of dopexamine and dobutamine for increasing oxygen delivery in high-risk surgical patients. Anasth & Int Care 23:478–484
8. Smithies M, Yee TH, Jackson L, Beale R, Bihari D (1994) Protecting the gut and the liver in the critically ill: effects of dopexamine. Crit Care Med 22:789–795
9. Shoemaker W, Appel P, Kram H, Waxman K, Lee TS (1988) Prospective trial of supranormal values of survivors as therapeutic goas in high risk surgical patients. Chest 94:1176–1186
10. Boyd O, Grounds RM, Bennett ED (1994) A randomized clinical trial of the effect of deliberate perioperative increase of oxygen delivery on mortality in high-risk surgical patients. JAMA 270:2699–2707
11. Packer M, Carver J, Rodeheffer R, Ivanhoe R, Dibianco R, Zeldis S, Hendrix G, Bomner W, Elkayam U, Kukin M (1991) Effects of oral milrinone on mortality in severe congestive heart failure. N Engl J Med 325:1468–1475
12. Packer M (1993) The development of positive inotropic agents for chronic heart failure: how have we gone astray? J Am Coll Cardiol 22 (4 Suppl):119A–126A
13. Remme WJ (1993) Inodilator therapy for heart failure. Early, late, or not at all? Circulation 87 (5 Suppl):IV97–107
14. Shipley JB, Hess ML (1995) Inotropic therapy for the failing myocardium. Clin Cardiol 18:615–619
15. Feldman AM, Bristow MR, Parmley WW, Carson PE, Pepine CJ, Gilbert EM, Strobeck JE, Hendrix GH, Powers ER, Bain RP, White BG (1993) Effects of vesnarinone on morbidity and mortality in patients with heart failure. N Engl J Med 329:149–155
16. Hamilton MA (1993) Prevalence and clinical implications of abnormal thyroid hormone metabolism in advanced heart failure. Ann Thor Surg 56:S48–53
17. Holland FW II, Brown PS Jr, Weintraub BD, Clark RE (1991) Cardiopulmonary bypass and thyroid function: a "euthyroid sick syndrome." Ann Thorac Surg 52:46–50
18. Clark RE (1993) Cardiopulmonary bypass and thyroid hormone metabolism. Ann Thor Surg 56:S16–23
19. Novitzky D, Cooper DKC, Chaffin JS, Greer AE, DeBault LE, Zuhdi N (1990) Improved cardiac allograft function following triiodothyronine therapy to both donor and recipient. Transplantation 49:311
20. Novitzky D, Cooper DKC, Barton CI, Greer A, Chaffin J, Grim J, Zuhid N (1989) Triiodothyronine as an inotropic agent after open heart surgery. J Thorc Cardiovasc Surg 98:972–978
21. Davis PJ, Davis FB (1993) Acute cellular actions of thyroid hormone and myocardial function. Ann Thor Surg 56:S35–42
22. Dyke CM, Ding M, Abd-Elfattah AS, Loesser K, Dignan RJ, Wechsler AS, Slater DR (1993) Effects of triiodothyronine supplementation after myocardial ischemia. Ann Thorac Surg 56:215–222

Heart-Lung Interactions*

M. R. Pinsky

Introduction

The primary goal of cardiovascular and respiratory systems is to supply adequate amounts of O_2 to the tissues to meet their metabolic demand. Since a primary role of critical care resuscitative efforts is to insure the adequacy of O_2 delivery in stress states, an understanding of cardio-pulmonary physiology and the effects of disease and therapeutic interventions on cardio-pulmonary status is central to the management of the critically ill patient.

The majority of problems associated with heart-lung interactions center on the effects of ventilation on the circulation. Ventilation can be spontaneous, partially assisted or totally supported by mechanical devices. Spontaneous inspiration decreases intrathoracic pressure (ITP), whereas positive-pressure inspiration increases ITP. Assisted ventilation has a variable effect on ITP, sometimes decreasing ITP (especially during early inspiration when triggered by spontaneous inspiratory efforts) and sometimes increasing ITP (especially at end-inspiration). All forms of ventilation cyclically increase lung volume in a tidal fashion above some end-expiratory value. Thus, changes in ITP and lung volume can occur in the same or opposite directions during ventilation depending on both ventilatory effort and mode of ventilation. Since changes in lung volume reflect a common aspect of all forms of ventilation, any hemodynamic differences that occur between spontaneous and positive-pressure breaths reflect effects of changing ITP and the energy necessary to create these changes.

Heart-lung interactions can be broadly grouped into interactions which involve four basic concepts (Table 1). Although addressed separately, these processes often co-exist. The four basic concepts are:
a) inspiration increases lung volume above end-expiratory volume;
b) spontaneous inspiration decreases ITP;
c) positive-pressure ventilation increases ITP; and
d) ventilation is exercise, it consumes O_2 and produces CO_2 and thus may stress normal adaptive circulatory mechanisms.

* This work was supported in part by the Veterans Administration.

Table 1. Hemodynamic effects of ventilation

Mechanical

A) *Increasing lung volume*
  1. autonomic tone
    - Vt < 12 ml/kg vagal withdrawal: cardiac acceleration
    - Vt > 15 ml/kg sympathetic withdrawal: cardiovascular depression
  2. end-expiratory lung volume
    - recruit to FRC: decrease pulmonary vascular resistance
    - hyperinflation above FRC: increase pulmonary vascular resistance
  3. compression of the heart in the cardiac fossa
B) *Intrathoracic pressure (ITP)*
  1. decreasing ITP
    - increase venous return (flow limited)
    - increase LV afterload
  2. increasing ITP
    - decrease venous return (primary effect)
    - decrease LV afterload (secondary effect, except in heart failure)

Metabolic

A) *Increase oxygen consumption (VO_2), work cost of breathing*
  1. limit blood flow to non-respiratory muscles
  2. limited ventilatory reserve in heart failure
B) *Increase CO_2 production (VCO_2)*
  1. increase ventilatory load on respiratory muscles

Hemodynamic Effects of Changes in Lung Volume

Lung inflation alters autonomic tone and pulmonary vascular resistance and, at high lung volumes interacts mechanically with the heart in the cardiac fossa to limit absolute cardiac volumes. Each of these processes is important in determining the hemodynamic response to mechanical ventilation.

Autonomic Tone

The lungs are richly enervated with autonomic fibers that mediate multiple homeostatic processes. Numerous cardiovascular reflexes are centered within this network. Inflation-incluced chronotropic responses act through vagally-mediated reflex arcs [1, 2]. Lung inflation at small tidal volumes (< 10 ml/kg) increases heart rate, via Vagal withdrawal. Larger tidal volumes (> 15 ml/kg) decrease heart rate via sympathetic withdrawal. Inspiration-associated cardio-acceleration is referred to as respiratory sinus arrhythmia [3] and denotes normal autonomic tone [4]. Loss of respiratory sinus arrhythmia commonly occurs in dysautonomic states, such as diabetic peripheral neuropathy, and the reappearance of respiratory sinus arrhythmia precedes return of peripheral autonomic control [5]. However, some degree of respiratory-associated heart rate change is intrinsic to the heart itself and persists even following cardiac denervation, as occurs following cardiac transplantation [6], suggesting that mechano-receptors in the right atrium can alter sino-atrial tone.

Independent of these phasic reflex arcs, ventilation also alters global endocrine function as it relates to the control of intravascular fluid balance. Both positive pressure ventilation and sustained hyperinflation stimulate hormonally-controlled fluid retention. Lung distention by compressing the right atrium increases sympathetic tone inducing fluid retention by inhibiting secretion of atrial nateretic peptide [7], plasma norepinephrine levels and plasma rennin activity [8, 9]. As a practical application of this process, patients with congestive heart failure reduce their plasma atrial naturetic peptide activity following exposure to nasal continuous positive airway pressure (CPAP) in parallel with improvements in global blood flow [10, 11].

Pulmonary Vascular Resistance

The major determinants of the hemodynamic response to increases in lung volume are mechanical in nature [12, 13, 17]. Lung inflation, independent of changes in ITP, primarily affects cardiac function and cardiac output by altering right ventricular (RV) afterload and both RV and LV preload [18]. RV afterload can be estimated as maximal RV systolic wall stress [19], which, by the LaPlace equation, is a function of RV end-diastolic volume and systolic RV pressure [20]. Since both the RV and pulmonary arteries both sense ITP as their surrounding pressure, changes in ITP will not alter the pressure gradients between the RV and pulmonary artery. Accordingly, systolic RV pressure can be defined as pulmonary arterial pressure (Ppa) minus ITP (transmural Ppa). Transmural Ppa may increase if pulmonary arterial flow increases; pulmonary vasomotor tone increases; pulmonary vascular resistance increases due to passive lung inflation; and pulmonary outflow pressure increases. All processes that increase transmural Ppa increase the RV afterload, impeding RV ejection [21]. If the RV does not empty as much as before, RV stroke volume will decrease [22] and RV end-systolic volume will increase [19]. As systemic venous blood flow continues RV end-diastolic volume will also continue to increase, increasing right atrial pressure (Right atrial pressure) as the RV overdistends. Since Right atrial pressure is also the back pressure for systemic blood flow, if Right atrial pressure increases due to RV overdistention, systemic venous return will also decrease [23] decreasing cardiac output.

If regional P_AO_2 decreases below 60 mmHg, local pulmonary vasomotor tone will increase, reducing local blood flow [24]. This process is called hypoxic pulmonary vasoconstriction. Hypoxic pulmonary vasoconstriction optimizes ventilation to perfusion matching when regional impairments in ventilation exist. However, if alveolar hypoxia occurs throughout the lungs, then overall pulmonary vasomotor tone increases, increasing pulmonary vascular resistance and impeding RV ejection [19]. Importantly, acute lung injury induces alveolar instability and collapse, decreasing lung volumes [25, 26]. Accordingly, pulmonary vascular resistance is often increased in patients with acute lung injury because of the resultant hypoxic pulmonary vasoconstriction. Thus, if PEEP recruits collapsed lung units hypoxic pulmonary vasoconstriction will be reduced, pulmonary vascular resistance will decrease, and RV ejection will improve.

Changes in lung volume also affect pulmonary vascular resistance, independent of changes in vasomotor tone [27–29]. The pulmonary circulation can be considered to consist of two populations of vessels that sense a different pressure surrounding them [28]. The small pulmonary arterioles, venules, and capillaries sense alveolar pressure as their surrounding pressure and are called alveolar vessels. The large pulmonary arteries and veins sense interstitial pressure as their surrounding pressure and are called extra-alveolar vessels. Interstitial pressure is usually similar to ITP. Extra-alveolar vessels, like airways, are acted upon by the radial interstitial forces of the lung that keep them patent [27, 30, 31]. As lung volume increases, the radial interstitial forces increase, increasing the diameter of extra-alveolar vessels. And, as lung volume decreases, the radial interstitial traction decreases, and extra-alveolar vessels decrease their cross-sectional diameter, increasing pulmonary vascular resistance [27, 32]. The collapse of small airways induces alveolar hypoxia which is the primary process increasing pulmonary vasomotor tone in this setting.

As lung volume increases above functional residual capacity (FRC) pulmonary vascular resistance will increase because alveolar resistance rises [31, 32]. Alveolar resistance increases because the extravascular pressure gradient between the large vessels and the alveolar vessels increases to a level above which this pressure gradient exceeds intralumenal pressure. The heart and extra-alveolar vessels sense ITP as their surrounding pressure, therefore, whereas the alveolar vessels sense alveolar pressure as their surrounding pressure, a extralumenal transpulmonary pressure gradient exists between the extra-alveolar and alveolar vessels. Since the extravascular pressure gradient equals transpulmonary pressure (alveolar pressure minus ITP), as lung volume increases the extravascular pressure gradient from large to small pulmonary vessels also increases. Thus, if transpulmonary pressure increases enough to exceed intralumenal pressure, the pulmonary vasculature will collapse where extra-alveolar vessels pass into alveolar loci, decreasing their cross-sectional area, increasing pulmonary vascular resistance. If the cross-sectional area of the pulmonary capillaries is already reduced, as may occur in the setting of chronic obstructive lung disease, then the addition of abnormal hyperinflation can create significant pulmonary hypertension and may precipitate acute RV failure (acute cor pulmonale) [33] and RV ischemia [34]. Canada et al. [35] demonstrated in a dog model of unilateral lung injury that PEEP decreased pulmonary vascular resistance in the injured lung, but it increased pulmonary vascular resistance in the normal lung.

Ventricular Interdependence

Changes in RV end-diastolic volume directly alter LV diastolic compliance. If RV volumes are increase, then LV diastolic compliance decreases [36]. This process is referred to as ventricular interdependence. Since both ventricles share a common intraventricular septum, if RV end-diastolic volume increases, then the septum shifts into the LV decreasing LV diastolic compliance [37]. Although RV dilation is not common during positive pressure ventilation, in the fluid-resuscitated patient, RV volumes can increase with pulmonary hypertension [38] and may decrease with LV diastolic compliance.

Mechanical Heart-Lung Interactions

As lung volumes increase the heart is compressed between the two expanding lungs, which increases the pressure surrounding the heart. The chest wall and diaphragm can move away from the expanding lungs, but the heart is unable to be displaced out of the cardiac fossa, thus, juxtacardiac ITP may increase more than lateral chest wall pleural pressure during positive pressure ventilation [39–41]. This compressive effect of the inflated lung can be seen with either spontaneous hyperinflation [42] or positive-pressure-induced hyperinflation with PEEP [43, 44]. This compression of the LV is not the same as ventricular interdependence because in ventricular interdependence LV diastolic compliance is decreased but with external compression it is the increase in ITP that decreases LV volume without any change in diastolic compliance [45, 46].

Hemodynamic Effects of Changes in Intrathoracic Pressure

The heart lies within the thorax, and as such is a pressure chamber within a pressure chamber. Therefore, changes in ITP will affect the pressure gradients for both systemic venous return to the RV and systemic outflow from the LV, independent of the heart itself. Increases in ITP, by increasing right atrial pressure and decreasing transmural LV systolic pressure, will reduce these pressure gradients decreasing intrathoracic blood volume. Using the same argument, decreases in ITP will augment venous return and impede LV ejection, thereby increasing intrathoracic blood volume.

Systemic Venous Return

Blood flows back to the heart from the periphery through low pressure-low resistance venous vessels. The pressure gradient for venous return is equal to the upstream venous pressure relative to right atrial pressure. This upstream venous pressure is referred to as mean systemic pressure, is a function of total blood volume, peripheral vasomotor tone, and blood flow distribution [47, 48]. During the ventilatory cycle mean systemic pressure does not change rapidly, while right atrial pressure does. Accordingly, variations in right atrial pressure represent the primary factor determining the fluctuation in pressure gradient for systemic venous return during ventilation [23, 49]. With increases in ITP, as seen with positive-pressure ventilation or hyperinflation during spontaneous ventilation, as right atrial pressure increases venous blood flow decreases [22, 23, 34,

50–56]. During spontaneous inspiration, the opposite flow pattern occurs [22, 52, 57–60].

Although decreases venous return in proportion to the increase in right atria pressure, the absolute decrease may be less than predicted by an isolated increase in right atrial pressure alone. Both positive-pressure ventilation and PEEP increase abdominal pressure tending to maintain mean systemic pressure relative to right atrial pressure constant [60–63]. Finally, when cardiac output is returned to pre-positive airway pressure levels by fluid resuscitation [63, 64] while positive airway pressure is maintained, liver clearance mechanisms increase above pre-PEEP visceral organ function returns to levels seen off positive airway pressure [65–67].

Based on a large body of clinical studies over 30 years plus the conceptual framework described above, the primary effect of changes in lung volume and ITP on cardiovascular function in subjects with normal baseline cardiovascular function is to alter RV filling by changing the pressure gradient for venous return. Thus, as described by Cournand et al. [68] this detrimental effect of positive pressure ventilation on cardiac output can be minimized by keeping both mean ITP and swings in lung volume as low as possible. Thus, prolonging expiratory time, decreasing tidal volume, and avoiding PEEP all minimize this decrease in systemic venous return to the RV [23, 52–55, 69, 70]. Similarly, intravascular fluid infusion or increased autonomic tone, by increasing upstream venous pressure [48, 71, 72], will also maintain venous blood flow and cardiac output, despite the addition of increased ITP [58].

Spontaneous inspiratory efforts decrease right atrial pressure accelerating venous return to the RV [13, 53, 57, 59]. This increased venous return is translated into an increase in RV stroke volume on the subsequent beat. The maximal increase in venous return is limited by collapse of the caval vessels as they enter the thorax as ITP becomes more negative [48, 73, 74]. This venous flow-limitation prevents massive RV volume overload during inspiratory occlusion strain maneuvers [75], which would otherwise push the subject into cor pulmonale [76].

Left Ventricular Afterload

LV afterload is determined by systolic wall tension which, by the LaPlace equation, is proportional to the product of transmural LV pressure and the radius of curvature of the LV. Under normal conditions maximal LV wall tension occurs at the end of isometric contraction when the product of LV end-diastolic volume and aortic diastolic pressure are maximal. This concept underscores the importance of diastolic hypertension in determining LV afterload, since even though arterial pressure increases during LV ejection, the LV radius of curvature decreases more, thus the normal LV unloads itself during ejection. However, in congestive heart failure, wherein LV volumes is constantly elevated, the radius of curvature of the LV does not decrease much during ejection, thus afterload increases during ejection. Accordingly, the systolic pressure responsiveness of patient sin heart failure. LV ejection pressure is the pressure equals intralumenal LV pressure minus pericardial pressure. When no aortic outflow obstruction exists and no pericardial volume restraint occurs, transmural LV systolic pressure can be approximated as arterial pressure relative to ITP. Thus, if arterial pressure were to remain constant as ITP increased, then LV afterload decrease. Similarly, if transmural arterial pressure were to remain constant as ITP increased but LV end-diastolic volume were to decrease because of the associated decrease in systemic venous return, then LV afterload would decrease. Decreases in ITP with a constant arterial pressure will increase LV transmural pressure and, thus, increase LV afterload, impeding LV ejection [77]. In support of this construct, Pinsky et al. [78] demonstrated in a canine model of acute ventricular failure and fluid resuscitation that increases in ITP increased cardiac output for a common transmural left atrial pressure. A similar beneficial response was seen in ventilator-dependent patients with severe LV failure [79].

Spontaneous ventilatory efforts against either an obstructive (bronchospasm) or restrictive (pulmonary fibrosis) load will decrease LV stroke volume and arterial pressure. This process of inspiration-associated decreases in arterial pressure is called pulsus paradoxus [80–84]. The mechanisms by which arterial pressure decrease during loaded spontaneous inspiration are complex and different depending on when in the strain maneuver it is analyzed. The immediate effect of the associated increase in RV end-diastolic volume is a transient intraventricular septal shift into the LV lumen plus pericardial volume restraint decreasing LV end-diastolic volume. Independent of this effect, increases in LV afterload will increase LV end-systolic volume [77]. If airway obstruction is sustained, arterial destruction can occur [85], which may create a hypoxia-induced impairment in LV diastolic compliance and contractile function [86].

Sudden increases in ITP will directly increase arterial pressure without changing transmural arterial pressure [77] or aortic blood flow [87]. If the increase in ITP is sustained then baroreceptor-induced decreases in peripheral vasomotor tone develop [88] decreasing arterial pressure [77] without altering the arterial pressure-flow relation [89]. Coronary perfusion pressure is not increased by ITP-induced increases in arterial pressure, whereas mechanical constraint from the expanding lungs may obstruct coronary blood flow. Thus, coronary hypoperfusion from a combined coronary compression and a decrease in coronary perfusion pressure may occur as a complication of increasing ITP [90–93].

Although increasing ITP will augment LV ejection by decreasing LV afterload, this effect has limited therapeutic potential, just as all afterload reducing therapies are limited by both the minimal end-systolic volume and the obligatory decrease in venous return. Thus, the potential augmentation of LV ejection by increasing ITP is limited under most conditions, because increasing ITP by reducing LV ejection pressure can only decrease end-systolic volume, but the decrease in venous return associated with the increase in ITP can stop venous blood flow. As ITP increases, all intrathoracic vascular pressures decrease as blood leaves the thoracic compartment, whereas stroke volume initially increases associated with an increase in arterial pressure equal to that in ITP. This cardiac augmentation later becomes preload-limited, such that stroke volumes do not increase further as ITP increases although filling pressures continue to decrease and arterial pressure continues to increase [93–97].

If simple manipulations of venous return and ejection pressure were the only forces determining heart-lung interactions as ITP varied, then mild increases in ITP and lung volume, as induced by the application of 5 cm H_2O positive end-expiratory pressure (PEEP) or continuous positive airway pressure (CPAP) would not induce much of a hemodynamic perturbation because the changes in ITP would be small. However, numerous clinical studies have consistently shown improvement in cardiac output with small levels of PEEP or CPAP. Furthermore, even when IPPV does significantly increase ITP, the decrease in LV end-systolic volume exceeds amounts predicted solely by the reduction in LV ejection pressure. Potentially, these observed changes reflect improve LV ejection efficiency. Although not proven, it seems reasonable to hypothesize that increasing ITP improves LV ejection by decreasing the degree to which asynchrony of shortening of parallel myocardial contractile elements. Improved synchrony of contraction should not alter contractility, as defined by the slope of the LV end-systolic pressure-volume relationship (ESPVR), but induce proportional decreases in both LV end-diastolic volume and end-systolic volume, such that the ESPVR is shifted leftward with volume on the x-axis. This shift of the ESPVR should decrease myocardial oxygen demand (MVO_2) increasing LV ejection efficiency (stroke work/MVO_2).

Theoretically, not only do increases in ITP unload the LV, but abolishing negative swings in ITP will also reduce LV afterload. This process is potentially more clinically relevant than increasing ITP for many reasons. First, many pulmonary disease states are associated with exaggerated decreases in ITP during inspiration. For example, in obstructive diseases large decreases in ITP occur due to increased resistance to inspiratory airflow [12, 75, 98]. Second, exaggerated decreases in ITP require increased respiratory efforts that increase the work of breathing, taxing a potentially stressed circulation. Finally, the exaggerated decreases in ITP only increase venous blood flow so far before flow-limitation develops [48]. Thus, abolishing markedly negative swings in ITP should selectively reduce LV afterload because venous return will remain constant. LV performance improves after the institution of positive-pressure ventilation in patients with combined cardiovascular insufficiency and respiratory distress [58, 97, 99–101]. Similarly, weaning patients from positive-pressure ventilation, by allowing the return of decreases in ITP, may precipitate acute LV failure and pulmonary edema in patients with borderline LV function [102, 103]. Weaning can be considered an exercise stress test, those who can not maintain the cardiac output will not wean successfully from mechanical ventilation. Furthermore, the institution of PEEP in patients with heart failure may further augment LV output by reducing LV afterload, despite the obligatory decrease in LV preload [58, 97, 99, 101, 104].

Ventilation as Exercise

Spontaneous ventilatory efforts are a form of exercise induced by contraction of the respiratory muscles. Blood flow to the respiratory muscles is believed to exceed the highest metabolic demand of maximally exercising skeletal muscle under normal conditions [105]. Thus, blood flow is not the limiting factor determining maximal ventilatory effort when cardiovascular function is normal. Although ventilation normally requires minimal O_2 delivery to meet its demand [105], in lung disease states where the work of breathing is increased the requirements for O_2 may increase to 25% or 30% of total O_2 delivery [69, 96, 105]. Furthermore, if cardiac output is limited, blood flow to both other organs and the respiratory muscles may be compromised, inducing both tissue hypoperfusion and lactic acidosis [106]. The institution of mechanical ventilation for ventilatory and hypoxemic respiratory failure may reduce metabolic demand on the stressed cardiovascular system increasing SvO_2 for a constant cardiac output and arterial O_2 content. Intubation and mechanical ventilation, when adjusted to the metabolic demands of the patient, may dramatically decrease the work of breathing, resulting in increased O_2 delivery to other vital organs and decreased serum lactic acid levels. If fixed right-to-left shunts exist, the obligatory increase in SvO_2 will result in an increase in the PaO_2, despite no change in the ratio of shunt blood flow to cardiac output.

References

1. Glick G, Wechsler AS, Epstein DE (1969) Reflex cardiovascular depression produced by stimulation of pulmonary stretch receptors in the dog. J Clin Invest 48:467–472
2. Painal AS (1973) Vagal sensory receptors and their reflex effects. Physiol Rev 53:59–88
3. Anrep GV, Pascual W, Rossler R (1936) Respiratory variations in the heart rate. I. The reflex mechanism of the respiratory arrhythmia. Proc R Soc Lond B Biol Sci 119:191–217
4. Taha BH, Simon PM, Dempsey JA, Skatrud JB, Iber C (1995) Respiratory sinus arrhythmia in humans: an obligatory role for vagal feedback from the lungs. J Appl Physiol 78 (2): 638–645
5. Bernardi L, Calciati A, Gratarola A, Battistin I, Fratino P, Finardi G (1986) Heart rate-respiration relationship: computerized method for early detection of cardiac autonomic damage in diabetic patients. Acta Cardiol 41:197–206
6. Bernardi L, Keller F, Sanders M, Reddy PS, Griffith B, Meno F, Pinsky MR (1989) Respiratory sinus arrhythmia in the totally denervated human heart. J Appl Physiol 67:1447–1455
7. Frass M, Watschinger B, Traindl O, Popovic R, Podolsky A, Gisslinger H, Flager S, Golden M, Schuster E, Leithner C (1993) Atrial natriuretic peptide release in response to different positive end-expiratory pressure levels. Crit Care Med 21:343–347
8. Payen DM, Brun-Buisson CJL, Carli PA, Huet Y, Leviel F, Cinotti L, Chiron B (1987) Hemodynamic, gas exchange, and hormonal consequences of LBPP during PEEP ventilation. J Appl Physiol 62 (1):61–70
9. Frage D, de la Coussaye JE, Beloucif S, Fratacci MD, Payen DM (1995) Interactions between hormonal modifications during Peep-Induced Antidiuresis and Antinatriuresis. Chest 107: 1095–1100
10. Wilkins MA, Su XL, Palayew MD, Yamashiro Y, Bolli P, McKenzie JK, Kryger MH (1995) The effects of posture change and continuous positive airway pressure on cardiac natriuretic peptides in congestive heart failure. Chest 107:909–915
11. Shirakami G, Magaribuchi T, Shingu K, Suga S, Tamai S, Nakao K, Mori K (1993) Positive end-expiratory pressure ventilation decreases plasma atrial and brain natriuretic peptide levels in humans. Anesth Analg 77 (6):1116–1121
12. Bromberger-Barnea B (1981) Mechanical effects of inspiration on heart functions: A review. Fed Proc 40:2172–2177

13. Brecher GA, Hubay CA (1955) Pulmonary blood flow and venous return during spontaneous respiration. Circ Res 3:40–214
14. Goldstein JA, Vlahakes GJ, Verrier ED, et al (1982) The role of right ventricular systolic dysfunction and elevated intrapericardial pressures in the genesis of low output in experimental right ventricular infarction. Circulation 65:513
15. Jardin F, Farcot JC, Boisante L, et al (1981) Influence of positive end-expiratory pressure on left ventricular performance. N Engl J Med 304:387
16. Jardin FF, Farcot JC, Gueret P, Prost JF, Ozier Y, Bourdarias JP (1984) Echocardiographic evaluation of ventricles during continuous positive pressure breathing. J Appl Physiol 56:619–627
17. Luce JM (1984) The cardiovascular effects of mechanical ventilation and positive end-expiratory pressure. J Am Med Assoc 252:807–811
18. Prec KJ, Cassels DE (1952) Oximeter studies in newborn infants during crying. Pediatr 9:756–761
19. Maughan WL, Shoukas AA, Sagawa K, Weisfeldt ML (1979) Instantaneous pressure-volume relationships of the canine right ventricle. Circ Res 44:309–315
20. Sibbald WJ, Driedger AA (1983) Right ventricular function in disease states: Pathophysiologic considerations. Crit Care Med 11:339
21. Piene H, Sund T (1982) Does pulmonary impedance constitute the optimal load for the right ventricle? Am J Physiol 242:H154–H160
22. Pinsky MR (1984) Determinants of pulmonary arterial flow variation during respiration. J Appl Physiol 56:1237–1245
23. Pinsky MR (1984) Instantaneous venous return curves in an intact canine preparation. J Appl Physiol 56:765–771
24. Madden JA, Dawson CA, Harder DR (1985) Hypoxia-induced activation in small isolated pulmonary arteries from the cat. J Appl Physiol 59:113–118
25. Hakim TS, Michel RP, Chang HK (1982) Effect of lung inflation on pulmonary vascular resistance by arterial and venous occlusion. J Appl Physiol 53:1110–1115
26. Quebbeman EJ, Dawson CA (1976) Influence of inflation and atelectasis on the hypoxic pressure response in isolated dog lung lobes. Cardiovas Res 10:672–677
27. Dawson CA, Grimm DJ, Linehan JH (1979) Lung inflation and longitudinal distribution of pulmonary vascular resistance during hypoxia. J Appl Physiol 47:532–536
28. Howell JBL, Permutt S, Proctor DF, et al (1961) Effect of inflation of the lung on different parts of the pulmonary vascular bed. J Appl Physiol 16:71–76
29. West JB, Dollery CT, Naimark A (1964) Distribution of blood flow in isolated lung; relation to vascular and alveolar pressures. J Appl Physiol 19:713–724
30. Lodato RF, Michel JR, Murray PA (1985) Multipoint pulmonary vascular pressure-cardiac output plots in conscious dogs. Am J Physiol 249:H351–H357
31. Lopez-Muniz R, Stephens NL, Bromberger-Barnea B, Permutt S, Riley RL (1968) Critical closure of pulmonary vessels analyzed in terms of Starling resistor model. J Appl Physiol 24:625–635
32. Hakim TS, Michel RP, Minami H, Chang K (1983) Site of pulmonary hypoxic vasoconstriction studied with arterial and venous occlusion. J Appl Physiol 54:1298–1302
33. Block AJ, Boyson PG, Wynne JW (1979) The origins of cor pulmonale, a hypothesis. Chest 75:109
34. Johnston WE, Vinten-Johansen J, Shugart HE, Santamore WP (1992) Positive end-expiratory pressure potentiates the severity of canine right ventricular ischemia-reperfusion injury. Am J Physiol (Heart Circ Physiol) 262:H168–H176
35. Canada E, Benumnof JL, Tousdale FR (1982) Pulmonary vascular resistance correlated in intact normal and abnormal canine lungs. Crit Care Med 10:719–723
36. Taylor RR, Corell JW, Sonnenblick EH, Ross Jr J (1967) Dependence of ventricular distensibility on filling the opposite ventricle. Am J Physiol 213:711–718
37. Brinker JA, Weiss I, Lappe DL, et al (1980) Leftward septal displacement during right ventricular loading in man. Circulation 61:626–633
38. Sibbald WH, Calvin J, Driedger AA (1982) Right and left ventricular preload, and diastolic ventricular compliance: Implications of therapy in critically ill patients. Critical Care State of the Art. Fullerton, Calif. Society of Critical Care, vol. 3

39. Gattinoni L, Mascheroni D, Torresin A, Fumagalli R, Vesconi S, Rossi GP, Rossi F, Baglioni S, Bassi F, Nastri G, Persenti A (1986) Morphological response to positive end-expiratory pressure in acute respiratory failure. Intensive Care Med 12:137–142

40. Tsitlik JE, Halperin HR, Guerci AD, Dvorine LS, Popel AS, Siu CO, Yin FCP, Weisfeldt ML (1987) Augmentation of pressure in a vessel indenting the surface of the lung. Ann Biomed Eng 15:259–284

41. Novak RA, Matuschak GM, Pinsky MR (1988) Effect of ventilatory frequency on regional pleural pressure. J Appl Physiol 65:1314–1323

42. Cassidy SS, Wead WB, Seibert GB, Ramanathan M (1987) Changes in left ventricular geometry during spontaneous breathing. J Appl Physiol 63 (2):803–811

43. Hoffman EA, Ritman EL (1987) Heart-lung interaction: effect on regional lung air content and total heart volume. Ann Biomed Eng 15:241–257

44. Olson LE, Hoffman EA (1995) Heart-lung interactions determined by electron beam X-ray CT in laterally recumbent rabbits. J Appl Physiol 78 (2):417–427

45. Cassidy SS, Robertson CH, Pierce AK, et al (1978) Cardiovascular effects of positive end-expiratory pressure in dogs. J Appl Physiol 4:743

46. Conway CM (1975) Hemodynamic effects of pulmonary ventilation. Br J Anaesth 47:761–766

47. Goldberg HS, Rabson J (1981) Control of cardiac output by systemic vessels: Circulatory adjustments of acute and chronic respiratory failure and the effects of therapeutic interventions. Am J Cardiol 47:696

48. Guyton AC, Lindsey AW, Abernathy B, et al (1957) Venous return at various right atrial pressures and the normal venous return curve. Am J Physiol 189:609–615

49. Kilburn KH (1963) Cardiorespiratory effects of large pneumothorax in conscious and anesthetized dogs. J Appl Physiol 18 (2):279–283

50. Chevalier PA, Weber KC, Engle JC, et al (1972) Direct measurement of right and left heart outputs in Valsalva-like maneuver in dogs. Proc Soc Exper Biol Med 139:1429–1437

51. Guntheroth WC, Gould R, Butler J, et al (1974) Pulsatile flow in pulmonary artery, capillary and vein in the dog. Cardiovascular Res 8:330–337

52. Guntheroth WG, Morgan BC, Mullins GL (1967) Effect of respiration on venous return and stroke volume in cardiac tamponade. Mechanism of pulsus paradoxus. Circ Res 20:381–390

53. Guyton AC (1963) Effect of cardiac output by respiration, opening of the chest, and cardiac tamponade. In: Circulatory Physiology: Cardiac Output and Its Regulation. Saunders, Philadelphia, PA, pp 378–386

54. Holt JP (1944) The effect of positive and negative intrathoracic pressure on cardiac output and venous return in the dog. Am J Physiol 142:594–603

55. Morgan BC, Martin WE, Hornbein TF, et al (1960) Hemodynamic effects of intermittent positive pressure respiration. Anesthesiology 27:584–590

56. Scharf SM, Brown R, Saunders N, Green LH (1980) Hemodynamic effects of positive pressure inflation. J Appl Physiol 49:124–131

57. Wise RA, Robotham JL, Summer WR (1981) Effects of spontaneous ventilation on the circulation. Lung 159:175–192

58. Braunwald E, Binion JT, Morgan WL, Sarnoff SJ (1957) Alterations in central blood volume and cardiac output induced by positive pressure breathing and counteracted by metraminol (Aramine). Circ Res 5:670–675

59. Morgan BC, Abel FL, Mullins GL, et al (1966) Flow patterns in cavae, pulmonary artery, pulmonary vein and aorta in intact dogs. Am J Physiol 210:903–909

60. Scharf SM, Brown R, Saunders N, et al (1979) Effects of normal and loaded spontaneous inspiration on cardiovascular function. J Appl Physiol 47:582–590

61. Fessler HE, Brower RG, Wise RA, Permutt S (1992) Effects of positive end-expiratory pressure on the canine venous return curve. Am Rev Respir Dis 146:4–10

62. Takata M, Robotham JL (1992) Effects of inspiratory diaphragmatic descent on inferior vena caval venous return. J Appl Physiol 72:597–607

63. Matuschak GM, Pinsky MR, Rogers RM (1987) Effects of positive end-expiratory pressure on hepatic blood flow and hepatic performance. J Appl Physiol 62:1377–1383

64. Brienza N, Revelly JP, Ayuse T, Robotham JL (1995) Effect of PEEP on liver arterial and venous blood flows. Am J Respir Crit Care Med 152:504–510

65. Sha M, Saito Y, Yokoyama K, Sawa T, Amaha K (1987) Effects of continuous positive-pressure ventilation on hepatic blood flow and intrahepatic oxygen delivery in dogs. Crit Care Med 15:1040–1417

66. Richard C, Berdeaux A, Delion F, et al (1986) Effect of mechanical ventilation on hepatic drug pharmacokinetics. Chest 90 (6):837–842

67. Dorinsky PM, Hamlin RL, Gadek JE (1987) Alterations in regional blood flow during positive end-expiratory pressure ventilation. Crit Care Med 15 (2):106–115

68. Cournaud A, Motley HL, Werko L, et al (1948) Physiologic studies of the effect of intermittent positive pressure breathing on cardiac output in man. Am J Physiol 152:162–174

69. Grenvik A (1966) Respiratory, circulatory and metabolic effects of respiratory treatment. Acta Anaesth Scand (Suppl)

70. Harken AH, Brennan MF, Smith N, Barsamian EM (1974) The hemodynamic response to positive end-expiratory ventilation in hypovolemic patients. Surgery 76:786–793

71. Magder S, Georgiadis G, Cheong T (1992) Respiratory variation in right atrial pressure predict the response to fluid challenge. J Crit Care 7 (2):76–85

72. Terada N, Takeuchi T (1993) Postural changes in venous pressure gradients in anesthetized monkeys. Am J Physiol 264:H21–H25

73. Scharf S, Tow DE, Miller MJ, Brown R, McIntyre K, Dilts C (1989) Influence of posture and abdominal pressure on the hemodynamic effects of Mueller's maneuver. J Crit Care 4 (1):26–34

74. Tarasiuk A, Scharf SM (1993) Effects of periodic obstructive apneas on venous return in closed-chest dogs. Am Rev Respir Dis 148:323–329

75. Stalcup SA, Mellins RB (1977) Mechanical forces producing pulmonary edema in acute asthma. N Engl J Med 297:592–596

76. Lores ME, Keagy BA, Vassiliades T, Henry GW, Lucas CL, Wilcox BR (1985) Cardiovascular effects of positive end-expiratory pressure (PEEP) after pneumonectomy in dogs. Ann Thorac Surg 40 (5):464–473

77. Buda AJ, Pinsky MR, Ingels NB, et al (1979) Effect of intrathoracic pressure on left ventricular performance. N Engl J Med 301:453–459

78. Pinsky MR, Summer WR, Wise RA, Permutt S, Bromberger-Barnea B (1983) Augmentation of Cardiac Function by Elevation of Intrathoracic Pressure. J Appl Physiol 54:950–955

79. Pinsky MR, Summer WR (1983) Cardiac Augmentation by Phasic High Intrathoracic Support (PHIPS) in Man. Chest 84:370–375

80. Blaustein AS, Risser TA, Weiss JW, Parker JA, Holman L, McFadden ER (1986) Mechanisms of pulsus paradoxus during resistive respiratory loading and asthma. J Am Coll Cardiol 8:529–536

81. Strohl KP, Scharf SM, Brown R, Ingram RH Jr (1987) Cardiovascular performance during bronchospasm in dogs. Respiration 51:39–48

82. Scharf SM, Graver LM, Balaban K (1992) Cardiovascular effects of periodic occlusions of the upper airways in dogs. Am Rev Respir Dis 146:321–329

83. Viola AR, Puy RJM, Goldman R (1990) Mechanisms of pulsus paradoxus in airway obstruction. J Appl Physiol 68 (5):1927–1931

84. Scharf SM, Graver LM, Khilnani S, Balaban K (1992) Respiratory phasic effects of inspiratory loading on left ventricular hemodynamics in vagotomized dogs. J Appl Physiol 73 (3):995–1003

85. Garpestad E, Parker JA, Katayama H, et al (1994) Decrease in ventricular stroke volume at apnea termination is independent of oxygen desaturation. J Appl Physiol 77 (4):1602–1608

86. Gomez A, Mink S (1992) Interaction between effects of hypoxia and hypercapnia on altering left ventricular relaxation and chamber stiffness in dogs. Am Rev Respir Dis 146:313–320

87. Butler J (1983) The heart is in good hands. Circulation 67:1163–1168

88. Shepherd JT (1981) The lungs as receptor sites for cardiovascular regulation. Circulation 63:1–10

89. Pinsky MR, Matuschak GM, Klain M (1985) Determinants of cardiac augmentation by increases in intrathoracic pressure. J Appl Physiol 58:1189–1198

90. Abel FL, Mihailescu LS, Lader AS, Starr RG (1995) Effects of pericardial pressure on systemic and coronary hemodynamics in dogs. Am J Physiol 268 (Heart Circ Physiol 37):H1593–H1605

91. Khilnani S, Graver LM, Balaban K, Scharf SM (1992) Effects of inspiratory loading on left ventricular myocardial blood flow and metabolism. J Appl Physiol 72 (4): 1488–1492
92. Satoh S, Watanabe J, Keitoku M, Itoh N, Maruyama Y, Takishima T (1988) Influences of pressure surrounding the heart and intracardiac pressure on the diastolic coronary pressure-flow relation in excised canine heart. Circ Res 63: 788–797
93. Beyar R, Goldstein Y (1987) Model studies of the effects of the thoracic pressure on the circulation. Ann Biomed Eng 15: 373–383
94. Cassidy SA, Wead WB, Seibert GB, Ramanathan M (1987) Geometric left-ventricular responses to interactions between the lung and left ventricle: positive pressure breathing. Ann Biomed Eng 15: 285–295
95. Scharf SM, Brown R, Warner KG, Khuri S (1989) Intrathoracic pressure and left ventricular configuration with respiratory maneuvers. J Appl Physiol 66 (1): 481–491
96. Shuey CB, Pierce AK, Johnson RL (1969) An evaluation of exercise tests in chronic obstructive lung disease. J Appl Physiol 27: 256–261
97. Grace MP, Greenbaum DM (1982) Cardiac performance in response to PEEP in patients with cardiac dysfunction. Crit Care Med 20: 358–360
98. Mitzner W, Gioia F, Weinmann GG, Robotham JL, Ehrlich W (1987) Interaction between high frequency jet ventilation and cardiovascular function. Ann Biomed Eng 15: 319–329
99. Peters J, Kindred MK, Robotham JL (1988) Transient analysis of cardiopulmonary interactions II. Systolic events. J Appl Physiol 64: 1518–1526
100. Rasanen J, Nikki P, Heikkila J (1984) Acute myocardial infarction complicated by respiratory failure. The effects of mechanical ventilation. Chest 85: 21–28
101. Rasanen J, Vaisanen IT, Heikkila J, et al (1985) Acute myocardial infarction complicated by left ventricular dysfunction and respiratory failure. The effects of continuous positive airway pressure. Chest 87: 158–162
102. Beach T, Millen E, Grenvik (1973) Hemodynamic response to discontinuance of mechanical ventilation. Crit Care Med 1: 85–90
103. Lemaire F, Teboul JL, Cinoti L, Giotto G, Abrouk F, Steg G, Macquin-Mavier I, Zapol WM (1988) Acute left ventricular dysfunction during unsuccessful weaning from mechanical ventilation. Anesthesiology 69: 171–179
104. Calvin JE, Driedger AA, Sibbald WJ (1981) Positive end-expiratory pressure (PEEP) does not depress left ventricular function in patients with pulmonary edema. Am Rev Resp Dis 124: 121–128
105. Roussos C, Macklem PT (1982) The respiratory muscles. N Engl J Med 307: 786–797
106. Kawagoe Y, Permutt S, Fessler HE (1994) Hyperinflation with intrinsic PEEP and respiratory muscle blood flow. J Appl Physiol 77 (5): 2440–2448

Physiology of Tissue Oxygen Delivery

J. Bakker

Introduction

Maintenance of adequate oxygen delivery to the cells to meet their ongoing demand is a crucial function of the cardio-respiratory system both in health and disease. Under normal conditions, oxygen delivery to the cells is controlled by the metabolic rate of the cells, that is oxygen delivery is a demand driven process [1–3]. In various pathological conditions the cardio-respiratory system may be unable to meet the oxygen demand of the tissues. Thus, manipulation of the bulk transport of oxygen (TO_2) is a frequent intervention in the intensive care patients. However TO_2 is only one part of the processes involved in the ultimate delivery of oxygen to the tissues (DO_2). The latter process essentially involves the following steps: Firstly oxygen is taken up from the atmosphere and diffuses from the alveolus to the capillary blood where it is transported bound to hemoglobin and, to a much lesser extent, dissolved in the plasma. Then, the cardiac output is distributed into the systemic circulation and ultimately delivered into the microcirculation. Finally oxygen is released from hemoglobin and diffuses from the intravascular space into the cells were it is utilized to maintain cell functions. These steps can be broken down to several detailed processes that will be discussed in this chapter. A good understanding of the physiology of the processes involved can help to understand and treat problems of tissue oxygenation in our critically ill patients.

Respiration

The major goal of respiration is to provide oxygen to the tissues and to remove carbon dioxide. As this subject is somewhat out of the scope of this chapter the 3 major processes involved will be briefly discussed.

Ventilation

Under normal conditions ventilation is facilitated by the downward and upward movement of the diaphragm. During heavy breathing, elevation and depression of the rib cage can increase the maximum anteroposterior thickness of the chest by about 20% and thus increase tidal volume. The lung is an elastic structure sliding freely within the pleural space. Only a small change in negative pleural pressure (-5 to -7.5 cm H_2O) during inspiration resulting in a slightly negative alveolar pressure (0 to -1 cm H_2O) is the main driving force for the flux of air into the lung [4]. During expiration these events are essentially reversed. The compliance of the lung, that is the extend to which the lung expands for a given rise in transpulmonary pressure (alveolar – pleural pressure), is an important factor in determining tidal volume. Lung compliance is determined by the elastic forces of the lung tissue itself (1/3) and the surface tension in the alveoli (2/3). Surfactant, a surface active agent consisting of a phospholipid, apoproteins and calcium, is crucial in reducing total surface tension in the lung thus preventing collapse of alveoli. Changes in the composition and activity of surfactant play an important role in the pathophysiology of the Adult Respiratory Distress Syndrome [5].

Diffusion

The difference between the partial pressure of oxygen between the two sides of the alveolo-capillary membrane (respiratory membrane) is the main driving force for the movement of the oxygen molecules through this membrane [6]. However, the net diffusion rate is also influenced by the solubility of oxygen, the cross sectional diffusion area, the diffusion distance and the molecular weight of oxygen [6]. These factors can be summarized by the Fick diffusion equation:

$$D = \frac{\Delta PO_2 \times A \times S}{\Delta d \sqrt{MW}} \qquad\qquad (Eq.\ 1)$$

As both the solubility and the molecular weight of oxygen are characteristics of the gas itself, this equation can be simplified to:

$$D = \frac{\Delta PO_2 \times A}{\Delta d} \times \frac{S}{\sqrt{MW}} \qquad\qquad (Eq.\ 2)$$

$$D = \frac{\Delta PO_2 \times A \times \beta}{\Delta d} \qquad\qquad (Eq.\ 3)$$

D = diffusion rate (O_2-flux); ΔPO_2 = pressure difference between two sides of the respiratory membrane; A = cross-sectional area of diffusion; S = solubility; Δd = diffusion distance; MW = molecular weight; β = diffusion coefficient.

Different disease processes can thus effect the diffusion of oxygen through the respiratory membrane. Disorders increasing the diffusion distance (e.g. interstitial edema and fibrosis) and decreasing the area of diffusion (e.g. alveolar collapse and flooding, emphysema) can have major impact on the oxygen diffusion capacity of the respiratory system. When oxygen uptake increases, as during exercise, the diffusion capacity is principally enhanced by an increase in both alveolar ventilation and perfusion. The latter is achieved by capillary recruitment and dilatation. This results in a better match of ventilation to perfusion (V_A/Q) [6]. However, as blood flow increases the contact time between the red cells and the alveolar space decreases. This could result in a decrease in arterial oxygen saturation. However, under normal circumstances, the uptake of oxygen is practically completed after passage of one third of the capillary leaving a substantial reserve capacity. Diffusion of oxygen also takes place at the capillary level in the tissues where oxygen molecules diffuse from the vascular space to the intracellular space. This will be discussed in more detail in the next section of this chapter.

Oxygen Transport in the Blood

Following the diffusion of oxygen through the respiratory membrane, oxygen is bound to hemoglobin in the red cell and subsequently transported to the tissues were it is released from the hemoglobin. Only a very small portion of the oxygen is transported dissolved in the plasma being linearly related to the partial pressure of oxygen following the law of Henry ($C = 0.003 \times PO_2$). By binding the oxygen to hemoglobin the blood can transport up to a 100 times more oxygen as could be transported dissolved in the plasma. Under normal conditions, 97% of the oxygen transported by the blood is bound to heme portion of the hemoglobin molecule. One hemoglobin molecule can bind 4 molecules of oxygen. Binding of the first oxygen molecule facilitates binding of the next one as the 3 dimensional shape of the hemoglobin changes thus exposing other binding sites. During the unloading of oxygen from the hemoglobin molecule at the tissue level, basically the reverse occurs. This gives rise to the sigmoid-shaped oxygen-hemoglobin binding and dissociation curve (ODC). Several factors can displace the oxygen-hemoglobin dissociation curve. This is best described by the effects of these factors on the P_{50}, the point at which 50% of the hemoglobin is saturated with oxygen. An increase in hydrogen ion concentration (decrease in pH), an increase in CO_2 concentration and an increase in temperature all increase the P_{50} (shift the ODC to the right) [7]. In the lungs the unbinding of H^+ and CO_2 increases the affinity for oxygen and shifts the ODC to the left (decrease in P_{50}), at the tissue level the reverse occurs. Also, increases in red cell 2,3-diphosphoglycerate (2,3-DPG) results in a right shift of the ODC (increase in P_{50}) [8]. Under normal conditions 2,3-DPG concentrations do not play a major role in the physiology of oxy-hemoglobin binding and dissociation. However, 2,3-DPG concentrations can be significantly decreased in banked blood resulting in a low P_{50} [9]. Although a low P_{50} could result in impaired DO_2, increased loading of oxygen and changes in regional blood flow following a decrease in P_{50} usually limit the negative effects on tissue oxygenation [10, 11].

Oxygen Transport and Delivery

The delivery of oxygen to the tissues is controlled by the oxygen demand (metabolic rate) of the tissues. Increases in oxygen demand are met by increases in blood flow and oxygen extraction [3, 12, 13]. An increase in oxygen extraction can be accomplished by capillary recruitment and increased microvascular flow and oxygen content. The cardio-respiratory system is integrated to deliver the required oxygen and remove the produced carbon dioxide. The integration of this system is schematized in Figure 1.

The bulk transport of oxygen (TO_2) is the product of cardiac output and the arterial oxygen content as denoted in the following equation:

$$TO_2 = CaO_2 \times CO \times \kappa \tag{Eq. 4}$$

where:

$$CaO_2 = (Hb \times SaO_2 \times 1.34) + (0.003 \times PaO_2) \tag{Eq. 5}$$

CaO_2 = arterial oxygen content; CO = cardiac output; κ = constant; Hb = hemoglobin level; SaO_2 = arterial oxygen saturation; PaO_2 = arterial oxygen pressure.

It should be realized that TO_2 is not equal to the actual delivery of oxygen to the tissues (DO_2). The distinction between TO_2 and DO_2 can be easily exemplified by

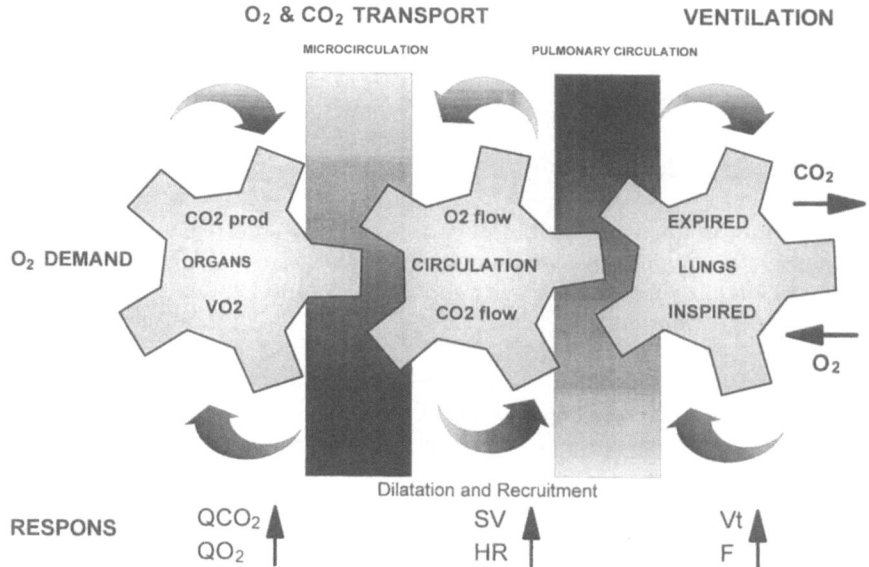

Fig. 1. The integration of oxygen delivery and carbon dioxide removal by the cardio-respiratory system. The system is driven by the oxygen demand of the tissues. An increase in demand is matched by an increase in delivery and an increase in oxygen uptake by the lungs.
Both dilatation and recruitment in the microcirculation of the tissues and lungs are important mechanisms to increase delivery and exchange.
QCO_2: total CO_2 flux; QO_2: total O_2 flux; *SV*: stroke volume; *HR*: heart rate; *Vt*: tidal volume; *F*: respiratory frequency

a patient on arterio-venous hemodialysis. The blood flow through the machine is not delivered to the tissues but would transverse directly into the venous system. Not only anatomical shunts but also virtual shunts contribute to the discrepancy between TO_2 and DO_2. A virtual shunt could be exemplified by an increased blood flow largely exceeding the metabolic needs of the tissue (excessive flow). Both forms of shunt probably play a role in the pathophysiology of sepsis and septic shock [14, 15].

In the following of this chapter principal determinants of oxygen delivery to the tissues and cells will be discussed.

Bloodflow Distribution

The major determinants of bulk blood flow (TO_2) are peripheral resistance and the pressure gradient as defined by Poiseuille's equation [12]:

$$R = \frac{8 \times \eta \times l}{\pi \times r^4} \qquad \text{(Eq. 6)}$$

R = resistance; η = blood viscosity; l = vessel length; r = vessel radius.

The total flow can thus be described by:

$$Q = \frac{\pi \times r^4}{8 \times \eta \times l} \times \Delta P \qquad \text{(Eq. 7)}$$

ΔP = pressure gradient.

The pressure gradient in the peripheral circulation almost equals the arterial pressure as the venous pressure is normally close to zero. From this equation it is clear that changes in blood viscosity and vascular tone, i.e. vessel diameter, have major effects on blood flow.

Viscosity. The viscosity of the blood is mainly the result of the large number of suspended red cells. The resistance to flow is the result of the adherence of red cells to the vascular wall resulting in a laminar flow pattern where the cells in the center of the vessel have the highest velocity whereas those close to the vessel wall hardly move [16]. Changes in viscosity can be induced by decreasing (hemodilution) or increasing (hemoconcentration) the number of red blood cells relative to the plasma volume. Although the hematocrit is related to the oxygen content and thus TO_2 (Eq. 4–5) the net gain of hemodilution or hemoconcentration on DO_2 is difficult to assess. Neural and humoral reflex responses influence the effects of changes in hematocrit on TO_2 and DO_2. Experimentally, increases in hematocrit from 30 to 55% do not significantly change TO_2 but have different effects on the distribution of blood flow [17]. Regional oxygen delivery to the kidneys and splanchnic organs seems to be more affected by changes in hematocrit than regional oxygen delivery to the heart and brain [17, 18]. Under normal conditions, due to the Fahraeus effect in the capillaries (the presence of a plasma layer between red cells and vascular endothelium), the capillary hematocrit can be about 50% of systemic hematocrit. When hemodilution does not drop systemic hematocrit below 17%, capillary hematocrit remains in the normal range [19]. During hemodilution, heterogeneity of capillary red cell distribution decreases (recruitment) probably related to an increase in red cell velocity [20]. Although, this could implicate an improvement of DO_2, differences in capillary structure could play a role in the different effects of hemodilution on various organs. Experimentally, hemodilution is associated with a decrease in regional TO_2 to stomach and intestine despite the increase in regional blood flow [17]. However in this setting, only intestinal VO_2 decreased whereas stomach VO_2 was maintained. The optimal hematocrit could therefore vary between different organs.

Regional and Microvascular Tone. Arteriolar tone represents the most important site of vascular resistance in most vascular beds. Changes in arteriolar tone can have major impact on regional blood flow as the peripheral resistance is primarily dependent upon the radius of the vessel (Eq. 6). Therefore vasoconstriction during a constant pressure gradient will result in a decrease in blood flow whereas vasodilatation under these circumstances will result in an increase in blood flow. In the Krogh concept of tissue oxygen exchange [21], pre-capillary sphincters regulate the number of perfused capillaries and thus the cross-sectional area of diffusion (Eq. 1–3). In this concept the capillaries are the smallest recruitable flow segments in the tissues. However, recent studies have shown that, at least in skeletal muscle, networks of capillaries perfused by a common feeder arteriole are the functional units of perfusion [22]. The architecture of the capillary network matches the structure of the associated tissue. For instance, in the skeletal muscle the capillary networks are arranged in parallel with the myofibrils [23]. Furthermore, the capillary density appears to be matched to the metabolic needs of the tissues and can be improved not only by exercise training but also by chronic hypoxia [24].

Regional blood flow is autoregulated by small changes in perfusion pressure. This autoregulation is brought about by several factors. Traditionally, metabolic and myogenic factors have been thought to control vascular tone in the arterioles. Myogenic tone (tension produced in response to an increase in stretch) can increase either direct, by an increase in arteriolar pressure or indirect by an increase in venous pressure both resulting in a decrease in arteriolar blood flow. In skeletal muscle myogenic tone is the major factor contributing to basal vascular tone. Metabolic factors couple oxygen demand to DO_2 and TO_2. Products of metabolism acting as loco-regional vasodilators increase blood flow proportional to the metabolic rate. Adenosine, prostaglandins, lactate, hydrogen ions, potassium, O_2 and CO_2 have all been identified as metabolic factors [25]. Recent data support the crucial role of the vascular endothelium and more specific its products (endothelium derived relaxing factor (EDRF), identified as nitric oxide (NO), endothelium-dependent hyperpolarizing factor (EDHF) and prostacyclin (PGI_2) in the regulation of DO_2 [26]. Changes in oxygen tension have been shown to elicit variations in vascular tone by direct actions on the vascular endothelium [27]. It has been shown that decreases in PaO_2 in the feeding arteriole with intact endothelium augments the production of EDRF/NO and PGI_2 [28, 29]. By studying the effects of endothelium and its products on oxygen extraction (O_2ER) of isolated skeletal muscle it has been shown that cyclooxygenase, NO and ATP-sensitive potassium channels play an important role in the regulation of TO_2 during hypoxia [30]. Not only chemical but also electrical communication between smooth muscle cells and endothelial cells seems to exist [31] resulting in so called: "myo-endothelial regulatory units". In these units, hyperpolarization generated in the capillaries in response to tissue hypoxia could be propagated upstream to induce dilatation. This process of signaling is potentially very effective as it does not require the production of metabolites "downstream" or the development of overt tissue hypoxia itself before adaptive increases in blood flow can occur [30].

Microcirculatory Oxygen Exchange

Oxygen is delivered to the microcirculation bound to hemoglobin. Following dissociation the oxygen diffuses through the red cell membrane to the plasma and subsequently into the cell cytosol. In similarity with the microcirculation of the lung, the driving force for the diffusion of oxygen is the PO_2 gradient between the vascular space and the cell cytosol. As the red cell hemoglobin does not equilibrate with tissue PO_2, the release of oxygen from the red cell occurs during the complete capillary transit time. The hemoglobin plays an important role in maintaining a relative constant PO_2 gradient for diffusion. At first hemoglobin facilitated dissociation minimizes the intra-red cell drop in PO_2 (3–4 mmHg during maximal VO_2) [32]. Also, hemoglobin facilitated dissociation maintains plasma PO_2 ($P_{pl}O_2$) and limits the drop in $P_{pl}O_2$ along the capillary. From this and Equation 3 it can be readily understood that decreases in red cell delivery to the microcirculation, decreases in red cell hemoglobin level and/or their oxygen content can limit DO_2. Furthermore, an increases in diffusion distance between the vascular space and the mitochondrion can also limit oxygen flux. This diffusion distance consists of plasma, endothelium, interstitium and cytosol. As this diffusion path is devoid of an oxygen carrier it is referred as the carrier free region (CFR). Oxygen transport through this CFR only occurs by free diffusion. In red cell skeletal muscle intracellular oxygen diffusion is facilitated by myoglobin. In resting dog skeletal muscle intracellular oxygen flux is predominantly related to the intracellular PO_2 gradient [33]. However, during exercise myoglobin facilitated oxygen diffusion plays a more important role [34]. Due to the shallow slope of the myoglobin-oxygen dissociation curve in the upper region, oxygen dissociation flux can increase rapidly with increases in VO_2.

Finally oxygen diffuses through the mitochondrial membrane to the site where oxygen is utilized (respiratory chain located in the mitochondrial innermembrane). The oxygen flux across the mitochondrial membrane is proportional to the oxygen flux across the CFR and related to the diffusion distance of the CFR and mitochondrial membrane thickness and the capillary exchange and mitochondrial exchange area [33]. Crude analysis yields a 20 to 100 fold greater PO_2 gradient across the CFR as across the mitochondrial membrane. It has been calculated that a PO_2 difference of 0.05 mmHg across the mitochondrial membrane is sufficient to support the required flux to maintain ATP synthesis [32]. However, cellular O_2-gradient requirements vary with the density and clustering of mitochondria within the cell. The non-uniform distribution of tissue PO_2 probably results from this mitochondrial clustering. The clustering if mitochondria could thus represent a regulatory mechanism to control cellular oxygen dependence [33].

Clinical Implications

Persistent tissue hypoxia is related to the development of organ failure and ultimate death. Despite these profound consequences and numerous publications on improving TO_2, optimizing actual delivery of oxygen to the metabolic active cells still represents a cumbersome clinical procedure. This relates to several factors associated with the (patho)physiology of adequate tissue oxygenation. At first adequate measures of tissue hypoxia in our critically ill patients are hard to define [35, 36]. From equation 6–7 it is evident that maintenance of an adequate pressure gradient is important to maintain tissue blood flow. However, experimentally optimal values are still hard to define [37, 38] and clinical targets vary widely [39–41].

Although increased blood lactate levels represent an attractive measure of tissue hypoxia in some clinical situations (hypovolemic and cardiogenic shock), its value in syndromes associated with alterations in metabolism and microcirculatory derangement (sepsis/septic shock, diabetes) are still controversial [42, 43]. The oxygen supply dependency phenomenon (increases in TO_2 being followed by increase in oxygen consumption) has been associated with poor outcome and the presence of tissue hypoxia [40, 44]. However the clinical relevance of this phenomenon and its correlation with the presence of tissue hypoxia are still a matter of ongoing debate [35, 45, 46]. Whereas PET scan and near infrared spectroscopy represent promising means of assessing tissue oxygenation, these procedures are difficult to perform in the critically ill patient. Secondly, increases in TO_2 are not necessarily associated with improved regional blood flow and tissue oxygen delivery [37, 47–50]. Moreover, the clinical measures of regional blood flow are limited. Gastric tonometry could represent a better measure of regional tissue hypoxia than global blood flow [51–53]. A low gastrointestinal pH (pHi) has been associated with multiple organ dysfunction [52] and poor outcome in critically ill patients [54, 55]. Also, treatment aimed at preserving a normal pHi is associated with improved outcome [55]. However, therapeutic interventions to improve a low pHi did not result in a decrease in mortality [55]. Although pHi can be influenced by specific therapy [49, 55, 56] its effect on outcome needs to be defined.

Urine output could also represent a measure of adequate regional blood flow. In critically ill patients, increases in blood pressure using norepinephrine has been associated with improved urine output and renal function [57–59]. Experimentally, a decrease in TO_2 following hemorrhage is associated with a decrease in renal DO_2 [60]. Treatment aiming at a blood pressure and cardiac output (TO_2) to preserve urine output could thus represent a valuable clinical goal.

Increases in TO_2 can be achieved by improving the determinants of TO_2 (Eqs. 4–5). This has been subject of many clinical and experimental studies [61]. Although rough clinical end-points have been suggested [41, 62–65], defining optimal levels of blood pressure, cardiac output, hemoglobin and arterial oxygen saturation still requires more clinical studies.

Conclusions

In optimizing tissue oxygen delivery in our critically ill patients we find ourselves often limited to increase global blood flow or arterial oxygen content. However, increasing the bulk flow of oxygen does not necessarily imply an increase of the actual delivery of oxygen to the metabolizing tissues. Many factors are involved in the process of tissue oxygen delivery whereas it seems that the capillary circulation forms the "bottleneck" of tissue oxygenation.

Although much is known about distribution of flow between and within organs during experimental conditions, human data are still very limited. Improved knowledge of physiological processes involved in the delivery of oxygen to the metabolizing cells can help to better understand the pathophysiology of tissue hypoxia and its treatment.

References

1. Granger HJ, Goodman AH, Cook BH (1975) Metabolic models of microcirculatory regulation. Federation Proc 34:2025–2030
2. Sheperd AP, Granger HJ, Smith EE, et al (1973) Local control of tissue oxygen delivery and its contribution to the regulation of cardiac output. Am J Physiol 225:747–755
3. Astrand P, Cuddy TE, Saltin B, et al (1964) Cardiac output during submaximal and maximal work. J Appl Physiol 19:268–274
4. Guyton AC, Hall JE (1996) Pulmonary Ventilation. In: Guyton AC, Hall JE (eds) Textbook of medical physiology. W. B. Saunders Company, Philadelphia, pp 477–489
5. Gregory TJ, Longmore WJ, Moxley MA, et al (1991) Surfactant chemical composition and biophysical activity in acute respiratory distress syndrome. J Clin Invest 88:1976–1981
6. Guyton AC, Hall JE (1996) Physical principles of gas exchange; diffusion of oxygen and carbon dioxide through the respiratory membrane. In: Guyton AC, Hall JE (eds) Textbook of medical physiology. W. B. Saunders Company, Philadelphia, pp 501–512
7. Kilmartin JV, Rossi-Bernardi L (1973) Interaction of hemoglobin with hydrogen ions, carbon dioxide, and organic phosphates. Physiol Rev 53:836–889
8. Benesch R, Benesch RE (1969) Intracellular organic phosphates as regulators of oxygen release by haemoglobin. Nature 221:618–622
9. Wranne B, Woodson RD, Detter RD (1972) Bohr effect: interaction between H^+, CO_2, and 2-3 DPG in fresh and stored blood. J Appl Physiol 32:749–754
10. Aberman A, Hew E (1985) Clarification of the effects of changes in P_{50} on oxygen transport. Acute Care 11:216–221
11. Woodson RD, Auerback S (1982) Effect of increased oxygen affinity and anemia on cardiac output and its distribution. J Appl Physiol 53:1299–1306

12. Guyton AC, Hall JE (1996) Local control of blood flow by the tissues, and humoral regulation. In: Guyton AC, Hall JE (eds) Textbook of medical physiology. W. B. Saunders Company, Philadelphia, pp 199–208
13. Weissman C, Kemper M (1991) The oxygen uptake-oxygen delivery relationship during ICU interventions. Chest 99:430–435
14. Dranzenovic R, Samsel RW, Wylam ME, et al (1992) Regulation of perfused capillary density in canine intestinal mucosa during endotoxemia. J Appl Physiol 72:259–265
15. Bakker J, Vincent JL (1993) The effects of norepinephrine and dobutamine on oxygen transport and consumption in a dog model of endotoxic shock. Crit Care Med 21:425–432
16. Guyton AC, Hall JE (1996) Overview of the circulation; Medical physics of pressure, flow, and resistance. In: Guyton AC, Hall JE (eds) Textbook of Medical Physiology. W. B. Saunders Company, Philadelphia, pp 161–170
17. Fan FC, Chen RYZ, Schuessler GB, et al (1980) Effects of hematocrit variations on regional hemodynamics and oxygen transport in the dog. Am J Physiol 238:H545–H552
18. Sheperd AP, Riedel GL (1982) Optimal hematocrit for oxygenation of canine intestine. Circ Res 51:223–240
19. Lindbom L, Mirhashemi S, Intaglietta M, et al (1988) Increase in capillary blood flow relative to hematocrit in rabbit skeletal muscle following acute normovolemic anemia. Acta Physiol Scand 134:503–512
20. Mirhashemi S, Messmer K, Arfors KE, et al (1987) Microcirculatory effects of normovolemic hemodilution in skeletal muscle. Int J Microcirc Clin Exp 6:359–370
21. Krogh A (1919) The number and distribution of capillaries in the muscles with calculations of oxygen pressure necessary for supplying the tissue. J Physiol London 52:409–415
22. Sweeney RE, Sarelius IH (1989) Arteriolar control of capillary cell flow in striated muscle. Circ Res 64:112–120
23. Delashaw J, Duling BR (1988) A study of the functional elements regulating capillary perfusion in striated muscle. Microvas Res 36:162–171
24. Yang HT, Ogilvie RW, Terjung RL (1994) Peripheral adaptations in trained aged rats with femoral artery stenosis. Circ Res 74:235–243
25. Skinner NS, Costin JC (1968) Tissue metabolites and regulation of local blood flow. Fed Proc 27:1426–1429
26. Vanhoutte PM (1989) Endothelium and control of vascular function. State of the art lecture. Hypertenstion 13:658–667
27. Jackson WF, Duling BR (1983) The oxygen sensitivity of hamster cheek pouch arterioles. Circ Res 53:515–525
28. Pohl U, Busse R (1989) Hypoxia stimulates release of endothelium-derived relaxant factor. Am J Physiol 256:H1595–H1600
29. Michiels C, Arnould T, Dieu M, et al (1993) Stimulation of prostaglandin synthesis by human endothelial cells exposed to hypoxia. Am J Physiol 264:C866–C874
30. Vallet B (1995) Vascular reactivity and tissue oxygenation. In: Vincent JL (ed) Yearbook of Intensive Care and Emergency Medicine. Springer Verlag, Heidelberg, pp 550–563
31. Song H, Tyml K (1993) Evidence for sensing and integration of biological signals by the capillary network. Am J Physiol 265:H1235–H1242
32. Clark A, Clark PAA (1986) The end-points of the oxygen path: transport resistance in red cells and mitochondria. Adv Exp Med Biol 200:43–47
33. Gayeski TE (1991) Principal determinants of tissue PO_2: Clinical considerations. In: Gutierrez G, Vincent J (eds) Update in Intensive Care and Emergency Medicine: Tissue oxygen utilization. Springer Verlag, Berlin, pp 56–70
34. Honig CR, Connett RJ, Gayeski TE (1992) O_2 transport and its interaction with metabolism; a systems view of aerobic capacity. Med Sci Sports Exerc 24:47–53
35. Pinsky MR (1994) Beyond global oxygen supply-demand relations: in search of measures of dysoxia [editorial]. Intensive Care Med 20:1–3
36. Vincent JL (1996) End-points of resuscitation: arterial blood pressure, oxygen delivery, blood lactate or …?. Intensive Care Med 22:3–5
37. Wang P, Ba ZF, Burkhardt J, et al (1992) Measurement of hepatic blood flow after severe hemorrhage: Lack of restoration despite adequate resuscitation. Am J Physiol 262:G92–G98

38. Bersten AD (1995) In defense of blood pressure. In: Vincent JL (ed) Springer Verlag, Berlin, pp 564–572
39. Shoemaker WC, Montgomery ES, Kaplan E, et al (1973) Physiologic patterns in surviving and nonsurviving shock patients. Use of sequential cardiorespiratory variables in defining criteria for therapeutic goals and early warning of death. Arch Surg 106:630–636
40. Bihari D, Smithies M, Gimson A, et al (1987) The effects of vasodilation with prostacyclin on oxygen delivery and uptake in critically ill patients. N Engl J Med 317:397–403
41. Boyd O, Grounds RM, Bennett ED (1993) A randomized clinical trial of the effect of deliberate perioperative increase of oxygen delivery on mortality in high-risk surgical patients. JAMA 270:2699–2707
42. Gutierrez G, Wulf ME (1996) Lactic acidosis in sepsis: a commentary. Intensive Care Med 22:6–16
43. Aduen J, Bernstein WK, Khastgir T, et al (1994) The use and clinical importance of a substrate specific electrode for rapid determination of blood lactate concentrations. JAMA 272:1678–1685
44. Bakker J, Vincent JL (1991) The oxygen supply dependency phenomenon is associated with increased blood lactate levels. J Crit Care 6:152–159
45. Pinsky MR (1995) Oxygen consumption-delivery relationships: Physiology and pathophysiology. Seminars in Respiratory and Critical Care Medicine 16:372–381
46. Vincent JL, De Backer D (1995) Oxygen uptake/oxygen supply dependency: fact or fiction? Acta Anaesthesiol Scand Suppl 107:229–237
47. Ruokonen E, Takala J, Kari A, et al (1993) Regional blood flow and oxygen transport in septic shock. Crit Care Med 21:1296–1303
48. Ruokonen E, Takala J, Kari A (1993) Regional blood flow and oxygen transport in patients with the low cardiac output syndrome after cardiac surgery. Crit Care Med 21:1304–1311
49. Marik PE, Mohedin M (1994) The contrasting effects of dopamine and norepinephrine on systemic and splanchnic oxygen utilization in hyperdynamic sepsis. JAMA 272:1354–1357
50. Silverman HJ, Tuma P (1992) Gastric tonometry in patients with sepsis. Effects of dobutamine infusions and packed red blood cell transfusions. Chest 102:184–188
51. Gutierrez G, Bismar H, Dantzker DR, et al (1992) Comparison of gastric intramucosal pH with measures of oxygen transport and consumtion in critically ill patients. Crit Care Med 20:451–457
52. Marik PE (1993) Gastric intramucosal pH. A better predictor of multiorgan dysfunction syndrome and death than oxygen-derived variables in patients with sepsis. Chest 104:225–229
53. Mohsenifar Z, Hay A, Hay J, et al (1993) Gastric intramural pH as a predictor of success or failure in weaning patients from mechanical ventilation. Ann Intern Med 119:794–798
54. Doglio GR, Pusajo JF, Egurrola MA, et al (1991) Gastric mucosal pH as a prognostic index of mortality in critically ill patients. Crit Care Med 19:1037–1040
55. Gutierrez G, Palizas F, Doglio GR, et al (1992) Gastric intramucosal pH as a therapeutic index of tissue oxygenation in critically ill patients. Lancet 339:195–199
56. Price K, Clark C, Gutierrez G (1992) Intravenous dobutamine improves gastric intramucosal pH in septic patients. Am Rev Respir Dis 145:A316 (Abstract)
57. Desjars P, Pinaud M, Bugnon D, et al (1989) Norepinephrine therapy has no deleterious renal effects in human septic shock. Crit Care Med 17:426–429
58. Hesselvik JF, Brodin B (1989) Low dose norepinephrine in patients with septic shock and oliguria: Effects on afterload, urine flow and oxygen transport. Crit Care Med 17:179–180
59. Redl-Wenzl EM, Armbruster C, Edelmann G, et al (1993) The effects of norepinephrine on hemodynamics and renal function in severe septic shock states. Int Care Med 19:151–154
60. Schlichtig R, Kramer DJ, Pinsky MR (1991) Flow redistribution during progressive hemorrhage is a determinant of critical O_2 delivery. J Appl Physiol 70:169–178
61. Bakker J (ed) (1995) Tissue oxygen delivery in the critically ill. IBERO, Houten Netherlands
62. Shoemaker WC, Appel PL, Waxman K, et al (1982) Clinical trial of survivors' cardiorespiratory patterns as therapeutic goals in critically ill postoperative patients. Crit Care Med 10:398–403
63. Hayes MA, Timmins AC, Yau EHS, et al (1994) Elevation of systemic oxygen delivery in the treatment of critically ill patients. N Engl J Med 330:1717–1722

64. Sibbald WJ, Doig GS, Morisaki H (1995) Role of RBC transfusion therapy in sepsis. In: Sibbald WJ, Vincent J (eds) Clinical trials for the treatment of sepsis. Springer Verlag, Berlin, pp 191–206
65. Reinhart K, Hannemann L, Kuss B (1990) Optimal oxygen delivery in critically ill patients. Int Care Med 16:S149–S155

Splanchnic Blood Flow

J. Takala

Introduction

The hepatosplanchnic region is functionally and metabolically a very active organ system. In this chapter, the expression "splanchnic" is used interchangeably with "hepatosplanchnic", and includes the liver and the organs drained by the portal circulation (the gut, the pancreas, and the spleen). Under normal conditions, metabolism of the splanchnic region represents roughly 20–35% of whole body energy expenditure and it receives similar fraction of whole body blood flow [1–4].

The various hepatosplanchnic functions are rarely vital for the immediate survival from an acute injury or disease. This probably explains, why the defense of splanchnic perfusion has a low priority, as compared to the blood flow to the heart and the brain. In contrast, the hepatosplanchnic region has a very important role in the regulation of circulating blood volume and systemic blood pressure [5]. This function of the splanchnic region may become vital in acute hypovolemia, when the splanchnic blood volume and flow are markedly reduced in order to defend the perfusion of the heart and the brain [6–8].

Acute reduction of splanchnic tissue perfusion can partially compensate for an acute hypovolemic episode, but prolonged hypoperfusion of the splanchnic region will inevitably lead to tissue injury and deterioration of the metabolic, absorptive, endo- and exocrine, and the host defense functions of the splanchnic organs. Since the splanchnic region is an important component of the host defense system due to its barrier function at the level of the gut mucosa and the abundance of lymphoid tissue and active macrophages in the gut wall, mucosa and spleen, it is an important source and target of inflammatory mediators. The activation of the various mediator networks can have a major impact on regional and local tissue perfusion via altered vasoregulation and changes in systemic cardiovascular performance [9, 10]. Under normal conditions, systemic hemodynamics have a direct impact on the blood flow to the splanchnic bed. Local and regional metabolic demands contribute to the physiologic control of splanchnic perfusion. Due to the prominent role of the liver in the whole body substrate flux and intermediary metabolism, metabolic changes in other regions of the body may also modify the splanchnic blood flow. Current concepts on the normal control of splanchnic blood flow are to a great extent based on experimental animal data, which can not necessarily be extrapolated to human physiology. There is very little human data on the changes in splanchnic perfusion and its regulation in the acutely ill patients requiring intensive care. Alterations in splanchnic perfusion due to various routine intensive care therapies, e.g. mechanical ventilation and vasoactive drugs, are superimposed on the complex and poorly understood interaction between the splanchnic blood flow, metabolic demands of the splanchnic and peripheral tissues, and the mediators of inflammation and vasoregulation.

Impaired splanchnic tissue perfusion has been suspected as one of the factors that may contribute to the development of multiple organ dysfunction and failure despite an apparently successful primary resuscitation and stabilization of vital functions in intensive care patients [11]. This concept has been difficult to evaluate, since routine monitoring of the adequacy of splanchnic blood flow in the clinical setting is not possible. The relatively recent introduction of gastrointestinal tonometry for gastric intramucosal pH (pH_i) or intramucosal pCO_2 monitoring by has provided a surrogate indicator of the adequacy of splanchnic tissue perfusion [12-20]. While some technical problems and physiologic limitations reduce the clinical value of gastrointestinal tonometry, results from several studies using this technique support the contribution of inadequate splanchnic tissue perfusion to subsequent development of multiple organ failure. Low gastric pH_i at admission to intensive care is associated with increased risk of subsequent organ dysfunction and death [16-19], whereas outcome is better in patients with normal pH_i at admission to intensive care and who either preserve normal pH_i or whose mucosal acidosis responds to treatment with fluids alone or in combination with vasoactive drugs [17, 20].

The explanation for the apparent association between inadequate splanchnic tissue perfusion and increased mortality and severe morbidity is evidently multifactorial. Inadequate mucosal perfusion increases the intestinal mucosal permeability. Splanchnic perfusion abnormalities may cause tissue hypoxia or dysoxia, inadequate gut mucosal barrier function, and local and regional ischemia and reperfusion, leading to the activation of inflammatory mediators [10, 21-23].

This chapter discusses briefly the basic physiology of splanchnic blood flow, reviews the methods available for the measurement of splanchnic blood flow in the clinical setting, and summarizes the relatively limited available human data on splanchnic blood flow in intensive care patients.

Normal Physiology of Splanchnic Blood Flow

The anatomy of the splanchnic vasculature is important for the physiologic control of blood flow and for the assessment of splanchnic perfusion abnormalities. Although some degree of anatomical variation is common, the arterial blood supply through the three main arteries is distributed roughly as follows:

1) The *celiac trunk* supplies via the *common hepatic* artery the liver, and parts of the stomach, duodenum, and the pancreas (tributaries right gastric and gastroduodenal artery). The two other main branches of the celiac trunk are the

splenic artery (supplying the spleen and parts of the stomach and pancreas), and the *left gastric artery* (supplying the rest of the stomach and the lower part of the esophagus)
2) The *superior mesenteric artery* and its tributaries supply the small intestine, cecum, ascending and most of transverse colon, and parts of the duodenum and the pancreas.
3) The *inferior mesenteric artery* and its tributaries supply the descending, sigmoid and parts of the transverse colon and the rectum.

With the exception of the arterial flow to the liver, all splanchnic arterial blood flow is drained via the portal vein to the liver. Thus, the blood flow through the hepatic veins represents the total hepatosplanchnic blood flow or the sum of the portal venous flow and the arterial blood flow to the liver.

The anatomy of the vasculature in the small intestinal villus makes the villi susceptible to tissue hypoxia. The tissue PO_2 decreases from the base of the villus to its tip, and the gradient is blood flow dependent. There are at least two possible mechanisms for this oxygen gradient, and these mechanisms may act in concert. The parallel course of the artery and the vein close to each other and the opposite direction of blood flow may create a countercurrent exchange of oxygen from the artery to the vein. Also, the higher metabolic activity of the absorptive cells at the tip may be responsible for the lower tissue PO_2. The lower PO_2 makes the tip vulnerable during any reduction of blood flow [24].

As pointed out earlier, 20–30% of cardiac output is normally directed to the hepatosplanchnic region (Table 1). The arterial blood flow to the liver is about 20% of the total hepatosplanchnic flow, and the remaining 80% is delivered via the portal vein. The splanchnic oxygen extraction at rest is comparable to or slightly higher than the whole body oxygen extraction [1–4].

Moderate increases in splanchnic metabolic demands result in proportional increases in blood flow with relatively constant oxygen extraction, unless the oxygen extraction is initially very low. In the latter case, splanchnic oxygen extraction tends to increase before blood flow increases. Perhaps the most common example of a physiologic, moderate increase in the splanchnic metabolic demand is food intake. The enhanced regional perfusion may be the result of an increase in or a redistribution of systemic blood flow or a combination of both [2, 3, 25, 26].

The splanchnic region adapts well to reduced blood flow by increasing the oxygen extraction. For example, splanchnic blood flow is reduced during acute hypo-

Table 1. Splanchnic and whole body blood flow and oxygen uptake at rest [1–4]

	Blood flow ($L/min/m^2$)	Oxygen consumption ($ml/min/m^2$)	Oxygen extraction fraction
Splanchnic	0.50–0.80	20–40	0.22–0.35
Whole body	2.5–4.0	110–150	0.22–0.30

volemia to defend the perfusion of the heart and the brain, and during strenuous exercise to meet the metabolic demands of the working muscle [6–8, 27, 28]. The critical level of oxygen extraction beyond which tissue injury and functional deterioration will occur is not known. The duration of exposure is certainly important and differences between the various organs are most likely to exist. The liver seems to be relatively well protected against hypoxia, whereas local and regional hypoxia may develop more easily in the gut. In experimental studies the critical oxygen extraction ratio for the gut is around 70% [29, 30].

Regulation of Gut Blood Flow

The mechanisms of gut blood flow regulation can be categorized to intrinsic and extrinsic mechanisms (Table 2) [26]. The perfusion of the intestinal wall is inhomogenous. Upto 90% of the gut blood flow goes to the mucosa and the submucosa. Depending on the cause of change in total gut blood flow, the perfusion of the various layers of the gut wall may be affected differently. Redistribution of blood flow within the intestinal wall may also occur without concomitant changes in the total blood flow to the gut.

When the local blood flow is insufficient to the metabolic needs, vasodilatation induced by the local metabolic control enhances the perfusion (Table 2) [26, 31]. When the vascular transmural pressure increases, the arterioles vasoconstrict (myogenic control). The interaction of the metabolic and myogenic control helps to maintain adequate tissue perfusion, and at the same time prevent large chang-

Table 2. Intrinsic and extrinsic control of intestinal blood flow [26, 31, 35, 36]

Intrinsic mechanisms	Response	Proposed signal/mediator (examples, others may also be involved)
Local metabolic control	Vasodilatation	Tissue PO_2, metabolites
Myogenic control	Arteriolar vasoconstriction	Increased vascular transmural pressure
Local reflexes	Vasodilatation	Gut luminal contents
Locally produced vasoactive substances	Vasodilatation	Nitric oxide, Adenosine

Extrinsic mechanisms	Response
Sympathetic innervation	Vasoconstriction
Circulating vasoactive substances catecholamines (physiologically most important)	Vasoconstriction (α-adrenergic) Vasoconstriction (β-adrenergic)
vasopressin	Vasoconstriction
angiotensin	Vasoconstriction
Systemic hemodynamic changes	Variable

es in the intestinal capillary pressure. Since the intestinal capillary permeability is relatively high, the control of the capillary pressure changes also reduces changes in transcapillary fluid flux. Nitric oxide is important in the maintenance of basal vasodilatation in the mesenteric vasculature [32, 33].

The gut has only a weak blood pressure-flow autoregulation, which is somewhat enhanced by feeding [26]. The weak autoregulation is reflected in reduced intestinal blood flow despite vasodilatation, when arterial pressure acutely decreases. In addition to arterial pressure also the venous outflow pressure influences the gut blood flow. During adequate tissue perfusion, increased venous outflow pressure causes arterial vasoconstriction via the myogenic control, whereas during inadequate tissue perfusion a similar change in venous pressure leads to vasodilatation and increased capillary density via the metabolic control.

The principal components of extrinsic gut blood flow regulation are sympathetic nervous activity, circulating vasoactive substances, and systemic hemodynamics (Table 2) [8, 26, 34, 35]. Sympathetic nervous activity reduces gut blood flow by increasing the vascular resistance, mostly in the arteries and arterioles. During prolonged stimulation, the blood flow tends to recover ("autoregulatory escape"). After the stimulation, a transient hyperemia follows [26]. Catecholamines are by far the most important circulating endogenous vasoactive substances. Norepinephrine with predominantly alpha-adrenergic activity increases the intestinal vascular resistance, whereas the effects of epinephrine are dose-dependent: vasodilatation at low doses and vasoconstriction at increasing doses. Although the pure pharmacological effects of adrenergic agent are predictable, their net effects on gut blood flow in vivo depend on the concomitant changes in systemic hemodynamics [26, 34]. The pharmacological effect of both vasopressin and angiotensin is intestinal vasoconstriction. Their role in normal control of intestinal blood flow is clearly minor as compared to catecholamines. Vasopressin and angiotensin may both be involved in the intestinal vasoconstriction in acute hypovolemia, and they may also modulate the response to sympathetic nerve stimulation and norepinephrine [8, 26].

A complex interaction between the various control systems enhances intestinal blood flow following food intake. Local reflexes, release of vasoactive gastrointestinal hormones, and metabolic control are all involved in the postprandial hyperemia [26, 36].

Regulation of Hepatic Blood Flow

The regulation of hepatic blood flow has unique characteristics because of the interaction between portal venous and hepatic arterial inflow. This hydrodynamic interaction, also called the hepatic arterial buffer response, aims at compensating any change in one of the inflows to the liver (portal venous or hepatic arterial) by a reciprocal change in the other [1, 3]. Adenosine is probably the principal mediator of this response [37]. The vascular resistance across the intestine and the hepatic arterial resistance are the primary determinants of the portal venous and hepatic arterial flows, respectively. The intrahepatic portal venous resistance has only a minor role. The hepatic arterial pressure-flow autoregulation is very weak and the hepatic portal venous bed lacks autoregulation [1, 3].

Increased sympathetic nervous activity increases both the hepatic arterial and portal resistance. The arterial vasoconstriction has similar autoregulatory escape as the intestinal vasoconstriction. The portal response differs substantially from the hepatic arterial and intestinal responses to sympathetic stimulation. The portal resistance increases relatively slowly but is sustained without any autoregulatory escape [3, 38].

Nitric oxide contributes to the regulation of the hepatic blood flow since it maintains basal vasodilatation both in the mesenteric vasculature and the hepatic artery [32, 33].

Measurement of Splanchnic Blood Flow in the Clinical Setting

The multivessel influx and efflux, and the mixing of portal venous and hepatic arterial blood within the liver make direct measurement of splanchnic blood flow impossible in patients (except during laparotomy). In contrast to cardiac physiology, the basics of splanchnic circulatory physiology have been extrapolated from experimental studies and never confirmed in normal man. New methods have allowed qualitative or at best semiquantitative assessment of local mucosal blood flow using laser Doppler techniques, and portal or hepatic arterial flow using ultrasound Doppler techniques. The problems that so far remain with these approaches include poor reproducibility (especially between users), lack of reference methods, poor applicability in a number of patients, and data interpretation.

Total hepatosplanchnic blood flow can be measured in the intensive care setting using the Fick principle [39]. The drawback of this method is that it does not differentiate between hepatic arterial and portal venous flow, and it gives no information of the local or within-organ distribution of blood flow within the hepatosplanchnic region. These measurements are currently used only for research purposes. Since new information on the physiology and pathophysiology of splanchnic blood flow in intensive care patients is accumulating [40–46], the theoretical basis, limitations, and practical aspects of these methods deserve consideration.

The hepatic uptake of indicator substances that are metabolized exclusively by the liver and distributed in the plasma is estimated either after a bolus injection of the indicator or during constant infusion and steady-state plasma concentration [39, 47, 48]. Indocyanine green is the indicator of choice. Since the hepatic extraction of the dye is never 100% and varies in an unpredictable fashion, hepatic venous catheterization is necessary for the measurement in order to take into account the fractional extraction of the indicator dye (Fig. 1). Less invasive modifications of this method, using only systemic blood sampling, have been proposed [47, 49, 50]. In these approaches, either a constant hepatic dye extraction has to be assumed or the extraction has to be estimated from pharmacokinetic models. Due to the variability of dye extraction between patients and the acute changes that occur in the dye extraction in response to common intensive care interventions (Figs. 1, 2), the assumption of a constant or predictable dye extraction is not valid [39]. Based on critical evaluation, the pharmacokinetic models are not valid for clinical application [47]. Accordingly, non-invasive methods can-

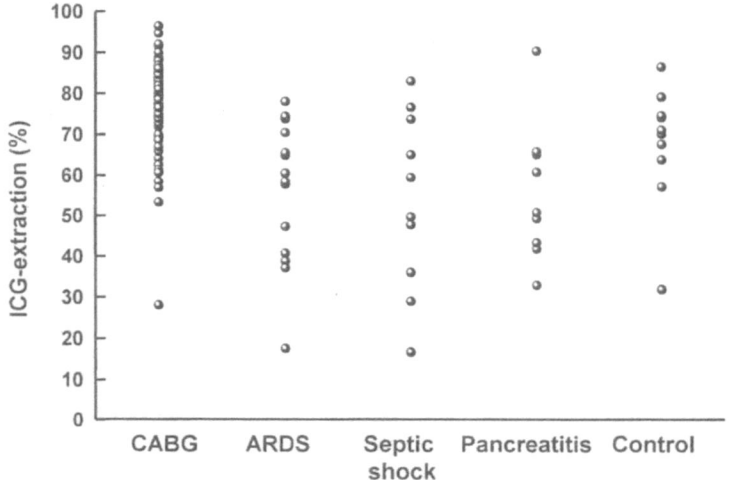

Fig. 1. Hepatic indocyanine green (ICG) extraction in different intensive care patient groups. *CABG:* postoperative coronary artery bypass patients; *ARDS:* patients with the acute respiratory distress syndrome; *Pancreatitis:* patients requiring intensive care due to severe acute pancreatitis; *Control:* preoperative patients scheduled for major abdominal surgery. (Redrawn from [39], with permission)

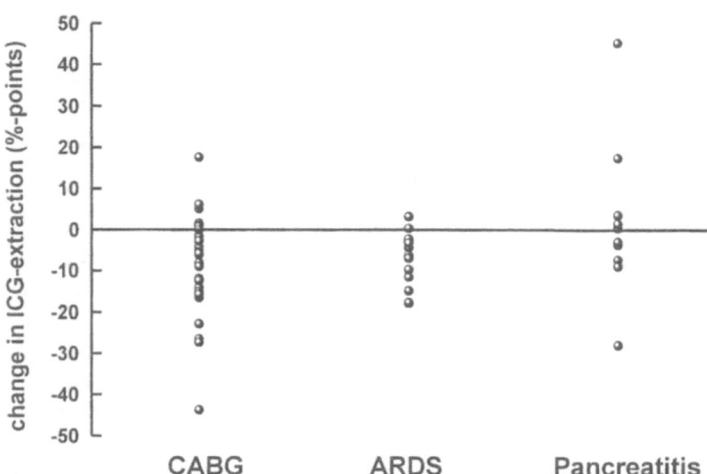

Fig. 2. Acute changes in hepatic ICG-extraction in response to an infusion of dobutamine. (From [39], with permission)

not replace hepatic venous catheterization for the measurement of splanchnic blood flow.

Both continuous infusion and bolus injection techniques in combination with hepatic vein blood sampling have been used in the measurement of splanchnic blood flow in intensive care patients, but so far, only the primed continuous infusion technique has been formally evaluated in this setting [39]. Intensive care patients are prone to have several factors that may interfere with the splanchnic blood flow measurement, including hemodynamic instability, positive pressure ventilation, and hepatic dysfunction. Other methodological problems, e.g. unstable dye extraction and lack of steady state dye concentration have also been reported [51].

We have used rather extensively the primed, continuous infusion of indocyanine green dye to study splanchnic blood flow in intensive care patients. The method can be modified to include simultaneous measurement of hepatosplanchnic and lower extremity blood flow, if the distribution of whole body blood flow is of interest. The method and its evaluation in the intensive care setting has been previously described in detail [39].

Briefly, catheters are inserted in the femoral artery for dye infusion, and in the ipsilateral femoral vein, a hepatic vein, and radial artery for blood sampling. The correct, non-wedged position of the catheter is verified with fluoroscopy using a small amount of contrast dye. After a priming dose, a constant infusion of indocyanine green (ICG) is commenced and continued for 30 minutes. Blood is sampled for the measurement of arterial, and hepatic and femoral vein ICG-concentrations after 20, 25, and 30 minutes of infusion. Plasma ICG-concentration is measured spectrophotometrically.

The hepatosplanchnic and femoral blood flows are calculated as follows:

total splanchnic blood flow =

infusion rate (L/min) $\times$ Ci/(Ca $-$ Chv) $\times$ (1 $-$ Hcr),

where Ci is the ICG-concentration of infusate (mg/L), and Ca and Chv are the ICG-concentrations in the artery and hepatic vein (mg/L), respectively;

femoral blood flow =

infusion rate (L/min) $\times$ (Ci $-$ Cfv)/(Cfv $-$ Ca) $\times$ (1 $-$ Hcr),

where Cfv is the ICG-concentration in the femoral vein (mg/L). This formula takes into account the effect of the rate of dye infusion into the femoral artery.

The mean coefficient of variation of both splanchnic and femoral blood flow within each 30-minutes period of measurement in 240 measurements was 6%, which is at least as good as the variability of routine cardiac output measurements using the thermodilution method [39].

Splanchnic Blood Flow in Intensive Care Patients

The number of studies on splanchnic blood flow in intensive care patients is limited, and they are either snapshots in non-standardized or poorly specified conditions, or deal with acute therapeutic interventions in very specific conditions [39–46, 51–58]. Only 10 of the studies have been published during this decade [39–46, 54, 58]. Hence, generalizations based on these data has to be made with caution. Also, repeated, longitudinal studies over the course of critical illness in the same patient are lacking, and nothing can be concluded about the pattern of changes in splanchnic perfusion during intensive care. What these studies have demonstrated is that data obtained from experimental studies or more stable patients should not be uncritically extrapolated to the intensive care patient.

Since most recent studies on splanchnic blood flow in intensive care patients have been published from the author's institution and have all been performed under standardized conditions [39–41, 43–46, 58], the following discussion will focus on summarizing the results of these published data, and also some previously unpublished data has been included for the purpose of illustration.

A concept of two distinct patterns of splanchnic blood flow abnormalities is evolving according to these studies, and both patterns put the splanchnic tissues at risk of a mismatch between tissue perfusion and metabolic demands.

Low Flow States and Hypovolemia

In conditions with low cardiac output without any major inflammatory stimuli (e.g. cardiogenic shock) the splanchnic blood flow decreases without changes in splanchnic metabolic demand [41, 43–46]. This pattern closely resembles the one observed in uncomplicated hypovolemia [8]. The hypovolemia-induced splanchnic vasoconstriction persists even after the blood volume and systemic hemodynamics have been restored. Since hypovolemia and acute blood volume changes are not uncommon in intensive care patients, it is conceivable that this may increase the risk of inadequate splanchnic perfusion [6].

Since the metabolic demands remain relatively unchanged, splanchnic oxygen extraction has to increase to compensate for the reduced splanchnic blood flow (Fig. 3). The slower the flow decreases or the hypovolemia develops, the better the physiological compensation mechanisms will develop and may maintain adequate tissue oxygenation despite markedly decreased flow. Normal vasoregulation is an important prerequisite for the maintenance of adequate tissue oxygenation.

For how long and how severe hypoperfusion a patient will tolerate, before tissue hypoxia is inevitable, is not known. Brief exposures to very low hepatic venous saturation (10–20%) without any major consequences have been observed after cardiac surgery [41, 44, 59, 60]. On the other hand, during liver resection, a perioperative hepatic vein saturation below 30% was associated with postoperative liver function abnormalities [61]. It is conceivable that the tolerance and response to low splanchnic blood flow can vary substantially between patients, and the previous disease history may also modify the response substantially.

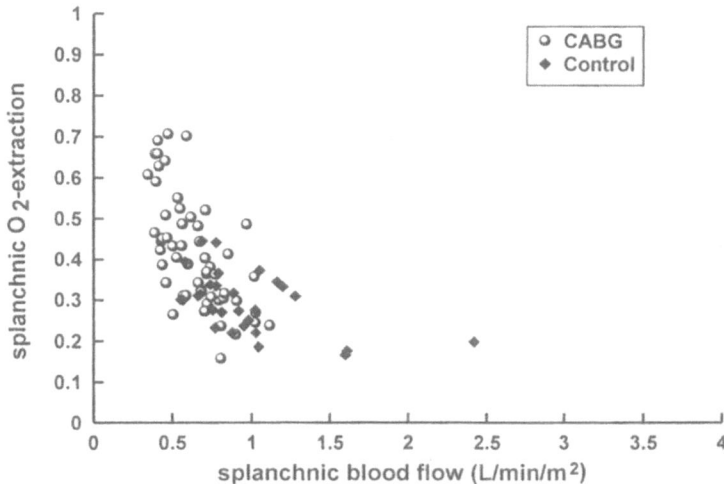

Fig. 3. Splanchnic blood flow and oxygen extraction after coronary artery bypass surgery and in preoperative patients scheduled for major abdominal surgery. (Redrawn from unpublished raw data obtained in conjunction with [43, 44, 46] and other unpublished data obtained by the author)

Splanchnic Blood Flow in Systemic Inflammatory Response Syndrome (SIRS)

A different pattern of splanchnic blood flow is observed in patients with severe infections and SIRS. The systemic blood flow in these patients may be either normal or hyperdynamic. The splanchnic blood flow may be normal or increased, but the hallmark of these conditions is a disproportionate increase in splanchnic oxygen consumption [40, 42, 51–57]. Accordingly, the oxygen extraction is also increased, even in hyperdynamic septic shock during hypotension (Fig. 4) [40]. Since vasoregulation is often impaired in SIRS and grossly impaired in septic shock, it is conceivable that splanchnic tissue hypoxia is a clinically relevant risk. Any deterioration of systemic hemodynamics due to myocardial depression or hypovolemia, or an increase in oxygen demand of any cause further puts the adequacy of tissue perfusion at risk.

Splanchnic Blood Flow Response to some Common Therapeutic Interventions

Sufficient blood volume is of paramount importance for the maintenance of adequate splanchnic tissue perfusion. The prolonged splanchnic vasoconstriction following restoration of blood volume has been demonstrated in healthy subjects [8]. Only indirect data on measurements of the effects of blood volume on splanchnic perfusion in intensive care patients is available. Restoration of splanchnic perfusion using gastric pH$_i$ as the endpoint strongly supports the primary importance of blood volume [17–20].

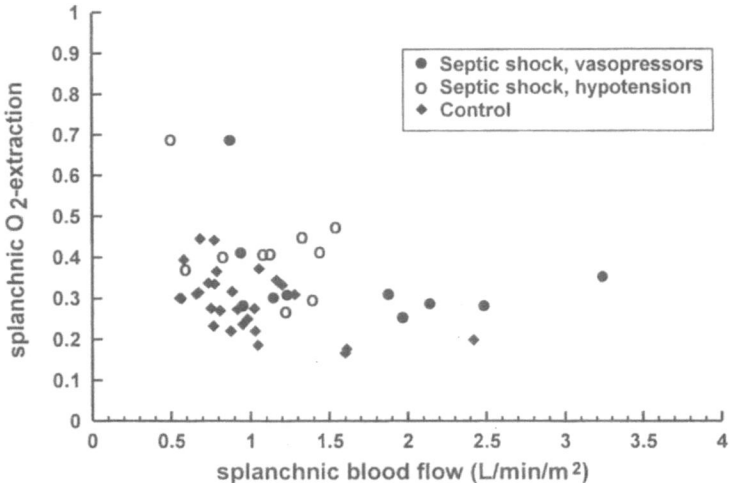

Fig. 4. Splanchnic blood flow and oxygen extraction in patients with septic shock, when volume resuscitated but hypotensive, and after hypotension had been treated with vasopressors, and in preoperative patients scheduled for major abdominal surgery. (Redrawn from unpublished raw data obtained in conjunction with [40] and other unpublished data obtained by the author)

Adrenergic Agents. Only limited data are available on the effects of adrenergic agents on splanchnic blood flow in humans. Several studies performed in the late '80s explored the effects of various vasoactive drugs on splanchnic blood flow in congestive heart failure and were summarised in a comprehensive review [62]. The results of these studies have often been extrapolated also to the intensive care setting. All those studies used systemic indocyanine green clearance to estimate the splanchnic blood flow. As discussed in the previous section on methods of blood flow measurements, this cannot be justified. Since the adrenergic agents can acutely modify the hepatic indocyanine green extraction, any flow response estimations without hepatic venous dye sampling are susceptible to serious errors, and the results are clearly not valid [39, 62]. The limited available data obtained with acceptable methodology will be briefly summarized in the following paragraphs.

In hyperdynamic septic shock, vasopressor doses of dopamine increased splanchnic blood flow, whereas norepinephrine has more variable effects [40]. In patients with septic shock and gastric mucosal acidosis, dopamine worsened gastric mucosal acidosis, while norepinephrine increased gastric mucosal pH despite the systemic hemodynamic effects of the two drugs were identical [63]. These seemingly controversial results are likely related to different effects at the level of microcirculation. Alternatively, dopamine and norepinephrine may have different local metabolic effects.

Both dobutamine and dopexamine consistently increased splanchnic blood flow immediately after cardiac surgery [41, 43, 44]. The changes in total splanchnic blood flow and gastric mucosal pH_i were opposite (Figs. 5, 6): both drugs low-

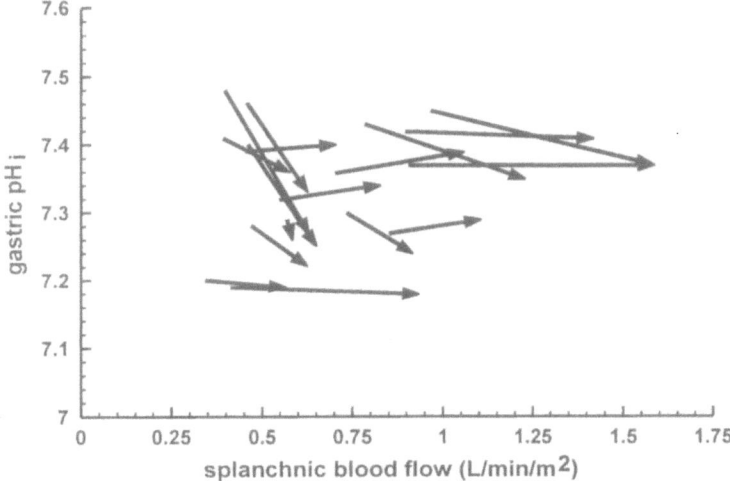

Fig. 5. Changes in splanchnic blood flow and gastric pH$_i$ in response to dobutamine after cardiac surgery. (Adapted from [44], with permission)

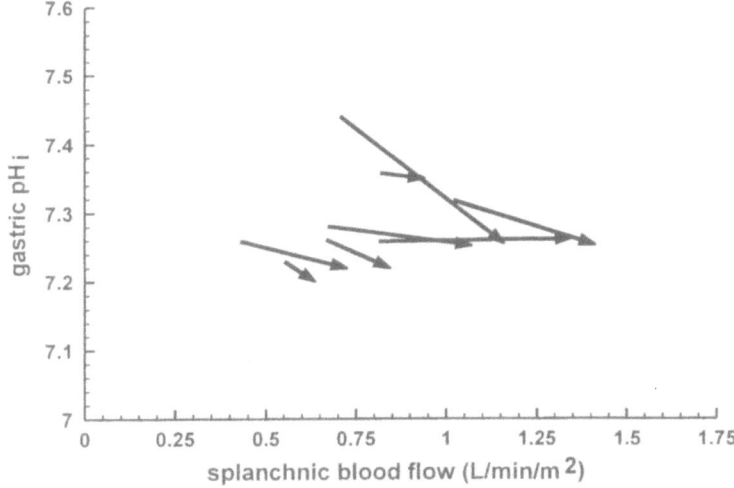

Fig. 6. Changes in splanchnic blood flow and gastric pH$_i$ in response to dopexamine after cardiac surgery. (Adapted from [43], with permission)

ered the gastric pH$_i$ or failed to correct the gastric mucosal acidosis despite major increases in splanhcnic blood flow [43, 44]. This pattern was even more prominent in patients with low cardiac output [44]. In contrast, dobutamine corrected gastric mucosal acidosis in patients with sepsis [64], demonstrating that the underlying disease can modify the splanchnic blood flow responses. Dopexamine has been believed to favor the distribution of blood flow to the splanchnic region. This was not the case in cardiac surgery patients: the increases in splanchnic blood flow induced by dobutamine and dopexamine were proportional to the increases in cardiac output and no redistribution of cardiac output was observed [41, 43, 44].

The worsening of the gastric mucosal acidosis or the failure to correct the acidosis despite increased splanchnic blood flow is probably related to a heterogeneous blood flow response within the splanchnic bed. This concept is supported by experimental studies, showing that the effects of vasoactive drugs on microcirculation may differ despite similar effects on blood flow distribution in major vessels [65]. Alternatively, the local metabolic demands may have increased.

Traditionally, the possible effects of adrenergic agonists on regional blood flow have been extrapolated from their relative adrenergic receptor activity. The accumulating data clearly demonstrates that the effects of sympathomimetic drugs on splanchnic blood flow in intensive care patients can neither be predicted from their pharmacological characteristics nor extrapolated from experimental models.

Non-Adrenergic Vasodilators. Data on the effects of vasodilators on splanchnic blood flow are very limited. Sodium nitroprusside increased hepatosplanchnic blood flow in parallel with cardiac output in postoperative cardiac surgery patients [46]. Despite the increase in splanchnic blood flow, gastric pH_i decreased slightly. After cardiac surgery, enalapril had no effect on either cardiac output or hepatosplanchnic blood flow, but reduced the gastric pH_i [58].

The available data suggest that also the effects of vasodilators may be modified by the underlying clinical condition. It seems likely that similar redistribution of blood flow as suggested for the adrenergic agents may also occur in response to non-adrenergic vasodilatation.

References

1. Bruns FJ, Fraley DS, Haigh J, Marquez JM, Martin DJ, Matuschak GM, Snyder JV (1987) Control of organ blood flow. In: Snyder JV, Pinsky MR (eds) Oxygen transport in the critically ill. Year Book Medical Publishers, Inc, Chicago, pp 87–124
2. Winsö O, Biber B, Gustavsson B, Holm C, Milsom I, Niemand D (1986) Portal blood flow in man during graded positive end-expiratory pressure ventilation. Intensive Care Medicine 12:80–85
3. Richardson PDI, Withrington PG (1981) Liver blood flow. Intrinsic and nervous control of liver blood flow. Gastroenterology 81:159–173
4. Granger HJ, Norris CP (1980) Intrinsic regulation of intestinal oxygenation in the anesthetized dog. American Journal of Physiology 238 (7):H836–H843
5. Rowell LB, Detry J-MR, Blackmon JR, Wyss C (1972) Importance of the splanchnic vascular bed in human blood pressure regulation. Journal of Applied Physiology 32:213–220
6. Takala J (1994) Splanchnic perfusion in shock. Intensive Care Medicine 20:403–404
7. Price HL, Deutsch S, Marshall BE, Stephen GW, Behar MG, Neufeld GR (1966) Hemodynamic and metabolic effects of hemorrhage in man with particular reference to the splanchnic circulation. Circulation Research 18:469–474
8. Edouard AR, Degrémont A-C, Duranteau J, Pussard E, Berdeaux A, Samii K (1994) Heterogenous regional vascular responses to simulated transient hypovolemia in man. Intensive Care Medicine 20:414–420

9. Matuschak GM (1994) Liver-lung interactions in critical illness. New Horizons 2:488–504
10. Matuschak GM (1995) Oxidative stress and oxygen-dependent cytokine production. In: Vincent J-L (ed) Yearbook of intensive care medicine. Springer-Verlag, Germany
11. Carrico CJ, Meakins JL, Marshall JC, Fry D, Maier RV (1986) Multiple organ failure syndrome. Archives of Surgery 121:196–208
12. Grum CM, Fiddian-Green RG, Pittenger GL, Grant BJB, Rothman ED, Dantzker DR (1984) Adequacy of tissue oxygenation in intact dog intestine. Journal of Applied Physiology 56: 1065–1069
13. Fiddian-Green RG, Amelin PM, Herrmann JB, Arous E, Cutler BS, Schiedler M, et al (1986) Prediction of the development of sigmoid ischemia on the day of aortic operations. Indirect measurements of intramural pH in the colon. Archives of Surgery 121:654–660
14. Fiddian-Green RG, Baker S (1987) Predictive value of the stomach wall pH for complications after cardiac operations: comparison with other monitoring. Critical Care Medicine 15:153–156
15. Doglio GR, Pusajo JF, Egurrola MA, Bonfigli GC, Parra C, Vetere L, Hernandez MS, Fernandez S, Palizas F, Gutierrez G (1991) Gastric mucosal pH as a prognostic index of mortality in critically ill patients. Critical Care Medicine 19:1037–1040
16. Gutierrez G, Bismar H, Dantzker DR, Silva N (1992) Comparison of gastric intramucosal pH with measures of oxygen transport and consumption in critically ill patients. Critical Care Medicine 20:451–457
17. Gutierrez G, Palizas F, Doglio G, Wainsztein N, Gallesio A, Pacin J, Dubin A, Schiavi E, Jorge M, Pusajo J, Klein F, San Roman E, Dorfman B, Shottlender J, Giniger R (1992) Gastric intramucosal pH as a therapeutic index of tissue oxygenation in critically ill patients. Lancet 339:195–199
18. Maynard N, Bihari D, Beale R, Smithies M, Baldock G, Mason R, McColl I (1993) Assessment of splanchnic oxygenation by gastric tonometry in patients with acute circulatory failure. JAMA 270:1203–1210
19. Mythen MG, Webb AR (1994) Intra-operative gut mucosal hypoperfusion is associated with increased post-operative complications and cost. Intensive Care Medicine 20:99–104
20. Mythen MG, Webb AR (1994) The role of gut mucosal hypoperfusion in the pathogenesis of post-operative organ dysfunction. Intensive Care Medicine 20:203–209
21. Deitch EA (1992) Multiple organ failure. Pathophysiology and potential future therapy. Annals of Surgery 216:117–134
22. Fink MP, Kaups KL, Wang H, Rothschild HR (1991) Maintenance of superior mesenteric arterial perfusion prevents increased intestinal permeability in endotoxic pigs. Surgery 110:154–161
23. Haglund U, Hulten L, Ahren C, Lundgren O (1975) Mucosal lesions in the human small intestine in shock. Gut 16:979–984
24. Lundgren O, Haglund U (1978) The pathophysiology of the intestinal countercurrent exchanger. Life Sciences 23:1411–1422
25. Brundin T, Wahren J (1991) Influence of a mixed meal on splanchnic and interscapular energy expenditure in humans. American Journal of Physiology 260:E232–E237
26. Granger DN, Richardson PDI, Kvietys PR, Mortillaro NA (1980) Intestinal blood flow. Gastroenterology 78:837–863
27. Rowell LB, Blackmon JR, Kenny MA, Escourrou P (1984) Splanchnic vasomotor and metabolic adjustments to hypoxia and exercise in humans. American Journal of Physiology 247: H251–H258
28. Rowell LB, Brengelmann GL, Blackmon JR, Twiss RD, Kusumi F (1968) Splanchnic blood flow and metabolism in heat-stressed man. Journal of Applied Physiology 24:475–484
29. Nelson DP, Samsel RW, Wood LDH, Schumacker PT (1988) Pathological supply dependence of systemic and intestinal O_2 uptake during endotoxemia. Journal of Applied Physiology 64:2410–2419
30. Zhang H, Spapen H, Manikis P, Rogiers P, Metz G, Buurman WA, Vincent J-L (1995) Tirilazad mesylate (U-74006F) inhibits effects of endotoxin in dogs. American Journal of Physiology 268:H1847–H1855
31. Granger HJ, Shepherd AP (1979) Dynamics and control of the microcirculation. Advances in Biomedical Engineering 7:1–61

32. Ayuse T, Brienza J, Revelly P, Boitnott JK, Robotham JL (1995) Role of nitric oxide in porcine liver circulation under normal and endotoxemic conditions. Journal of Applied Physiology 78:1319-1329
33. Mathie RT, Ralevic V, Alexander B, Burnstock G (1991) Nitric oxide is the mediator of ATP-induced dilatation of the rabbit hepatic arterial vascular bed. British Journal of Pharmacology 103:1602-1606
34. Bearn AG, Billing B, Sherlock S (1951) The effect of adrenaline and noradrenaline on hepatic blood flow and splanchnic carbohydrate metabolism in man. Journal of Physiology 115: 430-441
35. Shepherd AP, Granger HJ (1973) Autoregulatory escape in the gut: a systems analysis. Gastroenterology 65:77-91
36. Jensen MD, Johnson CM, Cryer PE, Murray MJ (1995) Thermogenesis after a mixed meal: role of leg and splanchnic tissues in men and women. American Journal of Physiology 268: E433-438
37. Lautt WW (1985) Mechanism and role of intrinsic regulation of hepatic arterial blood flow: hepatic arterial buffer response. American Journal of Physiology 249:G549-G556
38. Greenway CV, Oshiro G (1972) Comparison of the effects of hepatic nerve stimulation on arterial flow, distribution of arterial and portal flows and the blood content in the livers of anaesthetized cats and dogs. Journal of Physiology (London) 227:487-501
39. Uusaro A, Ruokonen E, Takala J (1995) Estimation of splanchnic blood flow by the Fick principle in man and problems in the use of indocyanine green. Cardiovascular Research 30: 106-112
40. Ruokonen E, Takala J, Kari A, Saxén H, Mertsola J, Hansen EJ (1993) Regional blood flow and oxygen transport in septic shock. Critical Care Medicine 21:1296-1303
41. Ruokonen E, Takala J, Kari A (1993) Regional blood flow and oxygen transport in low cardiac output syndrome after cardiac surgery. Critical Care Medicine 21:1304-1311
42. Steffes CP, Dahn MS, Lange MP (1994) Oxygen transport-dependent splanchnic metabolism in the sepsis syndrome. Archives of Surgery 129:46-52
43. Uusaro A, Ruokonen E, Takala J (1995) Gastric mucosal pH does not reflect change in splanchnic blood flow after cardiac surgery. British Journal of Anaesthesia 74:149-154
44. Parviainen I, Ruokonen E, Takala J (1995) Dobutamine-induced dissociation between changes in splanchnic blood flow and gastric intramucosal pH after cardiac surgery. British Journal of Anaesthesia 74:277-282
45. Uusaro A, Ruokonen E, Takala J (1996) Splanchnic oxygen transport after cardiac surgery: evidence for inadequate tissue perfusion after stabilization of hemodynamics. Intensive Care Medicine 22:26-33
46. Parviainen I, Ruokonen E, Takala J (1996) Sodium nitroprusside after cardiac surgery: central and regional hemodynamics. Acta Anaesthesiologica Scandinavica 40:606-611
47. Clements D, West R, Elias E (1987) Comparison of bolus and infusion methods for estimating hepatic blood flow in patients with liver disease using indocyanine green. Journal of Hepatology 5:282-287
48. Jorfeldt L, Juhlin-Dannfelt A (1978) The influence of ethanol on splanchnic and skeletal muscle metabolism in man. Metabolism 27:97-106
49. Grainger SL, Keeling PWN, Brown IMH, Marigold JH, Thompson RPH (1983) Clearence and non-invasive determination of the hepatic extraction of indocyanine green in baboons and man. Clin Sci 64:207-212
50. Skak C, Keiding S (1987) Methodological problems in the use of indocyanine green to estimate hepatic blood flow and ICG clearence in man. Liver 7:155-162
51. Wilmore DW, Goodwin CW, Aulick LH, Powanda MC, Mason AD, Pruitt Jr MD (1980) Effect of injury and infection on visceral metabolism and circulation. Annals of Surgery 192:491-500
52. Aulick LH, Goodwin Jr CW, Becker RA, Wilmore DW (1981) Visceral blood flow following thermal injury. Annals of Surgery 193:112-116
53. Dahn MS, Lange P, Lobdell K, Hans B, Jacobs LA, Mitchell RA (1987) Splanchnic and total body oxygen consumption differences in septic and injured patients. Surgery 101:69-80
54. Dahn MS, Lange P, Wilson RF, Jacobs LA, Mitchell RA (1990) Hepatic blood flow and splanchnic oxygen consumption measurements in clinical sepsis. Surgery 107:295-301

55. Gottlieb ME, Sarfeh IJ, Stratton H, Goldman ML, Newell JC, Shah DM (1983) Hepatic perfusion and splanchnic oxygen consumption in patients postinjury. Journal of Trauma 23: 836–843
56. Gump FE, Price JB Jr, Kinney JM (1970) Blood flow and oxygen consumption in patients with severe burns. Surgery, Gynecology and Obstetrics 130:23–28
57. Gump FE, Price JB Jr, Kinney JM (1970) Whole body and splanchnic blood flow and oxygen consumption measurements in patients with intraperitoneal infection. Annals of Surgery 171:321–328
58. Parviainen I, Rantala A, Ruokonen E, Takala J (1995) Failure of enalaprilat to reduce blood pressure in hypertensive cardiac surgery patients. Critical Care Medicine 23 (Suppl):A140
59. Landow L, Phillips DA, Heard SO, Prevost D, Vandersalm TJ, Fink MP (1991) Gastric tonometry and venous oximetry in cardiac surgery patients. Critical Care Medicine 19:1226–1233
60. Ruokonen E, Takala J, Uusaro A (1991) Effect of vasoactive treatment on the relationship between mixed venous and regional oxygen saturation. Critical Care Medicine 19: 1365–1369
61. Kainuma M, Nakashima K, Sakuma I, Kawase M, Komatsu T, Shimada Y, et al (1992) Hepatic venous hemoglobin oxygen saturation predicts liver dysfunction after hepatectomy. Anesthesiology 76:379–386
62. Leier CV (1988) Regional blood flow responses to vasodilators and inotropes in congestive heart failure. American Journal of Cardiology 62:86E–93E
63. Marik PE, Mohedin M (1994) The contrasting effects of dopamine and norepinephrine on systemic and splanchnic oxygen utilization in hyperdynamic sepsis. JAMA 272:1354–1357
64. Gutierrez G, Clark C, Brown SD, Price K, Ortiz L, Nelson C (1994) Effect of dobutamine on oxygen consumption and gastric mucosal pH in septic patients. American Journal of Respiratory and Critical Care Medicine 150:324–329
65. Giraud GD, MacCannell KL (1984) Decreased nutrient blood flow during dopamine- and epinephrine-induced intestinal vasodilation. Journal of Pharmacology and Experimental Therapeutics 230:214–220

Tissue Oxygenation

G. Berlot, A. Tomasini and M. Maffessanti

Introduction

The supply of oxygen to the cells is the most essential function developed in aerobic organisms, since its shortage is unavoidably associated with the failure of the cellular functions and, eventually, with the death of the entire organism. The goal of providing this essential stuff is accomplished via a complex interaction involving the cardiovascular system, the blood and the lungs.

A number of disturbances of this process have been described and are rewieved in other chapters. Whereas the underlying pathophysiologic mechanisms of some of these have been fully understood, the nature of others, and, for some of them, their very existence outside the research laboratory is still debated.

Cellular Respiration

Cellular respiration can be described as the transfer of electrons from organic compounds to the oxygen (O_2) [1, 2]. With this process, high-energy phosphates are produced, which provide energy to the cell. The oxidation of carbohydrates, aminoacids and fatty acids is associated with the production of Acetyl-CoA, which enter the trycarboxylic acid cycle, resulting in the production of CO_2 and four pairs of electrons. These latters are transferred from the cytosol into the mytochondria by the nicotinamide dinucleotide (NAD^+) and by the flavine-adenine dinucleotides (FAD^+). Once arrived into the inner mitochondrial membrane, the electrons move down a series of cytochrome-located redox reactions, each of whom is associated with a progressive reduction of energy level, until the final cytochrome reduces molecular O_2. During this process, adenosine-triphosphate (ATP) is produced, which is successively hydrolized to provide the fuel essential for the cellular functions. The hydrolysis of ATP is associated with the production of energy and the release of free H^+ and inorganic phosphate (Pi).

$$ATP + H_2O = ADP + Pi + H^+ + Energy$$

When O_2 is present in sufficient amounts, ADP, H^+ and Pi are reutilized to resynthetize ATP by the oxidative phosphorylation. The rate of ATP production is influenced by several factors, including the concentration of ADP, Pi and H^+ and the overall amount of the intramitochondrial phosphorylated adenine compounds (ATP, ADP and AMP). When they accumulate in the cytosol, these substances are transferred back to the mitochondria by different translocases. Hypoxia, and the related increase of intracellular H^+, induces an increase of the cytosolic concentrations of adenine nucleotides by favouring the movement of the ATP outward the mitochondria. The loss of ATP, in turns, reduces the rate of the oxidative phosphorylation and the rate of ATP production till a point beyond which it ceases completely. Once this treshold is reached, the cell must use anaerobic sources energy to survive, including glycolysis, the creatine kinase reaction and the adenylate kinase reaction. Actually, in hypoxic states, the cytosolic accumulation of the AMP stimulates the glycolysis, with the consequent production of lactate as a byproduct (Pasteur effect).

$$Glucose + 2\,Pi + 2\,ADP = lactate + 2\,ATP + 2\,H_2O + Energy$$

With this reaction, the net production of ATP is reduced in comparison with oxidative phosphorylation, in which 36 moles of ATP are supplied. Moreover, it increases the amount of cytosolic lactate.

The creatine-kinase reaction is another important source of source of ATP, occurring in the skeletal muscle, the heart and the brain:

$$[PCr] + [ADP] + [H^+] = [ATP] + [creatine].$$

In conditions of sustained hypoxia, the increase of cytosolic ADP stimulates the adenylate kinase reaction:

$$[ADP] + [ADP] = [ATP] + [AMP]$$

The subsequent demolition of AMP by the 5-nucleotidase determines the production of adenosine, which escapes from the cell and, once into the microvascular network, exerts a strong vasodilator effect, so providing a metabolic feed-back aimed to increase the blood flow in hypoxic areas. A the same time, the deamination of AMP with the subsequent formation of inosine monophosphate (IMP) leads to the production of inosine and hypoxanthine, which, in turns, are important sources of free oxygen radicals in the xanthine oxidase reaction. These latters can exert powerful direct and indirect cytotoxic effects by acting on the cellular membrane and on the DNA. In contrast, when the supply of O_2 is normal, the byproducts of adenosine metabolism are recycled in the mitochondria without a concomitant increase of the H^+.

Oxygen Carriage

The delivery of oxygen to the cells occurs by diffusion and by convection. The diffusive mechanism is involved in two different phases. The first occurs in the lungs, during the passage of the oxygen from the alveoli to the pulmonary capillaries, and is related on either the central venous hemoglobin concentration and saturation (SVO_2), and the cardiac output (CO). The other is located in the tissues, and is related to different locally acting mechanisms, including the tissue metabolism and the functional conditions of the capillary network [2].

Since the oxygen is transferred to the cells either bound to the hemoglobin (Hb) and as dissolved in the blood, the arterial blood content of O_2 (CaO_2) can be calculated according to the formula

$$CaO_2 = (Hb \times SO_2 \times 1.39) + (PaO_2) \times 0.0031$$

Where PO_2 = tension of the dissolved O_2; 0.0031 = solubility coefficient of O_2 in the plasma; Hb = hemoglobin concentration; SO_2 = hemoglobin O_2 saturation; 1.39 = ml of O_2 carried by 1 g of Hb.

In normobaric conditions, the amount of O_2 dissolved in the plasma is negligible; however, it increases to the point to supply all tissue O_2 needs when the subject is breathing hyperbaric oxygen.

The Hb is a complex molecule, which is compounded by 2α- and 2β-chains, each of whom is bound to heme residuals in a noncovalent linkage. Each heme contains an iron atom that reversibly binds O_2. This atom does not alter its valence during the O_2 loading and unloading but remains in the Fe^{++} (ferrous) state. However, the action of some substance (i.e. cyanide) can transform the Fe^{++} into Fe^{+++} (ferric) with the ultimate production of meta-Hb, which irreversibly binds O_2. As a consequence, the Hb-bound O_2 is no more unloaded to the cells. The binding and the release of each O_2 modifies the steric properties of the Hb molecule, which can be functionally considered as the union of two α-β-subunit. Actually, as the first O_2 molecule binds to a heme group of a α-chain, it determines a structural changes which is associated to an increased O_2 affinity of the next β-chain, which, in turn, binds another O_2 molecule. This causes another spatial rearrangement of the initial α-β-subunit, leading to the increased O_2 affinity of the other α-β-subunit.

Table 1

Increased affinity	Decreased affinity
Increased pH	Decreased pH
Decreased pCO_2	Increased pCO_2
Decreased temperature	Increased temperature
Decreased 2,3 DPG	Increased 2,3 DPG
Excess RBC pyruvate kinase	Reduced RBC pyruvate kinase
Phosphate depletion	Hyperphosphatemia
Abnormal hemoglobins	Anemia
Intoxications (Co-Hb, Met-Hb)	Hypoxemia
	Sickle cell disease

As a consequence, the affinity of the Hb for the O_2 progressively increases until a point, beyond which any further increase of the partial pressure of O_2 into the blood is no more associated with the increase of the Hb saturation. The functional properties of the Hb are of paramount importance in the process of tissue oxygenation. Within the pulmonary capillaries, at high O_2 concentrations, the binding of O_2 is facilitated, whereas at a peripheral level, where the O_2 tension is lower, the unloading is promoted.

Changes of the Hb binding capacity are associated with structural changes of its α- and β-subunits, which can be induced by different factors (Table 1).

As it appears, conditions normally present in ischemic regions, including a reduced pH and an increased CO_2 tend to reduce the Hb affinity in order to increase the oxygenation.

Oxygen Transport and Oxygen Consumption

The bulk of Hb-bound oxygen is carried to the various organs via a convective mechanism (DO_2), which is related either to the hemoglobin concentration and to the cardiac output [1, 2].

$$DO_2 = \text{Cardiac output (CO)} \times CaO_2.$$

Due to its small amount, the calculation of the CaO_2 usually does not take in account the dissolved oxygen (see above).

The oxygen consumption (VO_2) is approximatively equivalent to the mitochondrial production of ATP; actually, even in normal conditions, a small amount of O_2 is consumed in extramitochondrial sites not related to the production of energy [3]. The VO_2 can be invasively calculated with the reverse Fick's equation:

$$VO_2 = CO \times (CaO_2 - CvO_2),$$

where CvO_2 indicated the venous oxygen content.

Alternatively, VO_2 can be directly measured with the indirect calorimetry, using a metabolic cart which analyzes the inspiratory and expiratory concentration of O_2 and CO_2 [4, 5].

$$VO_2 = \left[\frac{(1 - FEO_2 - FECO_2) \times FIO_2}{(1 - FEO_2)} - FEO_2 \right] \times \dot{V}E$$

Where: FEO_2 = expiratory O_2; $FECO_2$ = expiratory CO_2; FIO_2 = inspiratory O_2; VE = minute volume.

To obtain accurate measurements, the FIO_2 must be stable and lower than 0.6, the system must be sealed and the inspiratory and expiratory branches must be separated.

The values of VO_2 obtained with the Fick's equation can be different from those obtained with the indirect calorimetry [6]. In a model of respiratory failure, the measured VO_2 was consistently higher than the calculated VO_2, and this difference has been attributed to the metabolism of phlogistic cells in the lung [7], whose VO_2 is not taken in account when using the Fick's equation. Similar results have been reported also in critically ill patients [7–9]. Recently, other investigators [10, 11], suggested that the VO_2 obtained with the Fick's equation is too inaccurate to be used for research purposes, and suggested that even in clinical conditions this technique should be used cautiously when therapeutic decisions are based on this value.

Each system has its advantages and disadvantages. The calculation of the VO_2 requires the insertion of a Swan-Ganz catheter and, more importantly, it cannot provide on-line informations. In turns, the direct measurement of the VO_2 can be influenced by high tidal volumes and oxygen concentration (FIO_2) [9].

DO_2/VO_2 Relationship

The relationship between the VO_2 and the DO_2, which is mathematically expressed by the oxygen extraction ratio (O_2ER), is of paramount importance for the tissue oxygenation. This relationship can be profoundly disturbed in some conditions, including sepsis and ARDS.

The VO_2/DO_2 relationship is biphasic (Fig. 1), and its alterations of can be better understood if one imagines to reduce progressively the DO_2.

In this circumstance, the VO_2 is initially maintained through an increase of O_2ER (segment B), till a critical point ($DO_{2\,crit}$) is reached below which the VO_2 becomes dependent upon changes of DO_2 (segment A) and anaerobic metabolism ensues, as indicated by the appearance of biochemical markers of tissue hypoxia, including the increase of the blood lactate value and of the gradient of CO_2 and pH between the arterial and the venous side [12, 13]. In humans, the value of the $DO_{2\,crit}$ remains undetermined: although Shibutani et al. [14] showed in patients subjected to progressive reduction of blood flow during cardio-pulmonary bypass that the VO_2 became dependent on DO_2 when it was reduced below 330 ml/min and Rashkin et al. [15] showed that in ARDS patients blood lactate levels were normal when DO_2 was higher than 8 ml/min/m^2, other authors failed to demonstrate in critically ill patients a value of DO_2 below which lactic acidosis ensued [16].

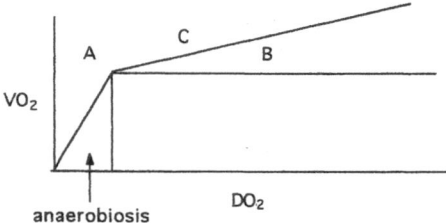

Fig. 1

In normal subjects facing a sudden increase of VO_2 (i.e. physical exercise), the increase of DO_2 is slighty higher than the increase of the O_2ER [17]. This response can be influenced by the underlying conditions: in patients after cardiac surgery, Routsi et al. [18] observed an increase of the DO_2 in patients able to increase their CO, whereas the others matched the enhanced oxygen needs by increasing the O_2ER. The tissue O_2ER is reduced in sepsis, as experimentally demonstrated by Zhang et al. [19] in model of cardiac tamponade in dogs given endotoxin. In critically ill septic patients, even if the resting O_2ER is typically reduced, tissue extractive capabilities are maintained till a very advanced phase, as demonstrated by Ronco et al. [20] in a group of dying patients undergoing the gradual withdrawn of the hemodynamic support.

There are relevant regional differences in O_2ER capabilities: in conditions of reduced systemic DO_2, VO_2 decreases in the muscles later than in the gut [21]. Several mechanism are responsible for the increased O_2ER, including (a) the hypoxia-induced production and release of vasodilating substances and (b) the activation of neurovascular reflexes, whose global effect consists in the opening of previously closed capillaries (capillary recruitment). When more and more capillaries are recruited, the intercapillary distance as well the distance between the capillaries and the cells decreases and the time spent by the red blood cell into the capillaries increases, thus allowing an enhanced O_2 unloading [1, 2].

Besides these factors, the muscle activity and the body temperature exerts a strong influence on the DO_2/VO_2 relationship and on the O_2ER. Hypothermia and muscle rest induce a reduction of the VO_2 due to a decrease of the cell metabolism, and paralysis and body cooling can be suited in critically ill febrile patients in order to reduce tissue oxygen needs [22, 23]. Experimentally, the value of the $DO_{2\,crit}$ decreases from 8–9 ml/min/kg at normothermia to 5–6 ml at 30 °C [5, 9]. The effects of hypothermia on the O_2ER are controversial, being reduced in some studies but normal in others [24, 25]. Besides O_2ER, a number of compensatory mechanism working in different timeframes have been developed in order to maintain the aerobic metabolism when the DO_2 is reduced (Table 2).

In critically ill patients, the reduction of the DO_2 can be so abrupt (i.e. cardiogenic or hemorrhagic shock) that these homeostatic responses can be partially or totally blunted or the tissue O_2ER capabilities can be impaired, at least at a regional level (i.e. sepsis and septic shock) [21]. As a consequence, anaerobic metabolism, albeit initially limited to some tissues, ensues [26]. Actually, several investigators demonstrated that in septic and ARDS patients in whom acute changes of DO_2 were induced in different ways, the VO_2, obtained with the Fick's equation, was dependent on DO_2 even when its values were higher than normal (Fig. 1, segment C) [27–31]. However, other investigators who measured the VO_2 with the indirect calorimetry, failed to demonstrate this abnormal VO_2/DO_2 dependency in similar groups of patients [32–34], and this discrepancy has been attributed to the mathematical coupling of VO_2 and DO_2 determined by acute variations of the CO, shared by both variables used in the Fick's equation [35]. Another possible explication is that patients with similar disease could have been studied in different phases of their clinical courses, and the conflicting results could be ascribed to the different hemodynamic conditions at the time of the

Table 2

Response	Mechanisms
In seconds	
> Ventilation	$PaCO_2$ or $[H^+]$ effects on the respiratory drive
> Cardiac output	Increased venous return due to peripheral vasodilation
	Myocardial sympathetic stimulation
Diversion of the blood flow	Vasodilation of more metabolically active tissues;
	vasoconstriction of resting areas
< Hb binding capacity	$\neq [H^+]$ during hypoxia (Bohr effect)
for the O_2 (P_{50})	
In hours	
< Hb binding capacity	Increased 2,3 DPG in blood red cells
for the O_2 (P_{50})	
Changes of blood volume	Increased plasma volume, reduced blood viscosity
In weeks	
Increased total Hb	Erythropoietin-induced bone-marrow stimulation

evaluation. Moreover, even the small doses of catecholamines used in some studies to increase the DO_2 might have influenced, via a thermogenic effect, the VO_2. Furthermore, it is possible that, due to the inter-organs differences in the O_2ER capabilities, the VO_2/DO_2 dependency could be present in some district (i.e. the gut) but not in others [36].

The reduction of the VO_2 observed either experimentally and clinically in conditions of reduced or maldistributed blood flow could also represent, at least in some regions, an adaptative, and probably time-limited, response to unfavourable conditions. Actually, Hotchkiss et al. [37], using sophisticated techniques, failed to demonstrate a bioenergetic deficit, in septic animals, despite an increase of plasma lactate concentration, which they attributed to derangements of its metabolism. This situation may be somewhat analogous to the phenomenon of the "hibernating myocardium". Experimentally, a prolonged reduction of oxygen availability to the myocardium by the sub-total occlusion of a coronary artery is associated with an early increase of the blood lactate levels measured distally to the occlusions followed by a gradual return to baseline [38, 39]. Other biological markers of tissue hypoxia, such as pH and pCO_2 in the blood distal to the occlusion shared the same pattern of an early alteration followed by a later return to the pre-occlusion values [38]. Using nuclear magnetic resonance (NMR) spectroscopy, Shafer et al. [40] demonstrated that the early peak of lactate is associated with a decrease in intracellular stores of adenosine triphosphate (ATP), and with an increase in inorganic phosphate, which remained high even when lactate had returned to the baseline. These biochemical changes are associated with decreased regional myocardial fiber shortening and a reduction of myocardial oxygen demand [38, 39]. This decrease of myocardial work in response to hypoxia is thought to be an adaptative mechanism aimed at maintaining the cells viable when the oxygen availability cannot match the oxygen requirements [41].

A similar reduction in cellular metabolism in response to reduced oxygen availability has been also observed in the brain or even in cell cultures [42] and may correspond to the so-called "oxygen conformism". Recently, Schumacker et al. [43] showed on isolated rat hepatocytes that a reduction in PO_2 was associated with a reduction in oxygen uptake, in the absence of significant lactate release. Yet, there was a significant reduction in ATP and an increase in NADPH concentrations. They raised the hypothesis that the cells may down-regulate some facultative metabolic activities to limit hypoxic damage.

Conclusions

Tissue oxygen metabolism depends on a complex interplay between the cardiovascular system, the respiratory apparatus and the blood. A number of adaptative mechanisms, working either centrally or peripherally have been developed to maintain an adequate energy production in the presence of a reduced oxygen availability and/or of increased oxygen needs.

References

1. Gutierrez G, Bismar H (1992) Oxygen transport and utilization. In: Dantzker DR (ed) Cardiopulmonary critical care, 2nd edition. WB Saunders, pp 199–229
2. Little RA, Denis Edwards J (1993) Applied physiology. In: Edwards JD, Shoemaker WC, Vincent JL (eds) Oxygen transport: principles and practice. WB Saunders, pp 21–40
3. Schumaker PT, Cain SM (1987) The concept of a critical oxygen delivery. Intens Care Med 13:223–229
4. Myburgh JA (1992) Derived oxygen saturations are not clinically useful for the calculation of oxygen consumption. Anaesth Int Care 20:460–463
5. Myburgh JA, Webb R, Worthley LIG (1992) Ventilation/perfusion indices do not correlate with the difference between oxygen consumption measured by the Fick principles and metabolic monitoring systems in critically patients. Crit Care Med 20:479–482
6. Hess D, Kacmarek R (1993) Techniques and devices for monitoring oxygenation. Resp Care 38:646–669
7. Light RB (1988) Intrapulmonary oxygen consumption in experimental pneumococcal pneumonia. J Appl Physiol 64:2490–2495
8. Takala J, Keinanen O, Vaisanen P, Kari A (1989) Measurement of gas exchange in intensive care: laboratory and clinical validation of a new device. Crit Care Med 17:1041–1047
9. Smithies MN, Royston B, Makita K, Konieczko K, Nunn JF (1991) Comparison of oxygen consumption measurements: indirect calorimetry versus the reverse Fick equation. Crit Care Med 19:1401–1406
10. Thrush DN (1996) Spirometric versus Fick-derived oxygen consumption: which method is better? Crit Care Med 24:91–95
11. Stock MC, Ryan ME (1996) Oxygen consumption calculated from the Fick equation has limited utility. Crit Care Med 24:86–90
12. Zhang H, Vincent JL (1993) Arteriovenous differences in pCO_2 and pH are good indicators of critical hypoperfusion. Am Rev Resp Dis 143:867–871
13. Bowles SA, Schlichtig R, Kramer DJ, Klions HA (1992) Arteriovenous pH and partial pressure of carbone dioxide detect critical oxygen delivery during progressive hemorrhage in dogs. J Crit Care 7:95–105
14. Shibutani K, Komatsu T, Kubal K (1983) Critical level of oxygen delivery in anesthetized man. Crit Care Med 11:640–644

15. Rashkin M, Boxkin C, Baughman R (1985) Oxygen delivery in critically ill patients. Relationship to blood lactate and survival. Chest 87:580–584

16. Astiz ME, Rackow EC, Kaufman B, Falk JL, Weil MH (1988) Relationship of oxygen delivery and mixed venous oxygenation to lactic acidosis in patients with sepsis ans acute myocardial infarction. Crit Care Med 16:655–660

17. Silance PG, Simon C, Vincent JL (1994) The relation between cardiac index and oxygen extraction in acutely ill patients. Chest 102:1190–1197

18. Routsi C, Vincent JL, Bakker J, De Backer D, Lejeune P, D'Hollander A, Le Clerc JL (1993) Relation between oxygen consumption and oxygen delivery in patients after cardiac surgery. Anesth Analg 77:1104–1110

19. Zhang H, Vincent JL (1993) Oxygen extraction is altered by endotoxin during tamponade induced stagnant hypoxia. Circ Shock 40:168–176

20. Ronco JJ, Fenwick JC, Tweedale MG, Wiggs BR, Phang T, Cooper DJ, Cunningham KF, Russell JA, Walley KR (1993) Identification of the critical oxygen delivery for anaerobic metabolism in critically ill septic and non septic humans. JAMA 270:1724–1730

21. Nelson DP, King CE, Dodd SL, Shumacker PT, Cain SM (1987) Systemic and intestinal limits of O_2 extraction in the dog. J Appl Physiol 63:387–392

22. Manthous CA, Hall JB, Kushner R, Schmidt GA, Russo G, Wood LDH (1995) The effect of mechanical ventilation on oxygen consumption in critically ill patients. Am J Resp Crit Care Med 151:210–214

23. Manthous CA, Hall JB, Olson D, Singh M, Chatila W, Pohlman A, Kushner R, Schmidt GA, Wood LDH (1995) Effect of cooling on oxygen consumption in febrile critically ill patients. Am J Resp Crit Care Med 151:10–14

24. Gutierrez G, Warley AR, Dantzker DR (1986) Oxygen delivery and utilization in hypothermic dogs. J Appl Physiol 60:751–757

25. Schumacker PT, Rowland J, Saltz S, Nelson DP, Wood LDH (1987) Effects of hyperthermia and hypothermia on oxygen extraction by tissues during hypovolemia. J Appl Physiol 63:1246–1252

26. Gutierrez G, Clark C, Brown SD, Price K, Ortiz L, Nelson C (1994) Effect of dobutamine on oxygen consumption and and gastric mucosal pH in septic patients. Am J Resp Crit Care Med 150:324–329

27. Haupt MT, Gilbert EM, Carlson RW (1985) Fluid loading increases oxygen consumption in septic patients with lactic acidosis. Am Rev Respir Dis 131:912–916

28. Gilbert EM, Haupt MT, Mandanas RY, Huaringa AJ, Carlson RW (1986) The effect of fluid loading, blood transfusion and catecholamine infusion on oxygen delivery and consumption in patients with sepsis. Am Rev Respir Dis 134:873–878

29. Vincent JL, Roman A, Kahn RJ (1990) Oxygen utake/supply dependency: effects of a short term dobutamine infusion. Am Rev Respir Dis 142:2–7

30. Fenwick JC, Dodek PM, Ronco JJ, Phang PT, Wiggs B, Russell JA (1990) Increased concentrations of plasma lactate predict pathologic dependence of oxygen consumption on oxygen delivery in patients with adult respiratory distress syndrome. J Crit Care 5:81–86

31. Kruse JA, Haupt MT, Puri VK, Carlson RW (1990) Lactate levels as predictors of the relationship between oxygen delivery and consumption in ARDS. Chest 98:959–962

32. Annat G, Viale JP, Carlisle P, Froment M, Motin J (1986) Oxygen delivery and uptake in the adult respiratory distress syndrome-lack of relationship when measured independently in patients with normal blood lactate concentrations. Am Rev Respir Dis 133:999–1001

33. Ronco JJ, Phang T, Walley KR, Wiggs B, Fenwick JC, Russell JA (1991) Oxygen consumption is independent of changes in oxygen delivery in severe adult respiratory distress. Am Rev Respir Dis 143:1267–1271

34. Vermeiy CG, Feenstra BWA, Adrichem WJ, Bruining HA (1991) Independent oxygen uptake and oxygen delivery in septic and postoperative patients. Chest 99:1438–1443

35. Bartlett RH, Dechert RE (1990) Oxygen kinetics: pitfalls in clinical research. J Crit Care 5:77–80

36. Nelson DP, Samsel RW, Wood LDH, Schumaker PT (1988) Pathological supply dependence of systemic and intestinal O_2 uptake during endotoxemia. J Appl Physiol 64:2410–2419

37. Hotchkiss RS, Karl I (1992) Reevaluation of the role of cellular hypoxia and bioenergetic failure in sepsis. JAMA 267:1503–1510

38. Fedele FA, Gewirtz H, Capone RJ, Sharaf B, Most AS (1988) Metabolic response to prolonged reduction of blood flow distal to a severe coronary stenosis. Circulation 78:729–735
39. Apstein CS, Gravino F, Hood WB (1979) Limitation of lactate production as an index of myocardial ischemia. Circulation 60:877–888
40. Shaefer S, Schwartz GG, Wisneski JA (1992) Response of high-energy phosphates and lactate release during prolonged regional ischemia in vivo. Circulation 85:342–349
41. Rahimtoola SH (1989) The hibernating myocardium. Am Heart J 117:211–221
42. Dyffey TE, Nelson SR, Lowry OH (1972) Cerebral carbohydrate metabolism during acute hypoxia and recovery. J Neurochem 19:959–977
43. Shumaker PT, Chandel N, Agusti AGN (1993) Oxygen conformance of cellular respiration in hepatocytes. Am J Physiol 265:L395–L402

Clinical Applications

Rationale for Hemodynamic Monitoring

J. A. Kellum

> When much blood is lost, the pulse becomes feeble, the skin extremely pale, the body covered with a malodorous sweat, the extremities frigid, and death occurs speedily.
> *Aulus Cornelius Celsus*, first century Roman savant [1]

Introduction

While the history of formal hemodynamic monitoring is relatively brief [2], an appreciation for the qualitative aspects of monitoring dates back to ancient times [1]. In one sense, hemodynamic monitoring is a natural extension of the physical examination, quantifying the various aspects of the physical assessment. For instance, methods to assess central venous pressure by examination of the neck veins were developed long before the routine use of central venous catheters. However, in the modern ICU's of today, hemodynamic monitoring is not used merely as a tool for the validation of the physical exam or for the periodic detailed assessment, but instead, on a continuous basis. Indeed, it is this feature that accounts for much of the utility of hemodynamic monitoring.

The Purpose of Hemodynamic Monitoring

There are four basic goals of hemodynamic monitoring. The first goal of monitoring is to identify patients at risk for organ injury. Patients with gross abnormalities of global hemodynamics, i.e. shock, are not difficult to identify; however many patients may have severe deficiencies in organ perfusion which are not easily detected by routine physical exam. In addition, even when patients are identified by other means, it is usually much later in the course when organ injury has already begun to occur. The ability of hemodynamic monitoring to alert the clinician to impending catastrophe, rather than merely to record it, speaks to the very reason that ICU's were developed in the first place. As we move into the next millennium, we are encountering a growing emphasis on cost containment, particularly in the United States. It is important to note that monitoring of large numbers of ICU patients permits a small number of intensivists to care for them and to be very selective and therefore cost-effective in the ordering of tests and therapies [2].

The second goal of monitoring is to identify patients who are already sustaining organ injury who require further diagnosis and treatment. Such patients generally require a higher level of monitoring than might have been used solely to identify patients at risk. For example, a patient who had been normotensive and making urine might have been monitored only non-invasively. However, if now the patient is hypotensive and remains so after a fluid challenge, more invasive monitoring may be required. Furthermore the cause of the abnormality must be sought. This is the third goal of monitoring; to characterize patients by hemodynamic subsets (i.e. cardiogenic, obstructive, hypovolemic, or distributive). Frequently, it is not enough simply to know that the blood pressure is low or that the right atrial pressure is normal. Such a scenario is compatible with a number of different clinical paradigms. In these situations the intensivist must apply other monitoring techniques to appropriately diagnose and treat the patient. Indeed, the final purpose of hemodynamic monitoring is to precisely titrate therapy to reestablish or to maintain normal physiologic function. In the ICU, it is rarely sufficient to make the diagnosis and prescribe therapy. Therapy must be titrated and diagnoses may change over time as the natural history of critical illness evolves or resolves.

Justification for Monitoring

Unfortunately, efficacy alone is no longer a justification for the use of any diagnostic or therapeutic modality. Each test or therapy must be proven to be superior to less expensive alternatives; and even then the cost must not outweigh the benefit. Fortunately, the fiscal justification for monitoring is relatively straight forward. The cost (both financial and medical) of allowing organ injury to occur or to be sustained is great compared to the small cost of monitoring [3]. Hence, it is likely that this modality will survive this new wave of cost-cutting. Still, the challenge for the intensivist will be to determine which patients require which level of monitoring and for how long.

A strong argument can also be made that physical findings are entirely insensitive when used to estimate hemodynamic parameters [4–5]. However, a diagnostic test cannot be justified solely on the basis of it's superiority to other methods. The information that the test provides must be useful (even crucial if the test is invasive). The information must impact the care of the patients so that changes in therapy are instituted. Such is the case for hemodynamic monitoring. The intensivist will approach two hypotensive patients in entirely different ways depending on their hemodynamic characteristics. The patient with a low cardiac output and high filling pressures may require inotropic support and diagnostic efforts focusing on the heart and great vessels; whereas the patient with a normal to high cardiac output and low filling pressures needs volume with perhaps vasopressor therapy and an investigation of the etiology of their distributive shock. The first patient's care may include an electrocardiogram, an echocardiogram and perhaps a coronary angiogram. In contrast, the second patient may need to have cultures drawn and to be begun on antibiotics. However, when the information that is provided by a given level of monitoring is no longer used to alter therapy, it should be discontinued.

In addition to these issues, there is a great deal of evidence now available that suggests that maintaining normal physiologic parameters improves outcome [5–9]. Unfortunately, it is often difficult to distinguish between the effects associated with treatment and the improved survival that is seen in patients who are healthy enough to achieve a "normal response". Furthermore, we must bare in mind the fact that these supportive measures simply keep patients alive long enough for them to recover from the underlying cause associated with their illness. In many cases this becomes a prolongation of the dying process when the underlying illness is incurable or the injury unrepairable. It has even been suggested that technology causes multiple organ dysfunction because it keeps patients alive and thus susceptible to ongoing organ injury [10]. Still, these data, taken collectively, argue strongly in favor of the use of hemodynamic monitoring and the titration of support to maintain normal physiologic parameters.

Some investigators have even advocated the use of inotropic agents to achieve supra-physiologic parameters [11–13]. In a clinical trial in high risk surgical patients, Shoemaker and coworkers [11] compared patients treated to achieve "normal" vs "supranormal" hemodynamic parameters (as defined prospectively). The investigators found a significant improvement in outcome and ICU length of stay for the "supranormal" group. However, in a similar study of patients with septic shock, Tuchschmidt and coworkers [12] found no difference in survival; although patients who reached the 4.5 L/min/m^2 cardiac index benchmark set by Shoemaker had a lower mortality (26% vs 60%). Boyd and coworkers [13] used dopexamine in high risk surgical patients to achieve high target oxygen transport. Although their results showed a decrease in 28 day mortality (5.7% vs 22.2%) for the treatment group, differences in oxygen transport between groups were not achieved. Interestingly, when target variables were achieved by aggressive use of dobutamine in a study by Hayes et al. [14], mortality was actually higher in the treatment arm (54% vs 34%). Finally, a large trial by Gattinoni et al. [15] evaluated the use of "supranormal" target variables in wide variety of patient types. Their results showed no difference in ICU or hospital mortality for any group. The authors concluded that therapy aimed at achieving a supranormal cardiac index cannot be justified.

Limitations and Complications

In addition to the potentially deleterious effects associated with increasing cardiac output to supranormal values, as seen in the Hayes study [14], monitoring alone is not without risk. Although noninvasive monitoring is almost risk free, all forms of monitoring, as for any diagnostic test, carry the risk that false positives will occur. In turn, these false positives may lead to incorrect treatment or further diagnostic testing which may itself lead to more treatment or more testing. The classic example of this occurs when healthy patients are routinely screened with a panel of laboratory tests [16]. Statistically, there is a high likelihood that the results of one of the tests will fall outside the normal range [17]. For this reason, even noninvasive monitoring should be limited to the population at risk.

When invasive hemodynamic monitoring is used instead of noninvasive techniques, the risks are far greater and differ by the type of monitoring and the site used. Infection remains the most frequent complication for all types and since the incidence increases with the duration of use (regardless of whether new lines are placed), it behooves the clinician to discontinue monitoring as soon it is no longer needed.

In addition to these complications, monitoring is associated with a number of limitations. Artifacts are commonly seen during pressure monitoring [2]. Table 1 lists some of the more common forms of artifact and their usual causes. Perhaps the most frequently described problems are with "catheter whip" and "damping". Strictly speaking, catheter whip occurs as a result of movement of the catheter tip such as when the pulmonary artery catheter is moved by the beating heart. This is in contrast to "underdamping" which is due to the dynamic response characteristics of the monitoring system [18]. The latter causes an accentuation of both the systolic and diastolic values away from the mean, while the former produces a chaotic or "noisy" signal which is difficult to interpret. "Overdamping" by contrast causes the signal to be diminished such that the systolic component appears lower and the diastolic appears higher. In general, damping does not distort the mean pressure.

Previously, Bellomo and Pinsky suggested four tests of the practical limitations of hemodynamic monitoring [19]. This list is shown in Table 2. While these rules

Table 1. Common forms of artifact and their causes. (Adapted from Nelson & Rutherford [2])

Signal characteristic	Artifact	Causes
Chaotic, "noisy"	Whip artifact	Catheter movement

Exaggerated	Underdamping	Harmonic amplification
		  tubing length
		  tubing diameter

Flattened	Overdamping	Air bubbles

		increased system compliance
		  compliant tubing
		  rubber ports
		  multiple stopcocks

Table 2. Requirements for the justification of hemodynamic monitoring. (Adapted form Bellomo & Pinsky [18])

1. Less invasive or otherwise less risky methods are unavailable or are unable to provide the required information.
2. The information obtained form monitoring is required to alter diagnosis, prognosis or treatment based on accepted physiologic principals.
3. The changes in treatment will result in improvements in patient outcome.
4. The changes in treatment will result in a more effective use of health care resources.

serve as useful guidelines, perhaps the most significant limitation to hemody-namic monitoring is lack of sensitivity and specificity for assessing changes in end organ function or tissue wellness. This problem has been illustrated by liken-ing monitoring to the inebriated motorist who looses his keys in the dark by his car only to be found searching for them 100 yards away, under a street light, be-cause that was where he could see [20]. Too frequently we concentrate our efforts on obtaining those data that are available rather than the data that are really needed. This is because global measures of oxygen supply and demand do not re-flect changes in regional blood flow. Unfortunately, regional markers themselves have yet to be shown superior to global markers in defining therapeutic effective-ness [21]. Still, hemodynamic parameters remain one of the most widely used methods of assessing tissue wellness. In general, two indices of tissue wellness are assessed, perfusion, and oxygen transport. Having considered what it is that we are measuring and the rationale for making these measurements in terms of their relation to physiologic variables, we must now consider the rationale for assess-ing these variables in the first place.

The Rationale for Assessing Perfusion

In much the same way that the body responds to changes in CO_2 by changing ventilation, organ blood flow is regulated in response to local metabolic demand. Thus, in health, the adequacy of perfusion is assured by the body's own physio-logic mechanisms; the exact mechanisms responsible for this are only partly understood. However, it is the dysfunction of these mechanisms that leads to the very common clinical signs of distributive shock. It is likely then that we can bet-ter understand this disease process by understanding the normal physiologic mechanisms which regulate organ blood flow and how disease alters them.

Determinants of Blood Flow Distribution

Blood flow to individual vascular beds is determined by three primary variables, 1) sympathetic tone (regional and global), 2) passive pressure-flow relationships, 3) local metabolic demand. Global autonomic tone provides the background "command and control" for the entire system, preserving flow to the vital organs by reducing flow to areas where it is not needed. When this control is impaired, some regions become ischemic while other areas maintain higher than needed flow. This point was demonstrated by Cain [22] who found that for hypoxic hy-poxia in the dog, the dysoxic threshold occurred at a higher global oxygen deliv-ery when α-adrenergic tone was blocked than when it was left intact. The effect of passive pressure-flow relationships was demonstrated by Kramer et al. [23] who showed that changes in mean arterial pressure induce blood flow redistribu-tion among organs. For example, as perfusion pressure decreases, the flow to var-ious beds also decreases but the magnitude differs significantly across organs. Furthermore, various stressors can alter this relationship in a nonuniform fashion. Finally, there is much recent work that has furthered our understanding of the effects on flow related to local metabolic demand; specifically with respect to adenosine [24]. This substance builds up as cells become hypoxic and are forced to fully hydrolyze their ATP stores. Since adenosine is both lipid soluble and a potent smooth muscle relaxing factor, it provides for an ideal mechanism whereby ischemic tissue can increase their relative share of global perfusion.

The Rationale for Assessing Oxygen Transport

In recent years, oxygen transport has received perhaps more attention than any other single monitoring variable. Nonetheless, despite numerous attempts to prove the clinical utility of this form of monitoring [6–8, 25] it remains unclear that it changes outcome. In part this may be due to the fact that assessing global oxygen transport does not tell us how individual organ systems are functioning. Furthermore, it is unclear that tissue oxygen delivery is really the limiting factor in determining organ-system function and viability in critically ill patients. However, if shock is the immediate systemic result of inadequate oxygen delivery to the tissues and if sustained tissue dysoxia results in organ-system dysfunction and death then therapy aimed at reversing tissue hypoperfusion would seem prudent. Indeed if loss of blood flow regulation occurs then a reasonable method to restore regional blood flow to hypoperfused vascular beds would be to increase global blood flow, accepting that increased non-nutrient blood flow may also occur. Such is our current practice given our relative inability to access specific organ dysoxia.

However, the future may be brighter. Certain technologic innovations are already in the early stages of evaluation which may unlock the secrets of regional monitoring. One significant example is gastric tonometry. This device allows for the measurement of mucosal pCO_2. As long as flow to the tissues is maintained, mucosal pCO_2 will approximate arterial pCO_2 and the difference between these values, the so called delta pCO_2, will be small (normally less than 40 mmHg) [26]. When the delta pCO_2 is significantly greater than this, for example > 100 mmHg, hypoperfusion almost certainly exists. Unfortunately, tonometry may be too insensitive to detect clinically significant changes in regional blood flow and too nonspecific to distinguish mild but important changes form normal [27]. Monitoring techniques for other aspects of tissue wellness are sorely needed. Targets for such research include bioenergetics, ion flux, white blood cell activation, and other aspects of the stress response. Without this knowledge clinicians will remain dependent on global markers to assess tissue wellness. However, clinicians will need to interpret data derived from these techniques in light of their limitations. Indeed, therapy aimed at a single global marker such as oxygen transport, arterial lactate or delta pCO_2 can be likened to the use of propranolol for tachycardia or aspirin for fever. Until a more comprehensive understanding of the mechanisms of injury and repair allows for the development of specific measures of tissue wellness, we will be forced to titrate resuscitative therapy by integrating the vast clinical, hemodynamic and laboratory data at our disposal.

References

1. Bellamy RF, Maningas PA, Wenger BA (1986) Current Shock Models and Clinical Correlations. Ann Emerg Med 15:1392–1395
2. Nelson LD, Rutherford EJ (1993) Principles of hemodynamic monitoring. In: Pinsky MR, Dhainaut J-F (eds) Pathophysiologic Foundations of Critical Care. Williams & Wilkins, Baltimore, pp 3–22
3. Polk SL, Roizen MF (1990) Cost-benefit analysis in monitoring. In: Blitt CD (ed) Monitoring in Anesthesia and Critical Care Medicine. Churchill Livingstone, New York, pp 65–77
4. Connors AF Jr, McCaffree DR, Gray BA (1983) Evaluation of right-heart catheterization in the critically ill patient without acute myocardial infarction. N Engl J Med 308:263–271
5. Moore CH, Lombardo TR, Allums JA, et al (1978) Left main coronary artery stenosis: hemodynamic monitoring to reduce mortality. Ann Thorac Surg 26:445–452
6. Shoemaker WC, Montgomery ES, Kaplan E, et al (1973) Physiologic patterns in surviving and non-surviving shock patients. Arch Surg 106:630–639
7. Hopkins JA, Shoemaker WC, Chang PC, et al (1983) Clinical trial of an emergency resuscitation algorithm. Crit Care Med 22:621–628
8. Shoemaker WC (1987) The role of oxygen transport patterns in the pathophysiology, prediction of outcome and therapy of shock. In: Bryan-Brown CW, Ayres SM (eds) New Horizons II: Oxygen Transport and Utilization. Fullerton, Society of Critical Care Medicine, p 65
9. Hinds C, Watson D (1995) Manipulating hemodynamics and oxygen transport in critically ill patients. NEJM 333:1074–1075
10. Pinsky MR, Matuschak GM (1990) Multiple systems organ failure: a unifying hypothesis. J Crit Care 5:108–114
11. Shoemaker WC, Appel PL, Kram HB, Waxman K, Lee TS (1988) Prospective trial of supranormal values of survivors as therapeutic goals in high-risk surgical patients. Chest 94: 1176–1186
12. Tuchsmidt J, Fired J, Astriz M, Rackow E (1992) Evaluation of cardiac output and oxygen delivery improves outcome in septic shock. Chest 102:216–220
13. Boyd O, Grounds RM, Bennett ED (1993) A randomized clinical trial of the effect of deliberate perioperative increase of oxygen delivery on mortality in high-risk surgical patients. JAMA 270:2699–2707
14. Hayes MA, Timmins AC, Yau EHS, et al (1994) Elevation of systemic oxygen delivery in the treatment of critically ill patients. N Engl J Med 330:1717–1722
15. Gattinoni L, Brazzi L, Pelosi P, et al (1995) A trial of goal-oriented hemodynamic therapy in critically ill patients. N Engl J Med 333:1025–1032
16. Robin ED (1983) A critical look at critical care. Crit Care Med 11:144–152
17. Meador CK (1965) The art and science of non-disease. N Engl J Med 272:92–101
18. Kleinman B (1989) Understanding natural frequency and damping and how they relate to the measurement of blood pressure. J Clin Monit 5:137–147
19. Bellomo R, Pinsky MR (1996) Invasive monitoring. In: Tinker J, Browne D, Sibbald W (eds) Critical Care – Standards Audit and Ethics. Arnold Publishing, pp 82–104
20. Bryan-Brown CW (1992) Pathway to the present: a personal view of critical care. In: Civetta JM, Taylor RW, Kirby RR (eds) Critical Care. JB Lippincott, Philadelphia, pp 5–12
21. Pinsky MR (1994) Beyond global O_2 supply-demand relations: in search of measures of dysoxia. Intensive Care Med 20:1–3
22. Cain S (1978) Effects of time and vasoconstrictor tone on oxygen extraction during hypoxic hypoxia. J Appl Physiol 45:219–224
23. Kramer DJ, Stein KL, Schlichtig RA, Armendariz E, Lanier A, Pinsky MR (1989) Pressure flow relationships in the superior mesenteric and hepatic arteries in endotoxic shock. Chest 96: 2933–2939
24. Berdenheur H, Schrader J (1986) Supply-to-demand ratio for oxygen determines formation of adenosine by the heart. Am J Physiol 250:H162–H173
25. Shoemaker WC, Kram HB, Appel PL, Fleming AW (1990) The efficacy of central venous and pulmonary artery catheters and therapy based upon them in reducing mortality and morbidity. Arch Surg 125:1332–1338

26. Schlichtig R, Bowles SA (1994) Distinguishing between aerobic and anaerobic appearance of dissolved CO_2 in intestine during low flow. J Appl Physiol 76:2443–2451
27. Kellum JA, Rico P, Pinsky MR (1996) Accuracy of pHi and delta PCO_2 for detecting gut hypoperfusion in acute canine endotoxemia. Am J Respir Crit Care Med 153:A659

Invasive Hemodynamic Monitoring

P. Rogers

The Intensive Care Unit utilizes 7.5% of hospital beds, yet consumes one-third of the total hospital budget [1]. Health care costs and resource utilization concerns have forced physicians to examine the patient care provided in the ICU. Protocols have been developed to "fast-track" patients, guidelines have been developed for diagnostic and therapeutic interventions, and evidence based treatment strategies have been invoked to reduce unnecessary procedures. The problem, is that there is little data to support which interventions should be performed and which are unnecessary. Invasive hemodynamic monitoring for example, has very little scientific data to support is widespread use [2, 3]. Equally concerning is the fact that many physicians using these interventions, have little understanding of the monitors and are often unable to apply the data to problem-solving [3–5].

If health care providers are going to effectively utilize invasive technology, such as hemodynamic monitoring, it is essential that they understand the goals and for such procedures. They should ensure that:

1. The information received cannot be acquired from less invasive and less risky monitoring;
2. The information improves accuracy of diagnosis, prognosis, and/or treatment;
3. The information results in improved patient morbidity and mortality;
4. The information results in more effective utilization and allocation of health care resources [2].

Healthcare professionals using these guidelines will find few clinical situations with a proven benefit [6, 7]. They will find many clinical situations which are probably appropriate but unproven [8–15]. More than likely they will find experience and training dictates their decision making. In any case, the provider must be able to interpret and apply the data to problem-solving. Because of the technical and physiologic limitations of hemodynamic monitoring, data obtained may not improve accuracy of diagnosis, prognosis or treatment and may lead to erroneous conclusions.

This chapter will review the goals of invasive monitoring focusing on arterial, central venous, and pulmonary artery catheterization. The technical and physiologic limitations will be described so that the data obtained can be appropriately applied to solving clinical problems and developing treatment strategies. Finally, the proven and probable indications for each of the invasive techniques will be reviewed so that the provider may feel confident utilizing or not utilizing this technology in the era of resource allocation and cost containment.

Goal of Monitoring

The goal of invasive hemodynamic monitoring is to evaluate the patient's cardiac status and to determine if adequate oxygen delivery is being provided to the tissues. If tissue requirement exceeds oxygen delivery, data acquired from the arterial, central venous and pulmonary artery catheters may be used to evaluate oxygen delivery (Table 1). Various components of cardiac output may be calculated and corrected to achieve a balance with oxygen consumption.

Technologic Consideration

Each of the intravascular catheters monitors pressure through a distal port which is percutaneously inserted into the vascular tree. The pressure generated is conducted through low compliance tubing and converted into an electrical signal by pressure-sensing diaphragm in the external transducers [16]. The accuracy of the data acquired, often depends on the reliability of the pressure monitoring system; the catheter, the tubing and the transducers [17].

The initial step in gathering accurate data is to ensure that the transducer is referenced and zeroed. The stopcock should be opened to atmosphere to the level of the right ventricle with the patient in the supine position since a 15 cm vertical change in transducer position will result in opposite charge of 10 mmHg blood pressure.

Hemodynamic data may also be distorted by the intrinsic dynamic response characteristics of the catheter-tubing-transducer setups [18]. Each component has its own natural frequency (FN in hertz) and damping coefficient. The range of damping coefficients (and natural frequency responses for a given system are shown in Figure 1. Optimal waveforms are produced only if the frequency and damping coefficient of the system are in the non-shaded areas marked adequate and optimal. At very low frequencies, there is no damping coefficient which is acceptable. As the frequency of the system increases, wider ranges of damping coefficients are acceptable. The natural frequency at which extension tubing begins to ring is described by the equation:

$$\text{Frequency} = \frac{1}{2\pi} \sqrt{\frac{\pi D^2}{4pL} \cdot \frac{\Delta P}{\Delta V}}$$

$\Delta P/V$ = compliance; D = diameter; L = length and P = density of solution [18].

To minimize distortion, the frequency of the monitoring system should be higher than the frequency of pulse pressure. Using short noncompliant tubing minimizes the ringing which tends to overestimate systolic pressures. Air bubbles

Table 1. Physiological variables derived from invasive monitoring

Unitary measures

Arterial pressure
Mean arterial pressure (MAP)
  Organ perfusion inflow pressure
Arterial pulse pressure and its variation during ventilation
  Left ventricular stroke volume changes and pulsus paradoxes
Arterial pressure waveform
  aortic valvulopathy, input impedance and arterial resistance

Central venous pressure (CVP)
Mean central venous pressure
  Pulmonary inflow pressure
Pulmonary artery pulse pressure and its variations during ventilation
  Right ventricular stroke volume, pulmonary vascular resistance changes during ventilation, and the degree of change in intrathoracic pressure

Pulmonary artery occlusion pressure (Ppao)
Mean Ppao
  Left atrial and left ventricular intralumenal pressure and by inference, left ventricular preload
Ppao waveform and its variation during occlusion and ventilation
  Mitral valvulopathy, atrial or ventricular etiology of an arrhythmia, accuracy of mean Ppao to measure intralumenal LV pressure, and pulmonary capillary pressure (Ppc)

Calculated measures
Calculated measures using multiple measured variables including cardiac output by thermo-dilution (Cotd), arterial and mixed venous blood gases (ABG and VBG, respectively)

Vascular resistances
Total peripheral resistance $= MAP/COtd$
Systemic vascular resistance $= (MAP - CVP)/COtd$
Pulmonary artery resistance $= (\text{mean } Ppa - Ppc)/COtd$
Pulmonary venous resistance $= (Ppc - Ppao)/COtd$
Pulmonary vascular resistance $= (\text{mean } Ppa - Ppao)/COtd$

Ventricular pump function
Left ventricular stroke volume (SVIv) $= COtd/HR$
Left ventricular stroke work (SWIv) $= (MAP - Ppao)/SVIv$
Preload-recruitable stroke work $= SWIv/Ppao$

Oxygen transport and metabolism
Global oxygen transport or delivery (DO_2) $= CaO_2/COtd$
Global oxygen uptake (VO_2) $= (CaO_2 - CvO_2)/COtd$
Venous admixture
Ratio of dead space to total tidal volume (Vd/Vt) $= PaCO_2/(PaCO_2 - PetCO_2)$

Right ventricular function using RV ejection fraction (Efrv) catheter-derived data
Right ventricular end-diastolic volume (EDVrv) $= SV/EFrv)$
Right ventricular end-systolic volume (ESVrv) $= EDVrv - SV$

HR: heart rate; *PaCO₂:* arterial carbon dioxide tension; *PetCO₂:* end-tidal carbon dioxide tension. Other abbreviations are explained in the table

should be flushed out of the system, and a continuous dilute heparin flush should be provided to prevent clotting within the system. Utilization of these techniques proves a frequency response of greater than 20 Hz [19].

Underestimation of pressure may result from signal damping. Damping within the system may be due to a kinked line, air bubbles, or clot on the catheter tip

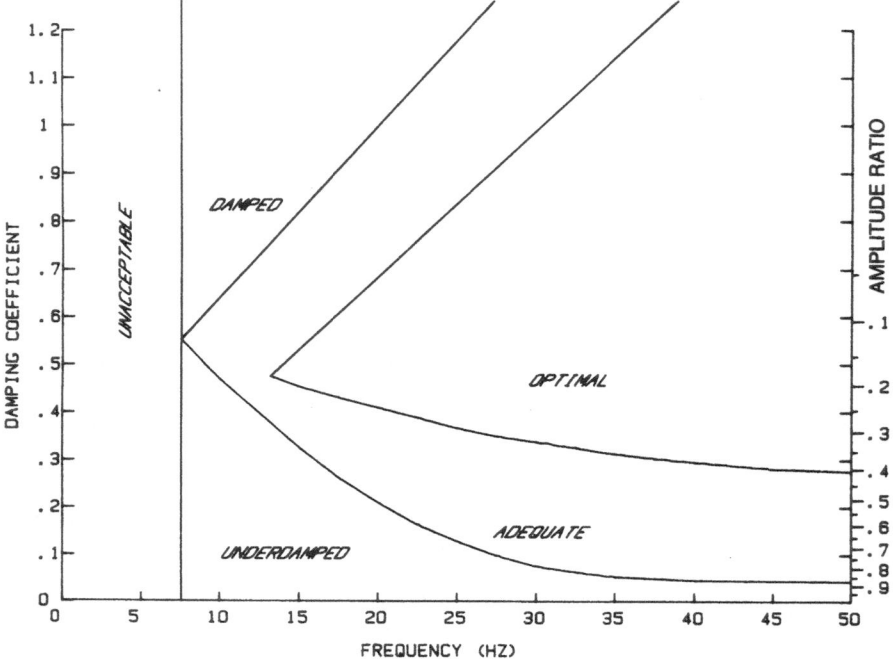

Fig. 1. The plot shows the range of damping coefficients and natural frequencies, outlining regions that indicate the type of distortion of the pressure wave

[19]. Frequency response and damping may be evaluated using the fast-flush dynamic response test [19]. The flush valve is opened and allowed to quickly closen, see Figure 2 for interpretation of fast flush testing.

A final technical consideration which may distort data is catheter whip artifact. Whip artifact is ringing of the pressure monitoring system due to movement of the catheter tip within the vasculature. Within the pulmonary artery, for example, the cardiac contraction is the driving force for this effect, and manifests itself as higher and lower pressures in phase with the cardiac cycle.

Since many of the diagnostic and therapeutic decisions made will be based on either direct or derived pressure data, it is essential that the data be accurate.

Recognition of "ringing", "signal damping", and "whip-artifact" will minimize incorrect data analysis.

Arterial Catheterization

Arterial catheterization is commonly performed in the critical care unit because the catheter it is easily inserted and provides useful data with minimal complications. Arterial catheters are generally placed for monitoring blood pressure, displaying arterial pressure wave forms, and providing easy accessibility to arterial blood for patients requiring frequent arterial blood gases or other laboratory in-

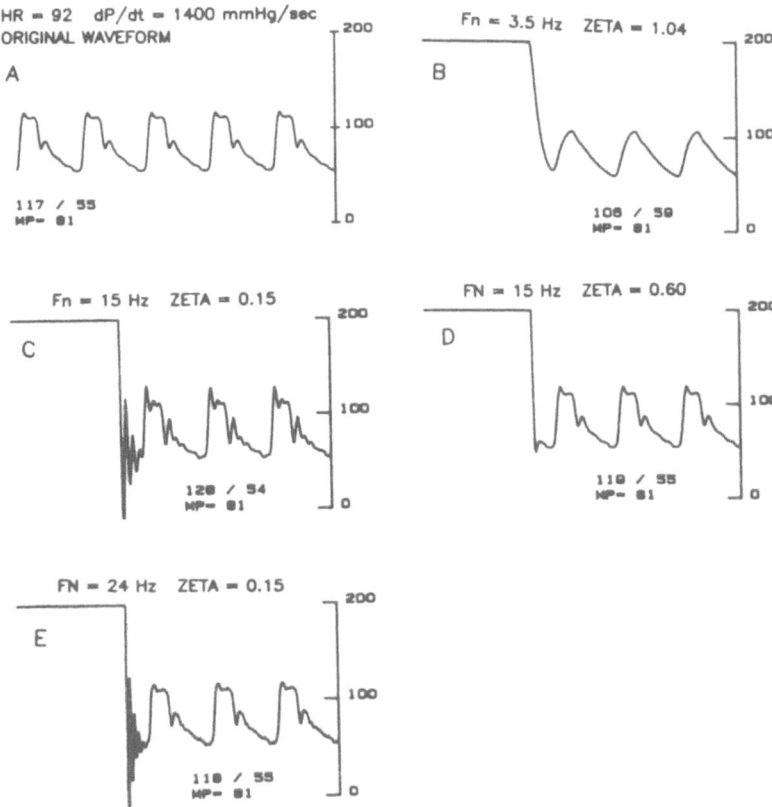

Fig. 2. Arterial pressure waveforms recorded with different pressure monitoring systems. The patient's heart rate is 92, with a maximum dP/dt of 1400 mmHg/sec. **A** The original patient waveform as it might be recorded with a catheter-tipped pressure transducer. The systolic pressure is 118 mmHg, diastolic is 55 mmHg, and mean pressure is 81 mmHg. **B** The same patient's arterial pressure waveform recorded with an overdamped plumbing system. Zeta is 1.04 and Fn is 3.5 Hz. The fast-flush signal (*upper left*) returns slowly to the patient's waveform. Systolic pressure is underestimated at 106 mmHg, diastolic pressure is overestimated at 59 mmHg, but mean pressure is unchanged at 81 mmHg. **C** Shows an underdamped condition with a low damping coefficient of 0.15 and a natural frequency of 15 Hz. After the fast-flush, the pressure waveform oscillates rapidly and returns to the original waveform shape quickly. Systolic pressure is overestimated at 128 mmHg, diastolic is almost the same as the original at 54 mmHg, and the mean pressure is unchanged at 81 mmHg. **D** Same as in C, but now a damping device has been inserted and adjusted. The waveform is optimally damped with a damping coefficient of 0.60 and a natural frequency of 15 Hz. **E** Shows an underdamped condition, but with high frequency of 24 Hz. The pressure waveform is only slightly distorted, and the pressures are close to the true pressures

formation. The catheter is inserted over a needle, although "Seldinger-type" guidewires may be used to assist threading a catheter into an artery which is either difficult to palpate or constricted. Small bore teflon catheters minimize the complication rate [20]. They are placed within the radial or femoral artery, although the brachial, axillary, or dorsalis pedis artery may be used [21–25]. Since the radial artery is superficial and has collateral circulation, thus missing the likelihood of ischemic complication, it is the most frequently cannulated. To further reduce the likelihood of ischemia, the presence of adequate collateral circulation may be assessed using the Allen test. To perform this test, the patient's wrist is grasped with both hands, occluding the radial and ulnar arteries. As the patient squeezes and relaxes, the skin distal to the occlusion, blanches. Patency of the radial artery is established by noting a return of color within 5 seconds of releasing of the ulnar artery. The patient must be awake and cooperative to achieve accurate results. Results may be difficult to interpret in patients with palor or jaundice [26].

Although the arterial catheter is small and usually inserted without difficulty, there are potential complications. A small arterial catheter relative to the vascular lumen will result in less thrombogenesis [27]. Higher incidence of vascular occlusion occurs with prolonged cannuation, small vessel size, and large catheter diameter. The incidence of clinically relevant thrombosis is less than 1% and manifests itself most commonly as necrosis of overlying skin, and not distal vascular insufficiency [28, 29]. Risk of infection has been reduced to less than 1% with the use of continuous flushing [30]. Rate of infection seems to correlate with duration of invascular catheter placement. One study found a 4% incidence of catheter related septicemia and 18% incidence of colonization patients who had catheters in place longer than 96 hours [31].

In addition to the technical considerations of setting up the arterial lines and transducers, there are important physiologic limitations to consider when analyzing and interpreting data gathered from arterial pressure monitoring. First, most monitors display systolic, diastolic and mean blood pressure. The mean arterial pressure (MAP) is the electrically averaged pressure-per-beat and is assumed to be major determinant of organ perfusion. Most systems alert the care providers to the possibility of hypoperfusion when a minimum mean pressure (often 60 mmHg) occurs. In response to loss of pressure, the carotid body baroreceptors alter vascular tone and increase pressure. While pressure is maintained, flow and ultimately oxygen delivery to individual organs may be inadequate. In addition, other determinants of perfusion such as organ perfusion pressure, intra-organ vascular resistance, and venous outflow pressure influence organ blood flow. Therefore, although the MAP remains above a arbitrary number of 60 mmHg, organs may be poorly perfused. Indirect markers of perfusion such as heart rate, respiratory rate, mental status, urine output, and capillary refill may give a better assessment of perfusion pressure than mean arterial pressure [2].

Another physiologic limitation is the occurrence of systolic pressure augmentation in lines placed in the distal arterial vasculature. As the pulse-pressure-wave form moves from the heart to the periphery the upstroke becomes steeper, and the systolic pressure becomes more peaked [17]. The more distal the pressure measurement is taken, the greater the increase in systolic pulse pressure. Systolic augmentation occurs because of reflection of the pulse-wave at the artery-arteriole junction back to the next pulse, augmenting the wave form moving from the heart [32]. As a result, peripheral pressures overestimate true central perfusion pressures. Again, other indirect markers may provide better assessment of perfusion.

Central Venous Catheters

Single or multilumen catheters may be percutaneously inserted with relative ease by a skilled clinician into the central venous system for the administration of phlebitic medications, fluid resuscitation, hyperalimentation, vasoactive drugs, and long term antibiotic regimens [2]. In addition, the central line may be used to transduce the venous pressure for diagnostic and therapeutic decisions. However, the reliability and efficacy of monitoring these pressures is poorly established [53]. Although a low central venous pressure value may affirm hypovolemia in a hemodynamically unstable patient, a normal or elevated central venous pressure does not ensure adequate left ventricular (LV) end-diastolic volume (EDV). In patients with normal cardio-pulmonary physiology, a central venous pressure may reflect LV EDP, and usually registers 2 mmHg less than the pulmonary artery occlusion pressure. However, hemodynamically unstable patients requiring intravascular monitoring rarely have normal cardiopulmonary physiology. Many will have cardiac abnormalities or pulmonary pathology that results in elevated central venous pressure despite a normal or low LV EDP [34]. Patients with right ventricular dysfunction, pulmonary artery hypertension, tension pneumothorax, cardiac tamponade, pulmonary embolism, chronic obstructive pulmonary disease with cor-pulmonale or hyperinflation secondary to inadequate exhalation time, may all have a normal or elevated central venous pressure with inadequate left ventricular end diastolic filling pressure and volume. Not only does the CVP correlate poorly with LV EDV, in one study of patients with normal cardiovascular physiology there was even poor correlation between CVP and right ventricular end diastolic volume [35]. Given the physiologic limitations of the central pressure monitoring, it is often difficult to assess left ventricular filling.

In experienced hands, the complication rate for central venous cannulation is very low. Carotid or subclavian artery puncture occurs approximately 2% of the time. Unrecognized carotid artery puncture may lead to hematoma formation with airway compromise. Patients with coagulopathy are more likely to develop hematomas, which are treated with compression and rarely require surgical evaluation or repair. Since the subclavian artery is not compressable, this approach should be used with caution in severly coagulopathic patients. Pneumothorax may occur in 0.2 to 0.3% of internal jugular vein cannulation attempts, and 3% of those with subclavian attempts. In either approach, the individual inserting the catheter must be aware of other potential complications including air embolism, ventricular dysrrhymias, and thoracic duct laceration.

Pulmonary Artery Catheter

In 1970 Swan and Ganz "rediscovered" the inflatable balloon-tip pulmonary artery catheter designed in 1953 by Lategola & Raher [36]. Initially the catheter was used to diagnose and treat myocardial infarctions [36]. However, in the last two decades, over 2 million PA catheters have been inserted. The catheter has been used to evaluate intracardiac pressures, to measure cardiac output, to sample venous oxygen saturation and to derive a number of hemodynamic variables from measured data which may aid in the diagnosis, treatment, and evaluation of interventions in hemodynamically unstable patients [36–40]. Despite the dramatic escalation in their use, there are no proven indications for pulmonary artery catheters and some clinicians have argued that the catheters should not be used at all because of the increased morbidity and potentially worsened outcome [3]. Although there are no proven indications for pulmonary artery catheter, there are several probably appropriate indications which are responsible for their widespread use [9, 10, 12, 13, 15] (Table 2). The data to support these indications, however, remain controversial. Equally concerning is that many physicians using these catheters do not use all the information, or lack the knowledge to interpret the information and apply it to problem-solving [4, 5]. It is clear that the data gathered must be interpreted with a thorough understanding of the limitations of each measurement including the intracardiac pressures, the occlusion pressure, the cardiac output, and the mixed venous oxygen saturation.

Intracardiac Pressures

The pulmonary artery catheter allows the clinician to continuously monitor central venous and pulmonary artery pressure, and to intermittently evaluate the pulmonary artery occlusion pressure (Ppao) [9, 36, 41]. The Ppao pressure is ob-

Table 2. Probable indications for pulmonary arterial catheterization

Data necessary for diagnosis
1. Distinguishing primary (non-cardiogenic) from secondary (cardiogenic) pulmonary edema
2. Diagnosis of acute ventricular septal defect
3. Diagnosis of acute cardiac tamponade

Data necessary for management
1. Vasoactive drug therapy for cardiogenic shock with or without acute mitral regurgitation
2. Cardiac dysfunction with ischemia requiring intra-aortic balloon counter-pulsation
3. Balancing fluid and vasoactive therapy in acute lung injury states (ARDS)
4. Assessing pulmonary pathology and response to ventilator therapy in acute lung injury states
5. To assess global cardiac output and systemic oxygen delivery
6. To direct vasodilator therapy in the management of pulmonary hypertension associated with acute cor pulmonale
7. To continuously monitor mixed venous oxygen saturation as an estimate of the adequacy of oxygen delivery to oxygen requirements in hemodynamically unstable patients

RIGHT HEART PRESSURES

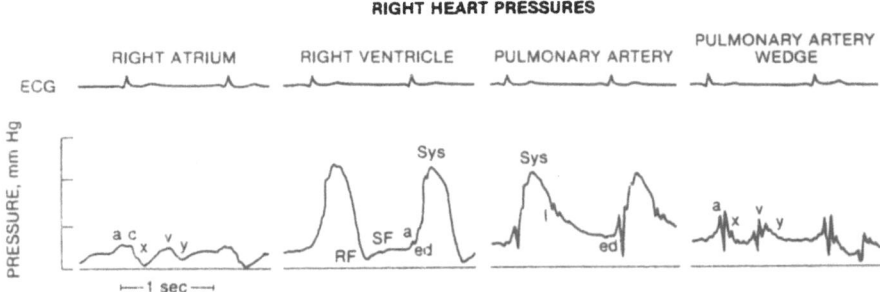

Fig. 3. Intracardiac pressure waveforms recorded with a fluid-filled catheter. *Sys* = peak systolic pressure; *ed* = end-diastolic pressure; *RF* = rapid filling wave; *SF* = slow filling wave; *a* = atrial systolic wave; *I* = incisura. Also shown are a, c, and v waves and the x and y descents

tained by inflating the balloon at the distal end of the catheter. Pulmonary artery flow directs the balloon into the distal vasculature, occluding the artery. The obstruction creates an equilibration of pressure between the balloon and the downstream vasculature near the left atrium (Fig. 3). In contrast to the Ppao, a true wedge pressure is obtained by advancing the catheter until it wedges in the vasculature [4]. The wedge pressure is usually several mmHg less than the occlusion pressure because collateral blood from other pulmonary arteries, and bronchial vessels are not sensed. In practice, the occlusion pressure is obtained and usually referred to as the "wedge pressure." A true "occluded" pressure occurs when the Ppao is less than the pulmonary arterial diastolic pressure (diastolic Ppa), left atrial pressure wave is present, and oxygenation saturation of sampled blood is arterial. To measure left atrial pressure accurately the pulmonary artery catheter must be positioned in zone III of the pulmonary vasculature otherwise alveolar pressure may be transmitted. If alveolar pressure is sensed, the Ppao will increase more than the PA diastolic pressure during a respiratory effort. If the Ppao increases the same or less than the diastolic Ppa, then pressure from the left atrium is being monitored [42]. In addition to accurate placement, the measurements must be taken at end-expiration so the effect of pleural pressure is not recorded [34]. Obviously, end-expiration will appear as different pressures depending on whether the patient is breathing spontaneously or with positive pressure ventilation. It is equally important, even if the catheter is correctly positioned and measured at end-exhalation to rule out other reasons for respiratory artifact. Patients who have an alveolar pressure greater than atmospheric at end exhalation may have a falsely elevated occlusion pressure [43]. Clinically, such positive alveolar pressures may be seen in two situations. First, patients with refractory hypoxemia treated with positive end-expiratory pressure (PEEP) may transmit a portion of that pressure to the occluded pressure. Second, patients with increased lung compliance and increased airway resistance, or patients with increased minute ventilation of any cause may have inadequate exhalatory time. As a result, hyperinflation or Auto-PEEP with positive alveolar pressure will develop. Hemodynamic instability due to increased intrathoracic pressures and inadequate venous return may develop [43]. Unrecognized, the reduced cardiac index and elevated occlusion pressure may be diagnosed as cardiogenic shock [43]. Anticipating patients with respiratory distress who may develop hyperinflation is the initial step in managing these patients. If Auto-PEEP is present, a brief trial of disconnection from the ventilator will demonstrate a fall in Ppao pressure and a return to normal cardiac index [43]. Likewise, Pinsky et al. described abruptly disconnecting patients from PEEP and measuring the lowest level the occlusion pressure reached within 1–3 seconds. They have termed this the "nadir wedge" and have demonstrated the maneuver can be done safely without respiratory compromise [44].

Other pressures which increase the pleural pressures can also be transmitted to the occlusion pressure. Two common clinical scenarios responsible for elevated pleural pressure are tense intraabdominal ascites and cardiac tamponade. In each instance systolic function is preserved, however, cardiac index is reduced due to inadequate filling. Although a high index of suspicion may suggest the diagnosis, evaluation of systolic function using transthoracic or transesophageal echocardiography may be required to differential [45].

In addition to the possibility that the occlusion pressure may reflect aveolar pressure as a result of placement in Zone I or II, secondary to PEEP or AutoPEEP, or the increased pleural pressure due to ascites or pericardial pressure, there is another physiologic liability that must be considered when interpreting the Ppao. The occlusion pressure is a pressure. It is not a direct measure of LV EDV, nor are pressure and volume linearly related on the diastolic filling curve. In fact, LV volume increases during diastole with little increase in pressure until the unstressed volume of the ventricle is reached. Accordingly, large changes in volume can occur with little change in pressure. At end-diastole, the pressure usually associated with an adequate filling volume is usually 8–10 mmHg, assuming normal LV diastolic compliance. In the event of reduced ventricular compliance a given volume produces a higher pressure [45, 46]. Depending on the degree of reduced compliance, a occlusion pressure of 10 mmHg may reflect only partial LV filling [45, 46]. A number of clinical scenarios may reduce LV compliance (Table 3) [46]. Since preload is a determinant of LV contractility, a Ppao of 10 mmHg in the noncompliant LV represents inadequate filling rather than decreased, the clinician may interpret a reduced cardiac index to be the result of reduced contractility. As with the previously mentioned scenarios, a high index of suspicion, a fluid challenge, and an evaluation of systolic function with an echocardiogram may be required [47].

Cardiac Output

A thermistor in the distal pulmonary artery catheter allows intermittent measurement of cardiac output [37]. A known volume of injectate at a given temperature is given through the proximal port. The change in blood temperature is

Table 3. Diagnoses associated with heart failure and normal systolic performance

Diagnosis

Disease states associated with normal systolic function and impaired ventricular diastolic performance
- Coronary artery disease
- Systemic hypertension
- Aortic stenosis
- Hypertrophic cardiomyopathy
- Infiltrative cardiomyopathies (amyloid, hemochromatosis)
- Idiotropathic restrictive cardiomyopathy

measured by the thermistor. Cardiac output is calculated by evaluating the area under the curve, which represents a change in blood temperature as a function of time [48, 49]. Good correlation has been reported between the thermodilution technique, dye dilution, Fick methodology, and electromagnetic flow meters [48, 49]. Accuracy in measurement depends on consistency of volume, a temperature of injectate, and correct computation constant. Usually cardiac output is averaged following multiple determinations, performed at random throughout the respiratory cycle [50, 51]. Using random bolus injections results in a 15–20% variation between the cardiac output obtained [49]. The variation is due to the fact that pulmonary artery, rather than aortic blood flow is being measured. Since pulmonary flow varies within the respiratory cycle, cardiac measurements may vary. Although, obtaining a measurement at a specific time in the respiratory cycle can decrease the measured variability to 5%, the technique is difficult, requiring a fixed ventilatory rate, a stable cardiovascular state, and a computerized injector timed to airway pressure [50].

In addition to the above technical limitations of obtaining a cardiac measurement, it is important to recall that cardiac output, and derived variables such as strokes work are dependent on adequate LV EDV. In the setting of hemodynamic instability, with depressed cardiac output, and stroke work, it is essential to first rule out inadequate filling volume [8]. As per the previous discussion on physiologic limitations of the pulmonary artery occlusion, this is not always obvious. The clinician must be aware of clinical settings that may give falsely high pressures when volume is adequate and consider echocardiography to evaluate systolic function and diastolic volume [47].

Mixed Venous Oximetry

The mixed venous oxygen saturation (SvO_2) can be measured either by sampling small aliquots of blood from the distal port, or if the catheter is equipped with fiberoptics, through continuous measurement using spectrophotometry [52, 53]. Spectrophotometry uses indwelling fiberoptic reflectance technology to continuously monitor dynamic changes and physiologic response to therapy. In comparison, intermittent SvO_2 measurement provides "snapshot" information of O_2 delivery and consumption at a given time.

The technology for continuous measurement of SvO_2 is based on reflection spectrophotometry. Light of specific wavelength is transmitted through one fiberoptic filament, is reflected in the blood stream, and transmitted back up another filament to a photodetector cell. Since hemoglobin and oxyhemoglobin absorb light differently, the reflected light is analyzed for percent saturation.

Several technical limitations of continuous monitoring should be noted. The system must be calibrated against the measure mixed venous O_2 saturation and repeated every six hours since base-line saturation drift can occur [54]. The system must be calibrated against the patient's hematocrit since different hematocrits have different calibration curves. The light intensity is displayed on the screen. Overwedging or abutment of the catheter against a vessel wall may increase the light intensity, while a kink in the catheter or a clot in the distal port may reduce light intensity. Either abnormality will result in inaccurate measurements.

In addition to technical considerations there are syndromes in which O_2 utilization rather than O_2 delivery is the problem. In these instances, tissue ischemia may be present in the presence of normal mixed venous oxygen levels, and the resulting normal SvO_2 may be misinterpreted.

The metabolic determinants of oxygen supply and dependency are complicated, and interpretation of SvO_2 requires an understanding of the complex physiology. The body maintains constant O_2 consumption across various oxygen deliveries. To maintain adequate consumption, oxygen extraction at the cellular level increases as O_2 delivery falls and mixed venous oxygen saturation falls [55]. Accordingly, a decrease in SvO_2 reflects either a decreased O_2 delivery or an increased O_2 consumption. A drop in SvO_2 should prompt the clinician to evaluate the patient's cardiac output as well as the oxygen content. Normal oxygen delivery values indicate the drop in SvO_2 is secondary to increased metabolic demands: listlessness, agitation, seizures, moving around the bed, respiratory work, either spontaneous or against the ventilator, are all causes of increased oxygen requirements and should respond to the SvO_2. In those patients who are sedated and paralyzed the SvO_2 is a useful parameter of hemodynamic status. The oxygen supply relationship described above represents normal physiology. However, SvO_2 results must be interpretated cautiously in patients with sepsis, acute respiratory distress syndrome (ARDS), end-stage liver disease, and certain drug toxicities such as cyanide poisoning [58]. In these patients oxygen utilization by the tissues is impaired, either by peripheral shunting as in the case of end-stage liver disease or by cellular dysfunction as in sepsis and ARDS [58]. Following the SvO_2 in these situations may result in misinterpretating the adequacy of the oxygen delivery to the tissues, since the venous saturation is normal or elevated.

Finally, there is controversy concerning the concept of "pathological oxygen supply-dependence." The hypothesis is that increasing O_2 delivery will improve oxygen consumption [12]. In other words, O_2 consumption is pathologically dependent on O_2 delivery. Several investigators have suggested that attempts to increase O_2 delivery to supraphysiologic levels will improve survival [12]. Antagonists of this rational argue that the observed co-variance reflects an artifact in the method of calculating O_2 delivery and O_2 utilization. These measures share two of the three variables, cardiac output and O_2 content. Mathematical coupling, rather than pathologic supply dependency results in the co-variance [56, 59]. When O_2 consumption is measured directly at the mouth, thereby eliminating mathematical coupling, there is no co-variance [59].

Complications of PA Catheters

Complications related to pulmonary artery cannulation including arterial puncture and hematoma, pneumothorax, air embolism, and ventricular arrhytmias are similar to those listed previously for central line insertion. Serious complications unique to pulmonary artery catheters are pulmonary artery perforation and pulmonary hemorrhage. Several risk factors for ruputure include a history of pulmonary artery hypertension and advanced age. Ruputure is usually related to distal migration of the balloon, resulting in overwedging on the monitor. Catheter placement should be checked radiographically, and balloon inflations performed by individuals who recognize overwedging on the monitor and increasing resistance to balloon inflation.

Conclusion

In an era of risk-benefit-cost-benefit analysis, it is prudent to use invasive hemodynamic monitoring in situations with proven or probably appropriate indications outlined in preceding text. In these instances hemodynamic monitoring provides a tool to monitor cardiovascular physiology and to titrate care and to evaluate response to therapy. As described, each of the three invasive monitors are associated with technical and physiologic liabilities which can lead to inaccurate data, or to inaccurate interpretation of the data. For the results of the monitors to be utilized effectively, the clinician must have a solid understanding of these technical and physiologic liabilities.

References

1. Snider GL (1994) Allocation of intensive care: the physicians role. Am J Resp Crit Care Med 150:575–580
2. Bellomo R, Pinsky MR (1996) Invasive hemodynamic monitoring. In: Tinker J, Browne D, Sibbald W (eds) Critical care – standards, audit, and ethics. Arnold Publishing, pp 82–104
3. Robin ED (1985) The cult of the Swan-Ganz catheter. Overuse and abuse of pulmonary flow catheters. Ann Intern Med 103:445–449
4. Connors AF, Dawson NV, McCaffrey DR, et al (1987) Assessing hemodynamic status in critically ill patients; do physicians use clinical information optimally? J Crit Care 2:174–180
5. Iberti TJ, Fischer EP, Leibowitz AB, et al (1990) A multicenter study of physician knowledge of the pulmonary artery catheter. J Am Med Assoc 264:2928–2932
6. Sturm JT, McGee MG, Fuhrman TM, et al (1980) Treatment of postoperative low output syndrome with intraortic balloon pumping. Experience with 419 patients. Am J Cardiol 45:1033–1036
7. Lefemine AA, Kosowsky B, Madoff I, et al (1977) Results and complications of intraaortic balloon pumping in surgical and medical patients. Am J Cardiol 40:416–420
8. Wiedemann HP, Matthay MA, Matthay RA (1984) Cardiovascular-pulmonary monitoring in the intensive care unit (Part 1). Chest 85:537–549
9. Raper R, Sibbald WJ (1986) Mislead by the wedge? The Swan Ganz catheter and left ventricular preload. Chest 89:427–434
10. Fein AM, Goldberg SK, Walkenstein MD, et al (1984) Is pulmonary artery catheterization necessary for the diagnosis of pulmonary edema? Am Rev Resp Dis 129:1006–1009
11. Robin ED (Editorial) (1987) Death by pulmonary-artery flow-directed catheter. Chest 92:727–731
12. Shoemaker WC, Appel PL, Kram HB, et al (1988) Prospective trial of supranormal valves of survivors as therapeutic goals in high-risk surgical patients. Chest 94:1176–1186
13. Gore JH, Goldberg RJ, Spodick DH, et al (1987) A community-wide assessment of the use of pulmonary artery catheters in patients with acute myocardial infarction. Chest 92:721–727
14. Tuman KJ, McCarthy RJ, Spiess BD, et al (1989) Effect of pulmonary artery catherization on outcome in patient undergoing coronary artery surgery. Anesthesiology 70:199–206
15. Rao TLK, Jacobs KH, El-Etr AA (1983) Reinfarction following anesthesia in patients with myocardial infarction. Anesthesiology 59:499–505
16. Lee AP (1981) Biotechnological principles of monitoring. Int Anesthesiol Clin 19:197–208
17. Bedford RF (1990) Invasive blood pressure monitoring. In: Bleit CD (ed) Monitoring in Anesthesia and Critical Care Medicine. Churchill Livingstone, NY, pp 93–134
18. Gardner RM (1981) Direct blood pressure measurement – dynamic responds requirements. Anesthesiology 54:227–236
19. Gold JP (1993) Aspects of physiologic monitoring. In: Barie PS, Shires GT (eds) Surgical Intensive Care. Little, Brown and Co, Boston, Toronto, London, pp 47–92
20. Bedford RF (1975) Percutaneous radial artery cannulation: increased safety using teflon catheters. Anesthesiology 42:219–222
21. Davis FM, Stewart JM (1980) Radial artery cannulation: a prospective study in patients undergoing cardiothoracic surgery. Br J Anaesth 52:41–47
22. Barnes RW, Foster EJ, Janssen GA, et al (1976) Safety of brachial arterial catheters as monitors in the intensive care unit-prospective evaluation with the doppler ultrasonic velocity detector. Anesthesiology 44:260–264
23. Adler DC, Bryan-Brown CW (1973) Use of the axillary artery for intravascular monitoring. Crit Care Med 1:148–150
24. Johnstone RE, Greenhouse DE (1973) Catheterization of the dorsalis pedis artery. Anesthesiology 39:654–655
25. Ersoz CJ, Hedden M, Lain L (1970) Prolonged femoral arterial catheterization for intensive care. Anesth Analg 49:160–164
26. Greehow DE (1972) Incorrect performance of Alless's test: ulnar artery flow erroneously presumed inadequate. Anesthesiology 37:356–357

27. Bedford RF (1977) Radial arterial function following percutaneous cannulation with 18 and 20 gauge catheters. Anesthesiology 47:37–39
28. Bedford RF, Wollman H (1973) Complications of percutaneous radial artery cannulation: an objective prospective study in man. Anesthesiology 38:228–236
29. Wyatt R, Graves I, Cooper DJ (1974) Proximal skin necrosis after radial artery cannulation. Lancet 2:1135
30. Shinozaki T, Deane R, Muzazan JE, et al (1983) Bacterial contamination of arterial lines: a prospective study. J Am Med Assoc 249:223–225
31. Band JD, Maki DG (1979) Infections caused by arterial catheters used for hemodynamic monitoring. Am J Med 79:735–741
32. O'Rourke MF, Taylor MG (1966) Vascular impedance of the femoral bed. Circ Res 18:126–139
33. Shoemaker WC, Kram HB, Appel PL, Fleming AW (1990) The efficacy of central venous and pulmonary catheters and therapy based on them in reducing mortality and morbidity. Arch Surg 125:1332–1338
34. Rajacich N, Burchard KW, Hagan FM, Singh AK (1989) Central venous pressure and pulmonary capillary wedge pressure as estimate of left atrial pressure: effects of positive end-expiratory pressure and catheter tip malposition. Crit Care Med 17:7–11
35. Reuse C, Vincent JL, Pinsky MR (1990) Measurement of right ventricular volume during fluid challenge. Chest 98:1450–1454
36. Swan HJC, Ganz W, Forrester JS, et al (1970) Catheterization of the heart in man with the use of a flow-directed balloon-tipped catheter. New Engl J Med 283:447–451
37. Weisel RD, Berger RL, Hechtman HB (1975) Current concepts: measurement of cardiac output by thermodilution. N Engl J Med 292:682–684
38. Kay H, Afshari M, Barash P, et al (1983) Measurement of ejection fraction by thermal dilution technique. J Surg Res 34:337–346
39. Swan HJC, Ganz W (1974) Guidelines for use of balloon-tipped catheter (letter). Am J Cardiol 34:119–120
40. Swan HJC, Ganz W (1975) Use of balloon flotation catheters in critically ill patients. Surg Clin North Am 55:501–509
41. Bouchard RJ, Gault JH, Ross J Jr (1971) Evaluation of pulmonary arterial end diastolic pressure as an estimate of left ventricular end diastolic pressure in patients with normal and abnormal left ventricular performance. Circulation 44:1072–1079
42. Teboul JL, Besbes M, Andrivet P, et al (1992) A bedside index asessing the reliability of pulmonary artery occlusion pressure measurements during mechanical ventilation with positive end-expiratory pressure. J Crit Care 7:22–29
43. Pepe PE, Marinii JJ (1982) Occult positive end-expiratory pressure in mechanically ventilated patients with airflow obstruction. Am Rev Resp Dis 126:166–170
44. Pinsky MR, Vincent JL, DeSmet JM (1991) Estimating left ventricular filling pressure during positive end-expiratory pressure in humans. Am Rev Resp Dis 143:25–31
45. Grossman W, McLaurin LP (1976) Diastolic properties of the left ventricle. Ann Int Med 84:316–326
46. Bonow RO, Udelson JE (1992) Left ventricular diastolic dysfunction as a cause of congestive heart failure: mechanisms and management. Am Int Med 117:502–510
47. Spirito P, Maron BJ (1988) Doppler echocardiography for assessing left ventricular diastolic function. Ann Int Med 109:122–126
48. Levett JM, Repogle RL (1979) Thermodilution cardiac output: a critical analysis and review of the literature. J Surg Res 27:392–404
49. Stetz CW, Miller RG, Kelly GE, Raffin TA (1982) Reliability of the thermodilution method in the determination of cardiac output in clinical practice. Am Rev Resp Dis 126:1001–1004
50. Jansen JRC, Schreuder JJ, Bogaard JM, et al (1981) Thermodilution technique for measurement of cardiac output during artificial ventilation. J Appl Physiol 51:84–91
51. Snyder JV, Powner BJ (1982) Effects of mechanical ventilation on the measurement of cardiac output by thermodilution. Crit Care Med 10:677–682
52. Muir AL, Kirby BJ, King AJ, et al (1970) Mixed venous oxygen saturation in relation to cardiac output in myocardial infarction. Br Med J 4:276–278

53. Kasnitz P, Druger GL, Yorra F, et al (1976) Mixed venous oxygen tension and hyperlactatemia. J Am Med Assoc 236:570–574
54. Oximetrix, Inc: Shaw catheter oximetry system instruction manual (1981) Mountain View, California, Oximetrix
55. Gutierrez G, Lund N, Bryan-Brown CW (1989) Cellular oxygen utilization during multiple organ failure. In: Pinsky MR, Mutuschak GM (eds) Multiple Systems Organ Failure. Crit Care Clin 5:271–287
56. Annat G, Viale JP, Percival C, et al (1986) Oxygen uptake and delivery in the adult respiratory distress syndrome. Am Rev Resp Dis 133:999–1004
57. Pepe PE, Culver BH (1985) Independently measured oxygen consumption during reduction of oxygen delivery by positive end-expriatory pressure. Am Rev Resp Dis 132:788–793
58. Danek SJ, Lynch JP, Weg JE, et al (1980) The dependence of oxygen uptake on oxygen delivery in the adult respiratory distress syndrome. Am Rev Resp Dis 122:387–395
59. Russell JA, Ronco JJ, Lockhart D, et al (1990) Oxygen delivery and consumption and ventricular preload are greater in survivors then in nonsurvivors of the adult respiratory distress syndrome. Am Rev Resp Dis 141:659–665

Analog Values from Invasive Hemodynamic Monitoring

A. Perel

The Value of Viewing the Analog Signals of Hemodynamic Parameters

The everyday practice of present day intensivists includes the monitoring and interpretation of an ever growing number of hemodynamic, as well as other, variables. A daily ICU flow sheet includes hundreds of numbers from various measuring devices. These numbers are used in the continuous decision making process that characterizes ICU clinical work. With the introduction of computerized patient data management systems, these numbers, being acquired and recorded automatically, achieve an even greater importance than before. We have all been trained to acquire, interpret and rely on these numbers. We should, however, be asking ourselves whether these numbers are accurate, what do they really mean, and is there additional information in our monitoring devices that we are prone to miss because it is not readily available in digital format?

Nearly all continuously measured parameters are displayed on our monitors as analog signals. These include one or more ECG leads (where the value of the analog signal is well appreciated), various pressures, concentrations of various gases (mainly CO_2), and more. The recognition and observation of these analog signals can be extremely informative as to the cardiac, and sometimes the respiratory, function of our patients. The analog signal may validate, explain, refute or add to the digital readout of the monitor in the same way that watching a person walk may complement information regarding his speed, number of steps, etc.

One of the main tasks in the care of critically ill patients and patients undergoing anesthesia and surgery, is the accurate estimation of effective intravascular volume and cardiac function. The assessment of preload is currently done mainly by measuring the central (CVP) and pulmonary capillary wedge (PCWP) pressures. The limitations of using these pressures as indicators of left ventricular (LV) end-diastolic volume, which is a true measure of preload, are well documented. It is mainly the clinically elusive and variable compliance of the heart chambers that prevents the assessment of end-diastolic volume from pressure measurement, to be consistently useful. The pulmonary artery catheter also enables the measurement of the cardiac output itself by the thermodilution method. However, when the cardiac output is low, its absolute value is uninformative as to the nature of the low flow state, e.g., hypovolemia versus heart failure. The accuracy and meaning of these frequently monitored physiological variables is beyond the scope of this chapter. What this chapter is going to concentrate on is the additional information that can be learned from the analog signals of some of the physiological parameters that are displayed on the screens of our monitors, with special attention to the information that can be derived from the respiratory variations in the analog signal of the arterial pressure.

Central Venous Pressure (CVP)

The CVP is a measure of right atrial pressure and therefore its analog signal reflects the phasic events that occur in the right atrium during the cardiac and respiratory cycles. For a detailed comprehensive review of the clinical value of monitoring the CVP waveform, the reader is referred to an excellent recent review by Mark [1]. The atrial contraction produces the a wave, which is later followed by the c wave that is caused by the upward motion of the tricuspid valve during isovolumic ventricular contraction. The c wave is followed by the x descent during atrial relaxation, which in turn is followed by the v wave, denoting systolic filling of the atrium. The ensuing y descent occurs after the opening of the tricuspid valve and the filling of the ventricle. In order to clearly view these fluctuations in the CVP waveform one has to switch the monitor's sweep speed to 50 mm/sec and use the 'freeze screen' option, which diminish the practicality of these observations.

More easily observed are the characteristic elevations of the CVP waveform during asynchronous atrial contraction and during tricuspid insufficiency. In the former situation, such as during nodal rhythm, the atrium contracts against a closed tricuspid valve, causing a typical "cannon" wave. In hypovolemic, mechanically ventilated patients who have such arrhythmia, the inspiratory decrease in venous return and atrial filling causes a typical decrease in the cannon wave, giving the CVP waveform a diamond shape appearance (Fig. 1). During tricuspid insufficiency, right ventricular contraction forces blood into the right atrium, creating a tall c-v wave which causes the displayed mean CVP value to overestimate right ventricular end-diastolic pressure.

The effect of changes in the intrathoracic pressure on the CVP waveform are of great interest to the clinician. Any change in the extravascular (pleural) intrathoracic pressure, such as during spontaneous or mechanical ventilation, will be transmitted to the great vessels within the chest. At the same time, however, the filling of these vessels and chambers will be changing as well, the result being that the interpretation of the analog signals of intrathoracic pressures is not always simple. For example, the typical increase in the CVP during a mechanical breath, may be associated with unchanging, or more often, decreasing pressure in the right atrium. In order to measure the true intravascular CVP, the pleural pressure has to subtracted from the measured CVP (e.g. by using a differential transducer), the result being a waveform of the transmural (filling) CVP. The estimation of the true filling pressure may pose a problem during the administration of considerable levels of PEEP, since the exact portion of the PEEP that is transmitted to the intrathoracic vessels and causes a falsely elevated CVP is not easy to assess, being dependent on the level of PEEP, as well as on the chest and lung compliances.

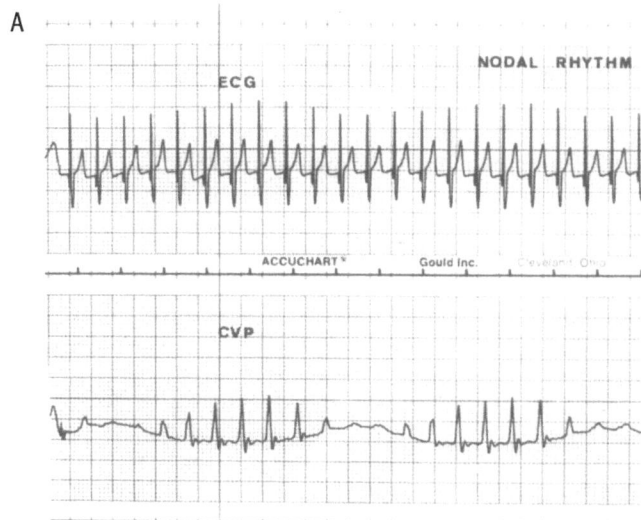

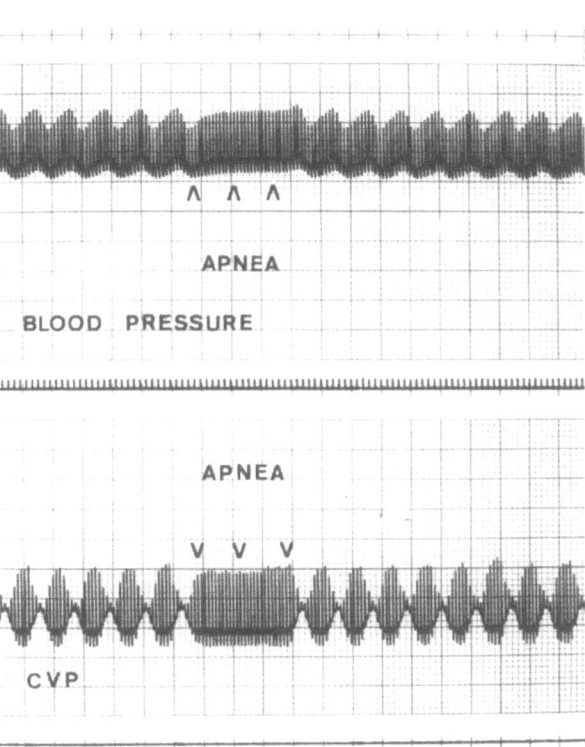

Fig. 1. A The CVP waveform (*lower panel*) during nodal rhythm in a mechanically ventilated hypovolemic patient. The CVP increases considerably with every atrial contraction (against the closed tricuspid valve), and decreases with every mechanical inspiration due to the emptying of the right atrium. **B** Lower speed recording producing the typical diamond shape appearance. Note significant decrease in the arterial pressure with every mechanical breath (dDown) denoting hypovolemia (see later in text)

The respiratory changes in the analog signal of the CVP are nevertheless a great source of information. For example, the degree by which the CVP rises during the mechanical breath is a close approximation of the inspiratory increase in pleural pressure. Thus, dividing the delivered tidal volume by that delta pressure will result in the approximate value of the chest wall compliance. Hence, exaggerated elevations of the CVP during mechanical ventilation should raise the suspicion that chest wall compliance is abnormally decreased (Fig. 2). During cardiac temponade there is elevation and equalization of the diastolic pressures of the right and left heart chambers, with a prominent x descent with an attenuated y descent (because the increased intrapericardial pressure prevents the fall in the right atrial pressure). Constrictive pericarditis is characterized by prominent x and y descents, creating an M shape trace. The trace of both right and left atrial pressures may acquire a square root shape ($\sqrt{}$) due to the rapid increase in the ventricular pressure during diastolic filling, in the presence of reduced ventricular compliance.

The degree of the inspiratory fall in the CVP with every spontaneous breath has been found to correlate with the response of the cardiac output to volume loading [2]. In patients in whom the CVP decreased by more than 1 mmHg with each inspiration, there was a positive increase in the cardiac output in response to

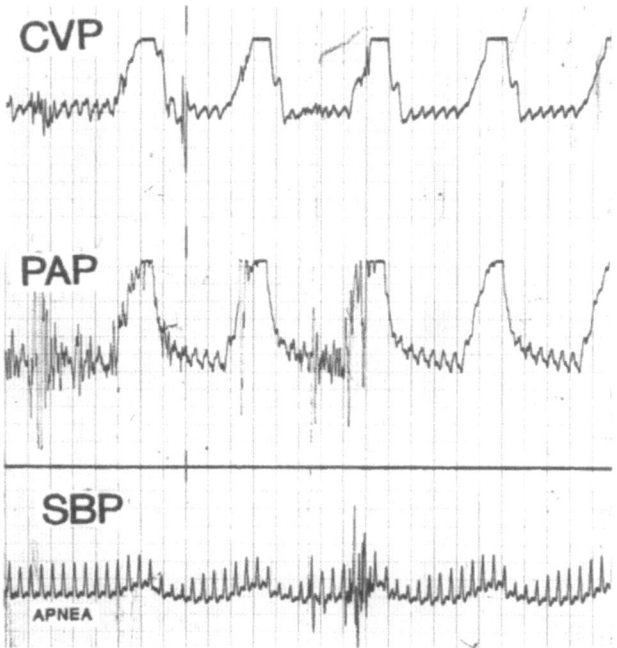

Fig. 2. The significant increases in the central venous pressure (CVP) and pulmonary artery pressure (PAP) with each mechanical breath are due to a greatly reduced chest wall compliance in a patient resuscitated following ruptured aortic aneurysm. Note also significant decreases in arterial pressure (see later discussion on SPV and dDown)

volume, while patients in whom the CVP decreased by less than 1 mmHg the cardiac output remained unchanged, denoting a flat left ventricular (Starling) function curve. This finding is based on the hypothesis that the inspiratory fall in the CVP means that the right heart is compliant and that it must be on the ascending limb of the cardiac function curve [2]. The main problem with the clinical usefulness of this observation is the variability of the inspiratory effort itself, and its total absence during controlled mechanical ventilation. During airway obstruction, for example, exaggerated negative pleural pressure swings may, in turn, cause considerable swings in the CVP waveform, which, together with other characteristic clinical signs, should call attention to the presence of this potentially dangerous disorder.

Pulmonary Artery Wedge Pressure (PCWP)

The analog signal of the PCWP is especially important since it serves for the identification of an accurate "wedging" position. Thus, under- or overinflation of the balloon, clotting of the lumen, or malpositioning, will be easily recognized by looking at the analog signal. In general, the PCWP waveform is similar to that of the CVP, and the main considerations in analyzing the CVP trace also apply to the analysis of the PCWP waveform. Thus, mitral insufficiency and asynchronous left atrial contraction associated with arrhythmias such as nodal rhythm, will produce abnormal elevations in the PCWP waveform during systole. The v wave may be augmented not only due to regurgitant flow, but may also increase as a result of reduced ventricular compliance. Significant elevations in the PCWP tracing may occur before the onset of ECG changes, indicating the development of myocardial ischemia [3]. These changes are due to endocardial ischemia with reduced left ventricular compliance. Later studies have not found the elevation of the PCWP to be a consistent early sign of ischemia.

The respiratory induced changes in the PCWP are also similar to those of the CVP waveform, namely, a decrease with every spontaneous breath and an increase during mechanical ventilation and PEEP. These changes in the PCWP can be quite significant, and therefore the digital pressure readout may be misleading. It is therefore important to identify the period of end expiration and to read the PCWP directly from the screen at that point. During partial ventilatory support, i.e., the presence of both spontaneous and mechanical breaths, the simultaneous observation of the airway pressure and the PCWP traces may be helpful in the determining the exact point of end-expiration. Modern monitors are equipped with a special cursor for facilitating the determination of the PCWP from its analog signal.

The Arterial Blood Pressure

The analog signal of the arterial pressure can be obtained directly from an arterial line, and, somewhat less accurately, with new devices that measure blood pressure continuously and non-invasively. The observation of the analog signal of the invasively measured arterial pressure is mandatory before any digital values are being considered. Such initial observation is necessary to determine whether the pressure waveform is damped (air, clot, kink) or under damped (caused by the physical properties of the measuring system and identified by a sharp pointed peak preceding the dicrotic notch). Thus, no therapeutic decision, based on the digital value of an invasively measured arterial pressure, should be taken before a good quality pressure waveform is observed.

The size and contour of the arterial waveform depend on many factors such as the stroke volume itself, the reflective waves produced by the periphery, vascular resistance and site of measurement. It is therefore very difficult to obtain meaningful clinical information from just observing the shape of the arterial pressure curve. Various attempts have been made to obtain the value of the cardiac output from the pulse contour of the arterial pressure, and some current monitors can indeed perform this task. However, at the present time, a thermodilution reference value of cardiac output is needed to calibrate the system because the individual shape of the arterial pulse is so variable. In addition, it was found that the ratio of the final amplitude to the initial amplitude of the pulse waveform during the stress phase of a Valsalva maneuver accurately predicted the PCWP, and the changes in the PCWP in response to medical therapy [4].

The Systolic Pressure Variation (SPV), dDown and dUp

Recent experimental and clinical studies have introduced a new method for assessing preload, based on the analysis of changes in the arterial pressure waveform during mechanical ventilation [5–7]. According to this method the changes in the systolic blood pressure (SBP) during one mechanical breath cycle can be clinically measured, and can be used for cardiovascular assessment.

The main hemodynamic effect of the increase in intrathoracic pressure during a mechanical breath is a transient decrease in right ventricular filling, leading eventually to a decrease in left ventricular (LV) stroke output and a decrease in systolic arterial pressure. This decrease in systolic pressure has been termed dDown (delta down), and is measured as the difference between the systolic pressure during a short apnea and the minimal value of the systolic pressure during the mechanical respiratory cycle (Fig. 3). The dDown has been shown in a series of experiments [5–7] to be a sensitive indicator of hypovolemia, since in this hemodynamic condition, the further decrease in venous return which occurs during the mechanical breath causes significant decrease in LV stroke output and in the arterial pressure. Thus, significant cyclic decreases in the arterial pressure with each mechanical breath should raise a strong suspicion of hypovolemia. Other possible reasons for this phenomenon include large tidal volumes, decreased chest wall compliance, air trapping, and hemodynamic conditions that reduce effective preload, such as unsynchronized atrial contractions during nodal rhythm.

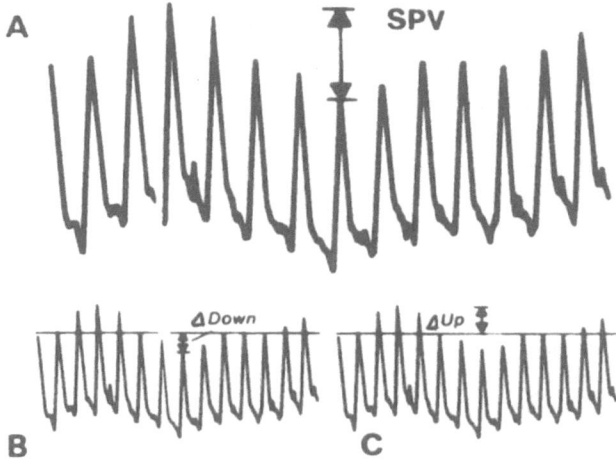

Fig. 3. The variations in the arterial pressure during one cycle of a mechanical breath. The early increase in the arterial pressure is termed the dUp (delta Up, measured as the difference between the peak systolic and the systolic pressure during a short apnea, represented as the solid horizontal line). The dDown (delta down) is the difference between the reference pressure and the minimal systolic pressure. The difference between the peak and trough systolic pressure is termed the Systolic Pressure Variation (SPV), which is the sum of the dUp and dDown

The absence of such decrease in pressure (i.e., dDown) is indicative of hypervolemia or congestive heart failure [8]. Although the venous return decreases during the mechanical breath in the presence of congestive heart failure as well, such decrease in preload does not affect LV output, since the LV functions on the flat portion of the Frank-Starling curve. Thus, lack of volume responsiveness is characterized by an absent dDown. On the other hand, hypervolemia and congestive heart failure are characterized by the prominence of the dUp (delta up), which is an increase in the systolic pressure (Fig. 3) which normally appears at the beginning of the mechanical breath and precedes the dDown [8, 9]. This early increase in systolic pressure following a mechanical breath is normally due to an increase in the pulmonary venous return as blood is squeezed from the lungs during inspiration. The magnitude of this early increase in LV preload is probably dependent on the pulmonary blood volume, being largest when the lung is in zone 3 conditions [10]. Another mechanism that is partly responsible for the augmentation of LV stroke output during early inspiration is the afterload reducing effect of the mechanical breath. Part of the airway pressure of the mechanical breath is transmitted to the LV and thoracic aorta, reducing the tension that the heart has to develop in order to eject blood (=afterload reduction) [11, 12].

Thus the arterial pressure normally responds in a bi-phasic manner to a mechanical breath. The dUp is a measure of LV stroke output augmentation, while the dDown is a measure of adequacy of fluid responsiveness. The Systolic Pressure Variation (SPV) is the total difference between the maximal and minimal systolic values during one cycle of a mechanical breath, and is the sum of the dUp and dDown. The clinical usefulness of such pressure waveform analysis has been recently demonstrated.

Coriat et al. [13] showed that in 21 patients that were recovering from vascular surgery, LV dimensions at end-diastole correlated well with the magnitude of both SPV ($r = 0.8$) and its dDown component ($r = 0.83$). Following baseline measurements, volume loading with two increments of 250 ml of 5% human albumin was performed in all but 3 patients. Each volume load caused a significant increase in the indexed end-diastolic area (EDa) and in the cardiac index (CI), and a concomitant significant decrease in the SPV (9 ± 4 to 6 ± 4 mmHg) and its dDown component (6 ± 4 to 3 ± 2 mmHg) (Fig. 4). The initial (preinfusion) dDown values showed a significant linear correlation to the increase in EDa and CI in response to the volume load. Thus the higher the initial dDown, the greater was the change in EDa and CI after volume loading. PCWP values failed to demonstrate any of the above correlations [13].

In another paper, Marik has demonstrated a remarkable correlation ($r = -0.84$) between PCWP values and the SPV in 226 ICU patients [14]. The correlation between the PCWP values predicted from the regression equation, and the actually measured PCWP values, was also highly significant. An SPV of ≤ 10 mmHg predicted a PCWP value of ≥ 12 mmHg with a predictive value of 89%. Similarly, an SPV ≥ 15 mmHg predicted a PCWP < 10 mmHg with a predictive value of 95%. The author concluded that a quite accurate estimate of PCWP, and hence of intravascular filling, can be obtained by the measurement of SPV.

THE SYSTOLIC PRESSURE VARIATION BEFORE

AND AFTER 500 ml OF 5 % ALBUMIN

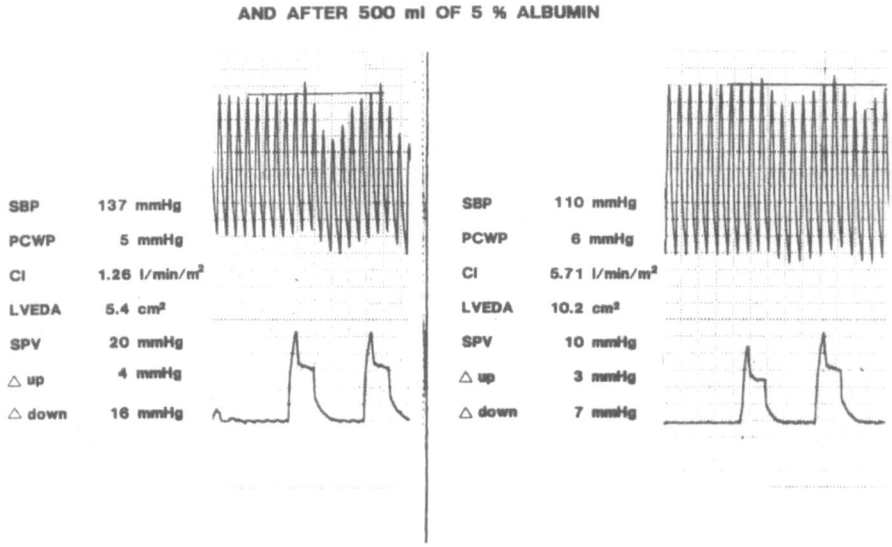

SBP	137 mmHg
PCWP	5 mmHg
CI	1.26 l/min/m²
LVEDA	5.4 cm²
SPV	20 mmHg
△ up	4 mmHg
△ down	16 mmHg

SBP	110 mmHg
PCWP	6 mmHg
CI	5.71 l/min/m²
LVEDA	10.2 cm²
SPV	10 mmHg
△ up	3 mmHg
△ down	7 mmHg

Fig. 4. The effect of volume loading on the Systolic Pressure Variation and the dDown. Note significant diminution of both values following volume loading

In a very recent paper Rooke et al. [15] have measured the SPV and dDown in anesthetized ventilated patients during blood withdrawal and subsequent volume replacement. They found that, in general, each 500 ml blood loss increased SPV by approximately 5 mmHg, the second 500 ml blood removal causing more dramatic changes than the initial blood removal. The SPV decreased by about 8.6 mmHg upon the first 500 ml volume replacement, decreasing from a mean of 19.6 mmHg after 1000 ml blood removal, to 3.8 mmHg after volume replacement. Their conclusion was that volume resuscitation appeared to be adequate when a fluid challenge reduced the SPV to 5 mmHg or less, and the dDown to 2 mmHg or less.

Technical Considerations

The SPV is simple to measure, being the difference between the maximal and minimal values of the systolic pressure during one mechanical breath, and can be measured from a strip chart recorder or from a "frozen" screen. However, relying solely on the SPV may be misleading, since it may include either a dominant dDown (this is true in the majority of cases), or a dominant dUp, the distinction between the two being very important since they represent very different volume states. For example, a septic hypervolemic patient may have a significant SPV which consists mainly of a dUp due to an inspiratory augmentation of LV stroke output. Interpreting the high SPV as a sign of hypovolemia may lead to unjustified fluid administration.

Thus measuring the dDown and dUp, in addition to the SPV, may offer additional useful information. However, some difficulties may be encountered in the determination of the reference (apnea) value of the systolic pressure, without which the dDown and dUp cannot be accurately determined. These difficulties include the fact that the short (5 seconds) apnea cannot be produced by disconnecting the ventilator due to possible changes in the end-expiratory airway pressure (and hence in venous return). In addition, the systolic pressure during the short apnea period can be used for the accurate determination of the dUp and dDown only during the first breath that follows the apnea. This is due to the low frequency changes in the arterial pressure (Meyer waves) that may change the value of the reference pressure. These technical difficulties demand a certain level of expertise in order to make optimal use of pressure waveform analysis.

The method is obviously restricted to patients who are on completely controlled mechanical ventilation with a fixed tidal volume. Large tidal volumes, decreased chest wall and increased lung compliance may exaggerate the magnitude of SPV, while very low lung compliance and increased chest wall compliance (e.g. open chest) may dampen the effect of the mechanical breath on LV output and arterial pressure.

The Respiratory Systolic Variation Test (RSVT)

We have recently developed a Respiratory Systolic Variation Test (RSVT) which may be done automatically and which may obviate the need for apnea as part of pressure waveform analysis. The test is based on the delivery of 4 successive mechanical breaths of increasing magnitude (0, 10, 20, and 30 cm H_2O). Normally, a larger tidal volume causes a greater decrease in venous return, and hence in LV stroke output and in the systolic pressure. A line of best fit is drawn between the 4 minimal systolic values (one after each breath) and the downslope calculated as the decrease in blood pressure for each increase in airway pressure (mmHg/cm H_2O) (Fig. 5). During hypovolemia, the gradual decrease in the venous return with the increasing tidal volume creates a very steep downslope. Hypervolemia and/or congestive heart failure are characterized by a very flat downslope due to the relative independence of LV output from a transient reduction in venous return. Hence the RSVT slope is similar in its qualities to the left ventricular function curve.

In a model of graded hemorrhage followed by retransfusion and further volume loading, in anesthetized ventilated dogs, we have found an RSVT slope of 0.12 ± 0.09 mmHg/cm H_2O during baseline, increasing to 0.79 ± 0.62 after 30% hemorrhage, and returning to 0.27 ± 0.37 mmHg/cm H_2O after retransfusion and volume loading [16]. In patients following vascular surgery [17] we have measured a mean baseline downslope of 0.32 ± 0.27, which decreased to 0.12 ± 0.24

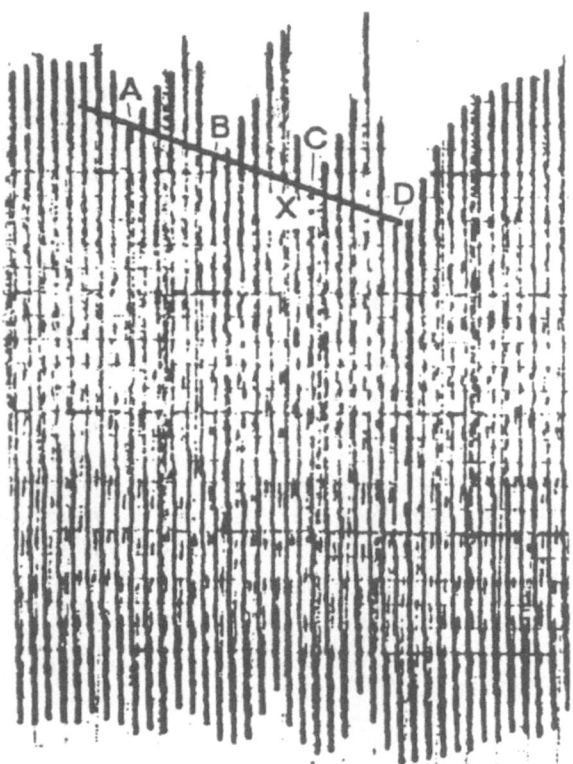

Fig. 5. The line of best fit that connects the 4 minimal systolic pressure values that are induced by the 4 incremental tidal volumes of the Respiratory Systolic Variation Test, is indicative of the responsiveness of left ventricular output to decreased venous return, and is an estimate of the left ventricular function curve

(p < 0.021) after the administration of 7 ml/kg of hetastarch. At the same time, cardiac output increased by 1.5 ± 1.1 L/min, indexed end-diastolic area increased by a mean of 3.2 cm², and PCWP increased by 4.1 ± 2.4 mmHg, all differences being significant (p < 0.01). The baseline (preinfusion) downslope of the RSVT correlated with the degree of increases in the cardiac output and the Eda. These preliminary data represent the possibility of using heart-lung interaction during mechanical ventilation as a very practical, generally available, non-invasive monitoring method. The derived data from such pressure waveform analysis are unique in that they reflect a dynamic parameter, i.e., the fluid responsiveness of the left ventricle.

The Plethysmographic Signal

The plethysmographic signal, produced by most pulse oximeters, is also a very useful analog signal in everyday clinical practice. The amplitude of the signal is a measure of peripheral vasodilatation, and its diminution is characteristic of vasoconstriction due to excess catecholamines, reduced cardiac output and hypothermia. The amplitude of the plethysmographic signal produced by pulse oximeters equipped with an automatic gain feature is of course quantitatively unreliable. Abnormally exaggerated decreases in the plethysmographic signal with each spontaneous breath is an important warning sign of airway obstruction in deeply sedated patients. In patients without arterial lines, the plethysmographic signal can be qualitatively analyzed for the presence of exaggerated SPV and dDown as early signs of hypovolemia (Fig. 6).

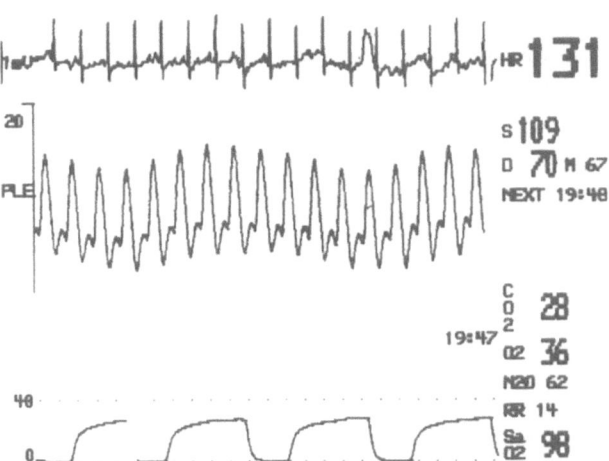

Fig. 6. Exaggerated respiratory induced variations in the plethysmographic signal (*middle panel*) in a hypovolemic patient

References

1. Mark JB (1991) Central venous pressure monitoring: Clinical insights beyond the numbers. J Cardiothorac Vasc Anesth 5:163–173
2. Magder S, Georgiadis G, Cheong T (1992) Respiratory variations in right atrial pressure predict the response to fluid challenge. J Crit Care 7:76–85
3. Kaplan JA, Wells PH (1981) Early diagnosis of myocardial ischemia using the pulmonary artery catheter. Anesth Analg 60:7–793
4. McIntyre KM, Vita JA, Lambrew CT, et al (1992) A noninvasive method of predicting pulmonary-capillary wedge pressure. N Eng J Med 327:1715–1720
5. Perel A, Pizov R, Cotev S (1987) The systolic pressure variation is a sensitive indicator of hypovolemia in ventilated dogs subjected to graded hemorrhage. Anesthesiology 67:498-502
6. Pizov R, Ya'ari Y, Perel A (1988) Systolic pressure variation is greater during hemorrhage than during sodium nitroprusside induced hypotension in ventilated dogs. Anesth Analg 67:170–174
7. Pizov R, Segal E, Kaplan L, et al (1990) The use of systolic pressure variation in hemodynamic monitoring during deliberate hypotension in spine surgery. J Clin Anesth 2:96–100
8. Pizov R, Ya'ari Y, Perel A (1989) The arterial pressure waveform during acute ventricular failure and synchronized external chest compression. Anesth Analg 68:150–156
9. Massumi RA, Mason DT, Vera Z, et al (1973) Reversed pulsus paradoxus. N Engl J Med 289:1272–1275
10. Brower R, Wise A, Hassapoyannes C, et al (1985) Effect of lung inflation on lung blood volume and pulmonary venous flow. J Appl Physics 58:954–963
11. Robotham JL, Cherry D, Mitzner W, et al (1983) A re-evaluation of the hemodynamic consequences of intermittent positive pressure ventilation. Crit Care Med 11:783–793
12. Pinsky MR, Summer WR (1983) Cardiac augmentation by phasic high intrathoracic pressure support in man. Chest 84:370–375
13. Coriat P, Vrillon M, Perel A, et al (1994) A comparison of systolic blood pressure variations and echocardiographic estimates of end-diastolic left ventricular size in patients after aortic surgery. Anesth Analg 78:46–53
14. Marik PE (1993) The systolic blood pressure variation as an indicator of pulmonary capillary wedge pressure in ventilated patients. Anaesth Intens Care 21:405–408
15. Rooke GA, Schwid HA, Shapira Y (1995) The effect of graded hemorrhage and intravascular volume replacement on systolic pressure variation in humans during mechanical and spontaneous ventilation. Anesth Analg 80:925–932
16. Perel A, Preisman S, Baer R, et al (1995) Respiratory Systolic Variation Test reflects preload during graded hemorrhage in ventilated dogs. Brit J Anaesth 74 (Suppl 1):A134
17. Perel A, Minkovich L, Abiad M, et al (1995) Respiratory Systolic Variation Test – A new method for assessing preload. Brit J Anaesth 74 (Suppl 1):A137

Non-Invasive Hemodynamic and Metabolic Monitoring

A. B. J. Groeneveld

Introduction

Monitoring of the circulation and metabolic status plays a central role in the management of critically ill patients. Mostly, monitoring is indicated in case of circulatory insufficiency, and consists of continuous or intermittent measurement of blood pressures and flows with help of arterial and central venous or pulmonary artery (PA) catheters, and of urinary flow via a bladder catheter. It has been doubted, however, whether the clinical benefits of insertion of a PA catheter, an invasive procedure not without risks, is outweighed by the detriments. This is mainly caused by the uncertainty whether hemodynamic variables are true indicators of the severity, course and outcome of the shock syndrome, whether some parameters are of greater significance than others, and whether treatment guided by presumed prognostically important variables indeed improves survival. Also, interpretation of PA catheter variables can be difficult, as, for instance, the filling pressures of the heart may hardly reflect end-diastolic volumes of the ventricles, which are more direct indicators of ventricular preload. Hence, non-invasive imaging techniques, such as nuclear angiography and echocardiography have been used to circumvent the complications of invasive procedures, and to estimate cardiac loading and contractility, in order to supplement invasive hemodynamic data in difficult to diagnose and to treat cases. Cardiac output can also be estimated by other non-invasive, mostly (semi)continuous means, some of which have been applied in the intensive care unit. Finally, non-invasive oximetry, indirect calorimetry and splanchnic tonometry may supplement clinical judgement on the basis of hemodynamic variables, by extending information on tissue oxygenation (Table 1).

Hemodynamic Monitoring

Pressure

Blood Pressure. Several manufacturers have designed and marketed automated noninvasive blood pressure measurement systems. They are usually semicontinuous and therefore cannot replace continuous measurements via arterial cannulas in the critically ill.

Table 1. Noninvasive techniques for hemodynamic monitoring of critically ill patients

	Global	Regional
Direct	Noninvasive blood pressure Echocardiography Doppler cardiac output Thoracic electrical impedance CO_2 rebreathing Pulse contour	Doppler fow velocity in renal/cerebral arteries
Indirect	Oxygen uptake Capnography	Tonometry Transcutaneous/pulse oxymetry/PCO_2 Toe-ambient temperature

Respiratory Variations in Arterial Pressure. The systolic variations in arterial blood pressure, caused by intermittent changes in venous return evoked by the ventilatory swings in intrathoracic pressure, can be used to evaluate some cardiac parameters [1]. In mechanically ventilated patients, for instance, positive pressure inflation is accompanied by a fall in arterial blood pressures, after a short lasting rise associated with a fall in left ventricular afterload. The severity of the pressure fall has been correlated with the extent of circulating volume depletion and echocardiographically determined underfilling of the heart [1, 2].

Blood Flow

1. Global
Various noninvasive methods are available for (semi)continuous cardiac output measurements [3, 4].

Doppler Flow Velocity and Echocardiography. Transthoracic or transesophageal/gastric Doppler ultrasonography/flow probes are methods to estimate cardiac output from ultrasound estimates of blood flow velocity and cross-sectional area [3–5, 7–16]. Either the aorta (root and descending), the mitral or the tricuspid orifice can be used as cross-sectional area [3, 10, 11, 14, 17]. The suprasternal route can also be used to estimate, preferably simultaneously, blood flow and cross-sectional area of the aortic root [6, 18]. There are two systems: continuous and pulsed Doppler systems [3]. The advantage of the latter is that it can be focused. It is controversial how these Doppler methods compare to the thermodilution cardiac output, particularly in artificially ventilated patients [3, 4, 6, 8–10, 14, 18, 19]. They may be less accurate and more prone to systematic and accidental errors than thoracic electric impedance, as compared to thermo-dilution cardiac output [6, 8, 18]. This variability may depend on the method used [5]. Some systems also allow fairly reliable estimations of transvalvular pressure gradients, ventricular filling and pressures in the pulmonary circulation [7, 19]. Nevertheless, many of the methods are highly dependent on an experienced physician.

Blood flow can also be estimated from changes in ventricular dimensions on twodimensional echocardiography [5, 12]. Twodimensional echocardiography can also be an essential adjunct, in selected patients, to conventional PA catheter derived variables, and may even replace PA catheterization [4, 11, 13, 15, 20, 21]. The route of choice is the transesophageal one since transthoracic imaging is often insufficient in critically ill patients with mechanical hyperinflation, surgical wounds, and others [13, 20-22]. The procedure is well tolerated and virtually without complications. It yields estimates of ventricular dimensions and contractility [12, 16]. Concerning the latter, the method is helpful in quantifying the extent and severity of myocardial infarction-induced wall motion abnormalities and in evaluating the myocardial depression of septic shock [16]. Conversely, evaluation of cardiac dimensions may be helpful, together with conventional hemodynamic variables, to differentiate between types of shock. For instance, hypovolemic shock is accompanied by small cardiac dimensions, cardiogenic shock by left ventricular wall motion abnormalities and septic shock by diffuse ventricular dilation [11, 13, 16, 21]. Echocardiography allows assessment of pericardial effusions and can be helpful to document right ventricular overload following pulmonary emboli in the right ventricular outflow tract and pulmonary arteries, thereby contributing to find the cause of obstructive shock. In fact, TEE can yield evidence for pulmonary embolism in otherwise unexplained circulatory compromise [22]. Other indications include thoracic trauma, dissecting aortic aneurysm, ventricular septal defect, endocarditis and valvular heart disease [15, 16, 23]. It can be used to evaluate to effect over various ventilatory modalities on cardiac loading and function [24]. Taken together, TEE may alter treatment in a substantial number of critically ill patients, independently of conventional hemodynamic variables [13, 15, 20]. Although transesophageal Doppler flow probes can remain in situ for some time, the methods mentioned cannot be performed for prolonged periods of time and necessitate experienced personnel.

Radionuclide Imaging. If a mobile gammacamera is available, cardiac dimensions and output can be assessed with help of ^{99m}Tc labeled red blood cells at the bedside of the critically ill patients [3, 4, 12, 25]. The first pass technique can be used for cardiac output estimations, even with help of a probe, and ECG-gated equilibrium scanning for evaluating biventricular dimensions and ejection fractions [3]. This has been done, mainly as a research tool to evaluate mechanism of disease and response to fluid loading and inotropic drugs [25]. The technique is relatively cumbersome and, obviously, cannot provide a continuous measurements.

A mobile probe system has been designed allowing for protein permeability measurements in the lungs, with help of labeled circulating protein and ^{99m}Tc labeled red blood cells, as an intravascular marker [26]. After injection, the radioactivy over the lungs (probe) and in blood (samples) can be followed in time and from these the so called pulmonary leak index can be calculated, an index that may be specific and sensitive for permeability changes in he pulmonary microvasculature. This measurement may certainly supplement hemodynamic and ventilatory variables in discriminating between hydrostatic and permeability pulmonary oedema in the course of the adult respiratory distress syndrome (ARDS) [26]. This may be important in view of different etiologic, therapeutic and prognostic implications among the types of oedema [26].

Thoracic Electrical Bioimpedance (TEI). This easy to use technique is still under active investigation [3, 12, 18, 27–31]. Various models have been used to extrapolate the measurements into various physiologic signals, since resistance and reactance, depend, among others, on hematocrit and the strength of the electric current [3, 27, 28, 32]. TEI then allows both thoracic blood and fluid volumes, cardiac output, and left ventricular ejection fraction estimations [3, 27, 32]. The TEI cardiac output may fairly correlate to cardiac output derived from thermodilution and other methods, but less in circulatory compromised and mechanically ventilated patients, so that the accuracy of the method remains somewhat controversial [18, 27–30]. The main advantage is the possibility for continuous monitoring, but the method is not widely applied yet, despite its technical simplicity. TEI can also be used to estimate body composition and volume status in critically ill, since a low body electric resistance is associated with a relative high total body water and low lean body mass, and vice versa [33]. Changes in hydration status are usually reflected by changes in impedance.

Thoracography. This method utilizes inductive plethysmography transducers placed around the chest, recording the oscillatory changes in cardiac volumes [34]. The (continuous) cardiac output derived by this method favorably compares to that derived from thermodilution and electrical impedance [34].

Pulse Contour Cardiac Output. This method utilizes the contour of the invasively or noninvasively measured arterial blood pressure to estimate cardiac output [35], after some assumptions. One of the disadvantages of the technique includes the need for calibration against a known method in each patients. The major advantage is the continuous availability of the estimate [35].

CO_2 Rebreathing Cardiac Output. A relatively unknown method to estimate cardiac output in critically ill patients is a modification of the CO_2 rebreathing technique, during which a sudden change in end-tidal PCO_2 is induced by hypoventilation of mechanically ventilated patients by means of introduction of dead space into the ventilatory circuit [12, 35, 36]. This change directly relate to the change in CO_2 elimination over the change in end-tidal PCO_2 if some constants are known [36]. The method highly correlates with thermodilution cardiac output [36].

2. Regional

Cerebral and Renal Blood Flow. The Doppler technique also allows assessment of renal blood flow velocity estimations [37]. Transcranial Doppler has been used for cerebral artery blood flow velocity assessments after head trauma, cerebral contusion, brain death, neurosurgery and subarachnoid hemorrhage, and for evaluation of effects of changes in PCO_2 and drugs on cerebral vessel tone, among others [38, 39].

Toe Temperature. The gradient between peripheral and core temperature has been viewed as an index of perfusion adequacy and has been found useful in cardiogenic shock [40]. In fact, the gradient significantly correlated with global indices of perfusion in this condition [40]. The gradient, however, only poorly correlated with global indices of perfusion, such as cardiac output and peripheral vascular resistance, during high flow (septic) shock, so that the clinical implications of the gradient remain obscure [40]. Nevertheless, the measure can be useful in monitoring blood flow of the legs, prior to and following arterial reconstructive surgery for vascular disease. There is no information regarding the prognostic and therapeutic significance.

Tissue Oxygenation

1. Global

Pulse Oxymetry. This non-invasive measure of oxygen saturation of arterial blood is performed in almost every patients on mechanical ventilation in the intensive care ward and may save arterial blood sampling and analyses [41, 42].

Oxygen Uptake. The measurement of oxygen consumption from in- and expiratory breath analysis is not routinely performed in the intensive care unit [35, 43–47]. It is a promising technique for evaluation of the effect of (therapy-induced) changes in hemodynamics on tissue oxygenation in shock, since it allows non-invasive, continuous and reliable assessment of oxygen consumption [35, 45–47]. It may therefore obviate PA catheterization and intermittent, and possibly less accurate determinations of oxygen consumption through measurements of arterio-mixed venous oxygen contents and cardiac output [43–47]. Relatively high inspiratory O_2 levels and some inhaled anesthetic gases may invalidate the measurements, however [43, 44].

2. Regional

Transcutaneous Oxygen Tension Monitoring [40]. The transcutaneous PO_2 reflects arterial PO_2 in case of adequate cardiac output and skin blood flow, but falls below this value in case of circulatory insufficiency. This has been used to monitor tissue oxygenation during circulatory failure and resuscitation. During cardiogenic shock and presumably selective cutaneous vasoconstriction transcutaneous PO_2 (thorax) correlated poorly with global indices of perfusion, however [40]. During septic shock, the variable correlated significantly to arterial pressure and left ventricular stroke work [40]. The transcutaneous PO_2 correlated well with the toe-ambient temperature gradient, particularly during hyperdynamic septic shock [40].

PCO$_2$ Measurements Related to Perfusion Adequacy

1. Global

Capnography. The end-tidal PCO$_2$ or CO$_2$ fraction, measured through capnography in exhaled breath, is a measure of arterial PCO$_2$ and dead space ventilation [48]. The latter is determined by perfusion of the lung. Hence, the end-tidal PCO$_2$ will rise and fall, respectively, during hypo- and hyperventilation, or during hyper- and hypoperfusion of the lungs, or combinations. Hypoperfusion of the lung may occur during low cardiac output (hypovolemic, hemorrhagic, traumatic shock, obstructive) shock and cardiopulmonary resuscitation [49]. Particularly in the latter, the end-tidal CO$_2$ fraction has been used as a noninvasive guide for resuscitation [49]. A low end-tidal PCO$_2$ (and increased dead space ventilation) is also a characteristic feature of regional pulmonary underperfusion in the course of pulmonary embolism. Finally, an increased dead space may occur during (mechanical ventilation for) chronic obstructive pulmonary disease and ARDS.

2. Regional

Tonometry. A recently developed method is splanchnic tonometry [50, 51]. A modified double lumen nasogastric tube, with a saline-filled balloon at its tip, is advanced into the stomach (or sigmoid colon in case of the sigmoid type tonometer). After a certain interval, to allow for equilibration of balloon saline and surrounding gastric mucosa PCO$_2$, the saline is aspirated and the PCO$_2$ is measured in a conventional blood gas machine. Together with the supplying arterial blood PCO$_2$ a PCO$_2$ gradient can be calculated that widens (elevated intramucosal PCO$_2$) in case of mucosal ischemia, independently of global tissue perfusion and oxygenation [52]. This principle is analogous to the Fick principle, where widening of the arterial-mixed venous PCO$_2$ gradient occurs during a fall in cardiac output for a given CO$_2$ production [51]. Some investigators used the blood bicarbonate content to calculate a so called intramucosal pH$_i$, but the composite nature of this variable, being influenced by both supplying blood acid-base and PCO$_2$ status and regional PCO$_2$, makes this index probably less suitable to reflect the oxygen supply demand balance of the gastrointestinal mucosa than the PCO$_2$ gradient [51, 52]. The necessity for acid secretion suppression prior to measurements remains controversial [50]. Nevertheless, the pH$_i$ has been shown to be of predictive value for outcome in critically ill patients as has been used as a guide for cardiovascular therapy to improve outcome [52].

Transcutaneous PCO$_2$ Measurements. There is a method to measure PCO$_2$ transcutaneously [28]. The PCO$_2$ may increase during shock.

Conclusion

A variety of noninvasive techniques are currently available on the intensive care unit for monitoring of hemodynamics and tissue oxygenation. Some of them are relatively simple but others require specialized equipment and personnel. The cost benefit ratio of some of these measures remains to be demonstrated, depending on the indication for which they should be used.

References

1. Perel A (1995) Cardiovascular assessment in ventilated patients by arterial pressure waveform analysis. Crit Care Intern 11/12:18–19
2. Coriat P, Vrillon M, Perel A, Baron JF, Le Bret F, Saada M, Viars P (1994) A comparison of systolic blood pressure variations and echocardiographic estimates of end-diastolic left ventricular size in patients after aortic surgery. Anesth Analg 78:46–53
3. Dobb GJ, Donovan KD (1987) Non-invasive methods of measuring cardiac output. Intens Care Med 13:304–309
4. Shephard JN, Brecker SJ, Evans TW (1994) Bedside assessment of myocardial performance in the critically ill. Intens Care Med 20:513–521
5. Goldstein M, Vincent J-L, Kahn RJ (1988) Evaluation of cardiac function by echo-Doppler studies in critically ill patients. Intens Care Med 14:406–410
6. Wong DH, Mahutte CK (1990) Two-beam pulsed Doppler cardiac measurement: reproducibility and agreement with thermodilution. Crit Care Med 18:433–437
7. Singer M, Bennett ED (1991) Noninvasive optimmization of left ventricular filling using esophageal Doppler. Crit Care Med 19:1132–1137
8. Lu C, Nicolosi GL, Burelli C, Cassin M, Zardo F, Brieda M, Cervesato E, Zanuttini D (1992) Limitations in the assessment of changes of cardiac output by Doppler echocardiography under various hemodynamic conditions. Am J Cardiol 70:1370–1374
9. Stoddard MF, Prince CR, Ammash N, Goad JL, Vogel RL (1993) Pulsed Doppler transesophageal echocardiographic determination of cardiac output in human beings: comparison with thermodilution technique. Am Heart J 126:956–962
10. Katz WE, Gasior TA, Quinlan JJ, Gorscan J (1993) Trangastric continuous-wave Doppler to determine cardiac output. Am J Cardiol 71:853–856
11. Jardin F, Valtier B, Beauchet A, Dubourg O, Bourdarias JP (1994) Invasive monitoring combined with two-dimensional echocardiographic study in septic shock. Intens Care Med 20:550–554
12. Wilson AF (1995) Noninvasive measurement of cardiac output. Cardiologia 40:551–559
13. Poelaert JI, Trouerbach J, De Buijzere M, Everaert J, Colardyn FA (1995) Evaluation of transesophageal echocardiography as a diagnostic and therapeutic aid in a critical care setting. Chest 1907:774–779
14. Feinberg MS, Hopkins WE, Davila-Roman VG, Barzilai B (1995) Multiplane transesophageal echocardiographic Doppler imaging accurately determines cardiac output measurements in critically ill patients. Chest 107:769–773
15. Alam M (1996) Transesophageal echocardiography in critical care units: Henry Ford Hospital experience and review of the literature. Progr Cardiovasc Dis 38:315–328
16. McLean AS (1996) Echocardiography in the intensive care unit. Intens Care World 13:12–17
17. Gorscan J (1995) Quantification of left ventricular function using transesophageal echocardiography. In: Vincent J-L (ed) Yearbook of Intensive Care and Emergency Medicine. Springer Verlag, Berlin Heidelberg New York, pp 575–592
18. Castor G, Klocke RK, Stoll M, Helms J, Niermark I (1994) Simultaneous measurement of cardiac output by thermodilution, thoracic electrical bioimpedance and Doppler ultrasound. Br J Anaesth 72:133–138
19. Sajkov D, Cowie RJ, Bradley JA, Mahar L, McEvoy RD (1993) Validation of new pulsed Doppler echocardiographic techniques for assessment of pulmonary hemodynamics. Chest 103:1348–1353
20. Khoury AF, Afridi I, Quinones MA, Zoghbi WA (1994) Transesophageal echocardiography in critically ill patients: feasibility, safety, and impact on management. Am Heart J 127:1363–1371

21. Kaul S, Stratienko AA, Pollock SG, Marieb MA, Keller MW, Sabia PJ (1994) Value of two-dimensional echocardiography for determining the basis of hemodynamic compromise in critically ill patients: a prospective study. J Am Soc Echocardiography 7:598–606
22. Patel JJ, Chandrasekaran K, Maniet AR, Ross JJ, Weiss RL, Guidotti JA (1994) Impact of the incidental diagnosis of clinically unsuspected central pulmonary artery thromboembolism in treatment of critically ill patients. Chest 105:986–990
23. Banning AP, Masani ND, Ikram S, Fraser AG, Hall RJC (1994) Transoesophageal echocardiography as the sole diagnostic investigation in patients with suspected thoracic aortic dissection. Br Heart J 72:461–465
24. Poelaert JI, Viser CA, Everaert JA, Koolen JJ, Colardyn FA (1993) Acute hemodynamic changes of pressure-controlled inverse ratio ventilation in the adult respiratory distress syndrome. A transesophageal echocardiographic and Doppler study. Chest 104:214–219
25. Schneider AJ, Teule GJJ, Groeneveld ABJ, Nauta JJP, Heidendal GAK, Thijs LG (1988) Biventricular performance during volume loading in patients with early septic shock, with emphasis on the right ventricle: a combined hemodynamic and radionuclide study. Am Heart J 116:103–112
26. Raijmakers PGHM, Groeneveld ABJ, Teule GJJ, Thijs LG. The diagnostic value of the ^{67}Gallium pulmonary leak index in pulmonary edema. J Nucl Med (In press)
27. White SW, Quail AW, De Leeuw PW, Traugott FM, Brown WJ, Porges WL, Cottee DB (1990) Impedance cardiography for cardiac output measurement: an evaluation of accuracy and limitations. Eur Heart J 11:79–92
28. Shoemaker WC, Wo CCJ, Bishop MH, Appel PL, Van de Water JM, Harrington GR, Wang X, Path RS (1994) Multicenter trial of a new thoracic electrical bioimpedance device for cardiac output estimation. Crit Care Med 22:1907–1912
29. Doehring L, Lum E, Dracup K, Friedman A (1995) Predictors of between-method differences in cardiac output measurement using thoracic electrical bioimpedance and thermodilution. Crit Care Med 23:1667–1673
30. Weiss S, Calloway E, Cairo J, Granger W, Winslow J (1995) Comparison of cardiac output measurements by thermodilution and thoracic electrical bioimpedance in critically ill versus non-critically ill patients. Am J Emerg Med 13:626–631
31. Jónsson F, Madsen P, Jørgensen LG, Lunding M, Secher NH (1995) Thoracic electrical impedance and fluid balance during aortic surgery. Acta Anaesthesiol Scand 39:513–517
32. Van der Meer NJM, De Vries PMJ (1995) Impedance cardiography: non-invasive monitoring of hemodynamics in the ICU. In: Vincent J-L (ed) Yearbook of Intensive Care and Emergency Medicine. Springer Verlag, Berlin Heidelberg New York, pp 615–628
33. Roos AN, Westendorp RGJ, Brand R, Souverijn JHM, Frölich M, Meinders AE (1995) Predictive value of tetrapolar body impedance measurements for hydration status in critically ill patients. Intens Care Med 21:125–131
34. Sackner MA, Hoffman RA, Krieger BP, Shaukat M, Stroh D, Sackner JD, Biziousky F, Brown J, Robinson JJ (1991) Thoracocardiography. Part 2: Noninvasive measurement of changes in stroke volume; comparisons to impedance cardiography. Chest 99:896–903
35. Stok WJ, Baisch F, Hillebracht A, Schulz H, Meyer M, Karemaker JM (1993) Noninvasive cardiac output measurement by arterial pulse analysis compared with inert gas rebreathing. J Appl Physiol 74:2687–2693
36. Bosman RJ, Stoutenbeek CP, Zandstra DF (1991) Noninvasive pulmonary blood flow measurement by means of CO_2 analysis of expiratory gases. Intens Care Med 17:98–102
37. Stevens PE, Gwyther SJ, Hanson ME, Boultbee JE, Kow WJ, Phillips ME (1990) Noninvasive monitoring of renal flow characteristics during acute renal failure in man. Intens Care Med 16:153–158
38. Petty GW, Wiebers DO, Meissner I (1990) Transcranial Doppler ultrasonography: clinical applications in cerebrovascular disease. Mayo Clin Proc 65:1350–1364
39. Berré J, De Backer D, Moraine J-J, Vincent J-L, Kahn RJ (1994) Effects of dobutamine and prostacyclin on cerebral blood flow velocity in septic patients. J Crit Care 9:1–6
40. Vincent J-L, Moraine J-J, Van der Linden P (1988) Toe temperature versus transcutaneous oxygen tension monitoring during acute circulatory failure. Intens Care Med 14:64–68
41. Schnapp LM, Cohen NH (1990) Pulse oximetry. Uses and abuses. Chest 98:1244–1250

42. Imman KJ, Sibbald WJ, Rutledge FS, Speechley M, Martin CM, Clark BJ (1993) Does implementing pulse oximetry in a critical care unit result in substantial arterial blood gas savings? Chest 104:542–546
43. Makita K, Nunn JF, Royston B (1990) Evaluation of metabolic measuring instruments for use in critically ill patients. Crit Care Med 18:638–644
44. Ronco JJ, Phang PT (1991) Validation of an indirect calorimeter to measure oxygen consumption in critically ill patients. J Crit Care 6:36–41
45. Ronco JJ, Fenwick JC, Tweeddale MG, Wiggs BR, Phang PT, Cooper DJ, Cunningham KF, Russell JA, Walley KR (1993) Identification of the critical oxygen delivery for anaerobic metabolism in critically ill septic and nonseptic humans. JAMA 270:1724–1730
46. Hanique G, Dugernier T, Laterre PF, Dougnac A, Roeseler J, Reynaert MS (1994) Significance of pathologic oxygen supply dependency in critically ill patients: comparison between measured and calculated methods. Intens Care Med 20:12–18
47. De Backer D, Moraine J-J, Berre J, Kahn RJ, Vincent J-L (1994) Effects of dobutamine on oxygen consumption in septic patients. Direct versus indirect determinations. Am J Respir Crit Care Med 150:95–100
48. Carlon GC, Ray C, Miodownik SS, Kopec I, Groeger JS (1988) Capnography in mechanically ventilated patients. Crit Care Med 16:550–556
49. Falk JL, Rackow EC, Weil MH (1988) End-tidal carbon dioxide concentration during cardiopulmonary resuscitation. N Engl J Med 318:607–611
50. Kolkman JJ, Groeneveld ABJ, Meuwissen SGM (1994) Effect of ranitidine on basal and bicarbonate-enhanced intragastric PCO_2: a tonometric study. Gut 35:737–741
51. Groeneveld ABJ, Kolkman JJ (1994) Splanchnic tonometry: a review of methodology, physiology and clinical applications. J Crit Care 9:198–210
52. Gutierrez G, Clark C, Brown SD, Price K, Ortiz L, Nelson C (1994) Effect of dobutamine on oxygen consumption and gastric mucosal pH in septic patients. Am J Respir Crit Care Med 150:324–329

Non-Invasive Estimation of the Effective Pulmonary Blood Flow and Gas Exchange from Respiratory Analysis

P. Christensen

Introduction

Monitoring of the effective pulmonary blood flow is important in the control of many intensive care therapies such as effect of drugs, optimization of PEEP level and ventilatory settings. A large number of methods have been developed for estimation of the effective pulmonary blood flow. However, only the indicator dilution combined with estimation of the pulmonary shunt have gained widespread use for clinical purposes. The drawback of the indicator dilution method is that it is an invasive method which require access to the pulmonary artery as well as a systemic artery. The increasing demands for noninvasive methods have led to the development of a number indirect methods of which the inert gas rebreathing method have gained most acceptance.

Methods Based on Oxygen and Carbon Dioxide

Breath-Holding Method

During a breath-holding period the alveolar partial pressure of carbon dioxide increases to a plateau value above the true mixed venous partial pressure of carbon dioxide. The change in P_ACO_2 during a breathholding period can be described by the following equation [1]:

$$P_ACO_2 = P_VCO_2 - SCO_2 (P_VCO_2 - P_ACO_2) \times e^{(-Kt)}$$

$$K = (SCO_2 \times Q \times (P_B - 47))/(V_1 + V_t)$$

where SCO_2 is the slope of the carbon dioxide dissociation curve, P_B the ambient pressure, V_1 the alveolar volume and V_t the lung tissue volume. Q is the effective pulmonary blood flow and P_VCO_2 is the true mixed venous partial pressure of carbon dioxide. P_VCO_2 is estimated from several breath holding maneuvers of increasing length. There exists several modifications of the breath-holding method some of which demands inspiration of carbon dioxide (to ensure that equilibrium can be reached). The breath-holding techniques are rarely used today, because of advances in sensor technology and the required maneuvers. The breath-holding techniques are considerably more sensitive to inhomogeneity in the distribution in ventilation than the rebreathing techniques.

Rebreathing Method

The derivation of the effective pulmonary blood flow from a recording of the partial pressure of carbon dioxide is in principle identical to the breath-holding algorithms [2]. The rebreathing maneuver is simple to learn and well suited for exercise studies. Furthermore, the rebreathing method is less sensitive to breath-by-breath variations in the emptying pattern of the lungs compared to the single-breath and breathholding methods. The algorithm for estimation of the effective pulmonary blood flow is based on the indirect Fick principle:

$$Q = (VCO_2)/(C_vCO_2 - C_aCO_2)$$

where Q is the effective pulmonary blood flow, VCO_2 the excretion rate of carbon dioxide. C_vCO_2 and C_aCO_2 are the content of carbon dioxide in the mixed venous blood and the arterial blood, respectively. Most modifications of the carbon dioxide rebreathing method use a mixture of carbon dioxide, oxygen and nitrogen. The carbon dioxide ensures the carbon dioxide equilibrium value is reached within the rebreathing period. From the recording of carbon dioxide during the rebreathing maneuver P_vCO_2 is estimated using algorithms similar the equation described above (see Breath-holding method). P_aCO_2 is estimated as the average of a number of end-tidal PCO_2 values recorded before the rebreathing maneuver. C_aCO_2 and C_vCO_2 are calculated from approximation of the carbon dioxide dissociation curves for arterial and venous blood, respectively. VCO_2 is often estimated from the mixed expired carbon dioxide concentration and a recording of the minute-volume. Thus, the simple rebreathing methods demand seperate maneuvers for calculation of P_vCO_2, P_aCO_2 and VCO_2. This has restricted the use of this method.

One Step Rebreathing Method

In 1976 Farhi et al. [3] reported at new rebreathing method that enabled determination of all variables needed to obtain cardiac output from a single rebreathing maneuver. This method takes into account that during a rebreathing maneuver readjustment of the lung tissue carbon dioxide content takes place. This problem is circumvented by hyperventilation during the rebreathing period. Thereby, causing an initial drop in PCO_2 and later during the rebreathing period reaching the initial PCO_2 level again, at this time T, the lung tissue content of carbon dioxide is identical to that at time 0. The algorithm corrects for errors caused by changes in the rebreathing bag volume at time 0 and T.

$$Q = V_{rb}(0) \times (P' - P_{rb}(0)/P_B - 47 - P_{eq}) \times (C_{eq} - C_c)) \times 1/T$$

where Q is the effective pulmonary blood flow, $V_{rb}(0)$ the initial rebreathing bag volume, p' the partial pressure that would result if the excess lung volume could be added to and mixed with the gas in the rebreathing bag, $P_{rb}(0)$ the partial pressure of carbon dioxide in the rebreathing bag at time 0. P_B is the barometric pressure, P_{eq} is the equilibrium partial pressure of carbon dioxide. C_{eq} and C_c are the content of carbon dioxide in the mixed venous blood and in the pulmonary capillary blood.

Farhi et al. (1976) showed that there is a systematic difference between the one step CO_2 rebreathing method and the acetylene method for estimation of cardiac output during both rest and exercise. This have been evaluated by Ohlson et al. [4] who found an acceptable correlation between the one step CO_2 rebreathing method and the direct Fick method.

The Partial CO_2 Rebreathing Method

In 1988 Capek and Roy [5] published a new CO_2 method based on partial rebreathing through an additional deadspace during a 30 sec period. The technique utilizes a differential form of the Fick equation thereby avoiding the need to estimate the absolute value of the mixed venous partial pressure of carbon dioxide. The average end-tidal carbon dioxide partial pressure and carbon dioxide excretion are estimated. Next an instrumental dead space is added for a short period of time assuming that no recirculation of blood takes place. From recordings of volume displacements and PCO_2 the new "steady-state" carbon dioxide excretion and end-tidal partial pressure of carbon dioxide can be calculated. The recorded end-tidal carbon dioxide values are corrected for the alveolar dead space. The carbon dioxide partial pressures are used to estimate the content of carbon dioxide. The slope of the carbon dioxide binding curve is corrected for influence of hemoglobin and the partial pressure of carbon dioxide. From the above data the effective pulmonary blood flow can be estimated:

$$Q = -(VCO_2(2) - VCO_2(1))/(C_{a2} - C_{a1})$$

where $VCO_2(1)$ and (2) are the carbon dioxide excretion before and at the end of the partial rebreathing period. C_{a1} and C_{a2} is the capillary blood content of carbon dioxide before and at the end of the partial rebreathing period. The method was compared to the thermal-dilution method in animal experiments. The results of the comparison showed that in 87% of the experiments the pulmonary capillary blood flow estimated by the partial rebreathing method was within 20% of the thermal-dilution values. Furthermore, the authors showed that the new method seems to be less sensitive to inhomogeneity in the distribution of ventilation/perfusion ratios. However, it should be noted that the method was evaluated using anaesthesized dogs during mechanical ventilation. Recently, Gama et al. [6] have published preliminary data of a study where the method have been successfully implemented in an intensive care environment. The advantage of the method is that the breathing pattern remain unchanged during the determination of the effective pulmonary blood flow.

Single-Breath Method

The single-breath method [7] for measurement of pulmonary blood flow has been the subject of numerous investigations during the past 30 years. The method is attractive due to its potential for providing noninvasive estimates of cardiac output on a breath by breath basis. The validity of the single-breath method is, however, debatable, because it depends on a number of assumptions that lack experimental verification. Furthermore, investigations comparing the single-breath method with invasive cardiac output methods have given contradictory results. Finally, a theoretical study has demonstrated extreme sensitivity of the estimated pulmonary blood flow to small random errors in the data measured using the single-breath method. These results have discouraged the use of the single-breath method.

The single-breath method estimates the pulmonary blood flow from the PCO_2 versus PO_2 curve recorded during a prolonged expiration. Analysis of a single-alveolus lung model shows that the pulmonary blood flow (Q), mixed venous PCO_2 ($PvCO_2$) and the rate of oxygen uptake (VO_2) are the only parameters that affect the PCO_2 versus PO_2 curve. If VO_2 is measured, the two other parameters (PBF and $PvCO_2$) can be determined by least squares curve fitting of the single-alveolus lung model to the experimental curve. The solution presented by Srinivasan [8] simplified the nonlinear data reduction procedure as the analytical expression for the PCO_2 versus PO_2 curve avoids the time consuming numerical integration procedures. This procedure is both theoretical and statistically ideal because it utilizes the expression for the PCO_2 versus PO_2 curve which can be derived from the alveolar model to fit the experimental data.

This expression is:

$$\frac{PO_2}{P_B} = 1 - \frac{PCO_2}{P_B} - K \frac{(\beta - PCO_2/P_B)^{(1-\alpha)/(\beta-\alpha)}}{(\alpha - PCO_2/P_B)^{(1-\beta)/(\beta-\alpha)}} \tag{1}$$

where P_B is the barometric pressure and K, α and β are the parameters to be estimated by the nonlinear curve fitting procedure. The effective pulmonary blood flow is related to α, β and VO_2 by the following equation:

$$Q = \frac{VO_2}{(1-\alpha)(1-\beta) S P_B}$$

where S is the slope of the CO_2 binding curve of blood.

However, the results obtained with the single-breath method shows a reproducibility no better than 15% (coefficient of variation on repeated estimates of the effective pulmonary blood flow) even in well trained heathy test subjects [9].

Estimation of Effective Pulmonary Blood Flow Using Inert Gases

Inert Gas Rebreathing Method

The rebreathing method for estimation of effective pulmonary blood flow [10] is based on the Bornstein modification of the Fick principle.

The rate of disappearance of inert gas from the lungs can be used to estimate effective pulmonary blood flow. In practice, a rebreathing bag is filled with a gas mixture containing an inert soluble gas (acetylene, freon-22 or nitrous oxide) and a poorly soluble gas (helium, argon or sulfur hexaphloride). Furthermore, if $C^{18}O$ is added to the gas mixture it will provide means to estimate the time at which the inert gas reaches the alveolar level of the airways and it also allows the diffusion capacity of the lungs to be estimated. The volume of the rebreathing bag has not been standardized, different investigators have used values ranging from 0.5–3.5 l. The gas mixture is rebreathed for a period that must be shorter than the recirculation time, during the rebreathing maneuver the concentrations of the gasses are measured by a mass spectrometer or a photoacoustic gas analyser.

Assuming complete gas mixing in the rebreathing system (rebreathing bag + lung) the disappearance curve for inert soluble was can be described by the expression:

$$F_X(t) = F_X(t_0) \times \exp\left(-(Q \times alfa_b/(FRC + (V_t \times alfa_t) + V_{rb})) \times t\right)$$

where $F_X(t_0)$ and $F_X(t)$ are the fractional concentration of inert solouble gas at the end of the first inspiration (t_0) and at time t. Q is the effective pulmonary blood flow, $alfa_b$ and $alfa_t$ are the solubility coefficients of the inert soluble gas in blood and lung tissue, FRC is the functional residual capacity corresponding to the initial lung volume, V_{rb} is the initial volume in the rebreathing bag and V_t the lung tissue volume.

The effective pulmonary blood flow was calculated from the following expression:

$$Q = A_X/alfa_b \times ((FRC + V_{rb}) \times 760/(P_B - 47) + (V_t \times alfa_t))$$

where A_X is the slope of a semilogarithmic plot of the relative fractional concentrations of inert soluble gas ($F_X(t)$) and time.

The rebreathing method have been used in large number of applications such as exercise study, effect of bronchodilatators, studies of regulation of the cardiovascular system. Recently, the inert gas rebreathing method have been used in several studies concerning evaluation of drug therapy and setting of artificiel ventilation in critically ill patients (both infants and adults) [11–13]. Furthermore, recent development in sensor technology [14], makes the method a promising tool for routine monitoring of the effective pulmonary blood flow in an intensive care environment.

Open Circuit Washin of Inert Gas

The open circuit method was published by Stout et al. in 1975 [15]. The method differs from the rebreathing methods published earlier in several respects,
1) the method do not require steady-state conditions,
2) the blood flow can be determined despite changes in FRC,
3) calculation of effective pulmonary blood flow is independent of the lung tissue volume,
4) in principle the method is capable of measuring both the effetive pulmonary blood flow and cardiac output, thus enabling estimation of right-left shunt.

The experimental procedure is simple the inspiration gas composition is changed to a gas mixture of an inert soluble gas, an inert insoluble gas, oxygen and balanced with nitrogen. This gas is inspired for a period of about 20 sec (assuming no recirculation during the measurement period). On Breath-by-Breath basis the inspired volume, expired volume, inert soluble gas uptake and end-tidal concentrations and blood flows are calculated. The physiological principle of the method is to estimated the uptake of the inert soluble gas during a non steady-state period with no recirculation, and correcting for incomplete mixing by an inert insoluble gas. The authors validated the method both theoretical and experimentally comparing with the direct Fick method. This comparison showed that the open circuit cardiac output was within $\pm 20\%$ of the direct Fick cardiac output. However, the method is rather sensitive to random measurement errors and uneven distribution of ventilation, compared to the inert gas rebreathing method [16].

Inert Gas Single-Breath Breath-Holding Method

Inert gas breath-holding methods for assesement of the effective pulmonary blood flow have required 2 or more breath-holding periods [17]. This has been a major drawback of the breath-holding method for estimation of acute changes in the effective pulmonary blood flow. Recently Kendrick et al. [18] have described a variant of the method which enables estimation of the effective pulmonary blood flow from a single breath-holding period (6 s–10 s). The breath-holding procedure is essential the same as for obtainment of carbon monoxide transfer factor and the algorithm is that described for the rebreathing method. Kendrick et al. found an acceptable agreement between the direct Fick method and the single-breath breath-holding method. The coefficient of variation of repeated estimates is appr. 10%. Thus, as other single-breath methods the technique must be expected to be sensitive to uneven distribution of ventilation.

Conclusion

There is a growing interest for estimation of the effective pulmonary blood flow in critically ill patients. Recently, development in gas analyzer and computer technology have made it possible to implement non invasive methods for estimation of the effective pulmonary blood flow based on analysis of gas exchange into the clinical environment. Of these the inert gas rebreathing method seems to be the most promising method.

References

1. Farhi LE, Haab P (1967) Mixed venous blood gas tensions and cardiac output by "bloodless" methods; recent developments and appraisal. Respir Physiol 2:225-233
2. Butler J (1965) Measurement of cardiac output using soluble gases. In: Fenn WO, Rahn H (eds) Handbook of Physiology. Respiration. Am Physiol Soc, sect 3, vol II, chapt 62: 1489-1503
3. Farhi LE, Nesarajah MS, Olszowka AJ, Metildi LA, Ellis AK (1976) Cardiac output determination by simple one-step rebreathing technique. Respir Physiol 28:141-159
4. Olhsson J, Wranne B (1986) Non-invasive assesment of cardiac output and stroke volume in patients during exercise: Evaluation of a CO_2-rebreathing method. Eur J Appl Physiol 55:538-544
5. Capek JM, Roy RJ (1988) Noninvasive Measurement of Cardiac Output Using Partial CO_2 Rebreathing. IEEE Trans Biomed Eng 35:653-661
6. Gama de Abreu M, Ragaller M, Quintel M, Albrecht DM (1996) Non-invasive, Semi-Continuous Pulmonary Capillary Blood Flow Measurement by a Partial CO_2 Rebreathing Technique. Intensive Care Med 22 (Suppl 3) S 362
7. Kim TS, Rahn H, Farhi LE (1966) Estimation of true venous and arterial PCO_2 by gas analysis of a single breath. J Appl Physiol 21:1338-1344
8. Srinivasan R (1986) An analysis of estimation of pulmonary blood flow by the single-breath method. J Appl Physiol 61: 198-209
9. Grønlund J, Christensen P, Hansen LG (1987) Single-breath – method for estimating pulmonary blood flow: Data reduction based on nonlinear curve fitting. Aviat Space Environ Med 58:1097-1102
10. Sackner MA, Greeneltch D, Heiman MS, Epstein S, Atkins N (1975) Diffusing Capacity, Membrane Diffusing Capacity, Blood Volume, Pulmonary Tissue Volume, and Cardiac Output Measured by a Rebreathing Technique. Am Rev Respir Dis 111:157-164
11. Bose CL, Lawson EE, Greene A, Mentz W, Friedman M (1986) Measurement of Cardiopulmonary Function in Ventilated Neonates with Respiratory Distress Syndrom Using Rebreathing Methodology. Pediatr Res 20:316-320
12. Steinhart CM, Burch KD, Brudno S, Parker DH (1989) Noninvasive determination of effective (nonshunted) pulmonary blood flow in normal and injured lungs. Crit Care Med 17:349-353
13. Christensen P, Andersen PK (1996) Clinical applicability of a rebreathing method for noninvasive estimation of effective pulmonary blood flow. Intensive Care Med 22 (Suppl 3) S 365
14. Clemensen P, Christensen P, Norsk P, Grønlund J (1994) A modified photo- and magneto-acoustic multigas analyzer applied in gas exchange measurements. J Appl Physiol 76: 2832-2839
15. Stout RL, Wessel HU, Paul MH (1975) Pulmonary blood flow determined by continuous analysis of pulmonary gas exchange. J Appl Physiol 38:913-918
16. Wendelboe Nielsen O, Hansen S, Grønlund J (1994) Precision and accuracy of a noninvasive inert gas washin method for determination of cardiac output in men. J Appl Physiol 76 (4): 1560-1565
17. Cander L, Forster RE (1959) Determination of pulmonary parenchymal volume and pulmonary capillary blood flow in man. J Appl Physiol 14:541-555
18. Kendrick AH, Rozkovec A, Papouchado M, West J, Laszlo G (1989) Single-breath breathholding estimate of pulmonary blood flow in man: Comparison with direct Fick cardiac output. Clin Science 76:673-676

Hemodynamic Assessment of the Critically Ill Patient Using Transesophageal Echocardiography

J. Gorcsan III

Introduction

Transesophageal echocardiography (TEE) has become an established tool to diagnose cardiac structure and function in patients who are critically ill. Mechanical ventilation, along with postoperative dressings and chest tubes may pose significant technical problems for the acquisition of echocardiographic data from the transthoracic approach. TEE can rapidly provide high quality diagnostic information with only minimal risk to the patient. Furthermore, TEE can be performed at the patient's bedside, without the need for transporting patients who may be hemodynamically unstable to an imaging laboratory, such as the radiology department [1]. This discussion will review the clinical assessment of cardiovascular physiology using transesophageal echocardiography in the intensive care unit setting and introduce recently developed echocardiographic methods to quantify left ventricular (LV) function which may be applied to the intensive care unit setting.

Assessment of Left Ventricular Volume

Rapid assessment of the LV volume status of the hypotensive patient is important for the rapid institution of corrective medical therapy. Although the balloon-tipped pulmonary artery (PA) catheter is the most widely used clinical reference standard for hemodynamic assessment in the critical care setting, particular situations exist where this device cannot be used or where it yields ambiguous information. The Frank-Starling relationship fundamentally relates LV filling with LV ejection, and the goal of clinical therapy of the hypotensive patient is to rapidly maximize this relationship. Although estimates of LV volume can be made from longitudinal imaging planes using TEE, this approach is limited by difficulties in imaging the LV apex [2]. Previous investigators have shown that measurement of the mid-ventricular short-axis area from the transgastric window with TEE can be used as a guide to estimate LV volume, and is a commonly used imaging plane for intraoperative monitoring (Fig. 1). Clements et al. were showed a significant correlation of LV end-diastolic area with end-diastolic volume estimated from simultaneous first pass radionuclide ventriculography (r = 0.85) in a series of 12 patients undergoing abdominal aortic aneurysm surgery [3]. They

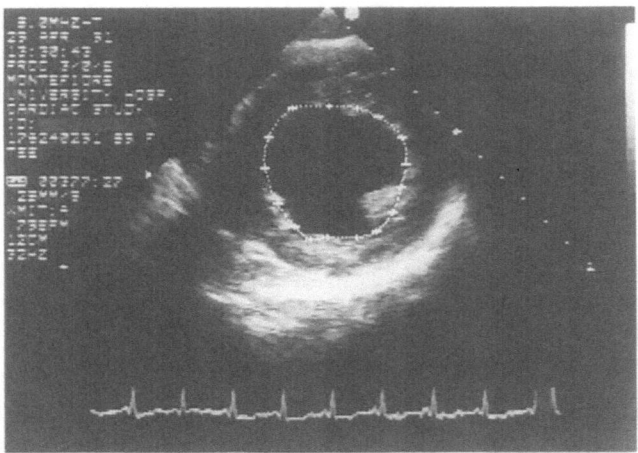

Fig. 1. Mid-ventricular short-axis TEE image with end-diastolic cavity area manually traced by off-line digital analysis system

also demonstrated a close relationship between end-systolic area by TEE and end-systolic volume ($r = 0.94$). Similar results were obtained by Urbanowitz and coworkers who showed a significant, but less close correlation of end-diastolic area with end-diastolic volume ($r = 0.74$) calculated from thermodilution stroke volume and radionuclide end-diastolic counts [4]. Unfortunately, the measurement of end-diastolic short-axis cross-sectional area cannot be reliably converted to absolute LV volume values. In addition, there is a wide range of values of LV short-axis areas in normal individuals. However, TEE can be useful to diagnose hypovolemia when measures of end-diastolic and end-systolic area are well below the normal range. TEE can rapidly differentiate between a small and hyperdynamic left ventricle which requires volume therapy, from a dilated and hypocontractile ventricle which requires inotropic support. Furthermore, measures of cross-sectional area by TEE can be helpful in following trends of volume status in individual patients. Cheung et al. demonstrated that LV short axis area measured by TEE was a sensitive indicator of changes in the total blood volume of patients undergoing cardiac surgery [5]. This was shown by incremental collections of the patients own blood which was readministered after bypass. Their study also showed that short-axis area was able to predict changes in preload in patients with both normal LV function and those with coronary artery disease with abnormal LV function. These studies combine to demonstrate the utility of TEE to assess LV volume status in selected clinical scenarios.

Estimation of Cardiac Output

Maintenance of blood flow to meet the metabolic requirements of the organism is essential to sustain life. The measurement of blood flow through the cardiovascular system is usually accomplished by the thermodilution cardiac output method in the intensive care unit setting. This method relates a change in the temperature of blood downstream from the site of an injection of a fluid bolus of know temperature to calculate cardiac output. Although reliable in many clinical settings, the thermodilution method requires insertion of a pulmonary artery catheter which may not always be possible or desirable. Furthermore, the thermodilution method is technically limited when the patient has significant tricuspid regurgitation or in the setting of low cardiac output where spurious mixing and unpredictable effects of the injectate on blood temperature may occur. Assessment of cardiac output by Doppler echocardiography has been well validated using the transthoracic approach [6, 7]. In situations where transthoracic echocardiographic data collection is technically limited, transesophageal Doppler echocardiography provides a less invasive alternate to pulmonary artery catheterization as a means to determine cardiac output. The Doppler technique fundamentally converts shifts in received ultrasound frequency to measures of blood velocity. To calculate flow at any point in the cardiovascular system and convert blood velocity data to stroke volume, two separate sets of measurements are performed. First, one needs to measure cross-sectional area of the selected site and second, one needs to integrate the Doppler blood velocity over the cardiac cycle. The integral of the spectral Doppler velocity over time, known as the flow velocity integral, is multiplied by cross-sectional area to determine stroke volume: flow velocity integral (cm) × cross-sectional area (cm^2) = stroke volume (cm^3 or ml). Stroke volume is then multiplied by heart rate to determine cardiac output. Accordingly, estimates of blood flow may be made at several sites within the heart and great vessels. The most simplified approach to the assessment of cross-sectional area is to choose a site where circular geometry may be assumed throughout the cardiac cycle. This was first demonstrated in the main pulmonary artery where cross-sectional area was calculated from the measurement of diameter: area = $1/4\,\pi$ (diameter)^2. TEE pulsed-Doppler or continuous-wave measures of pulmonary artery blood velocity were then made from a superior esophageal location [8, 9]. A limitation of this method was that the diameter of the pulmonary artery could not always be measured confidently, and that the technical quality of Doppler data may be interfered with by air in the traceal-broncheal tree. A second approach has been assessment of cardiac output from the mitral annular site [8]. Unfortunately, this method is limited by geometric changes that may occur in the mitral annular throughout diastole. The most favorable approach that has been described has been the site of the aortic valve. Doppler data may be acquired from a modified transgastric window where the transducer is angled steeply superior and slightly leftward to align to allow alignment of the ultrasound beam with blood flow across the aortic valve. The original method described by Katz et al. used a measurement of the diameter of the aortic annulus to calculate cross-sectional area assuming circular geometry and continuous-wave Doppler measure of blood velocity (Figs. 2, 3) [10]. In a consecutive series of 31 patients studied by this approach, technically adequate data were available in 88% of attempted studies. A significant correlation of Doppler-derived cardiac output measures with simultaneous thermodilution measures were observed

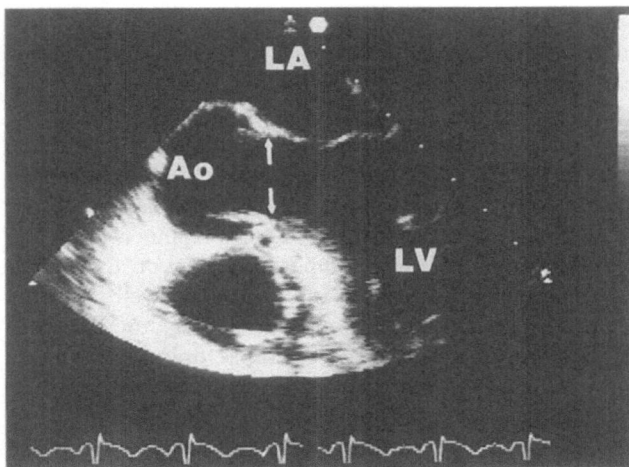

Fig. 2. Transesophageal image demonstrating measurement of aortic annulus (arrows). Ao = aorta, LA = left atrium, LV = left ventricle. Reprinted with permission from the American Journal of Cardiology, 1993; 71: 853–857

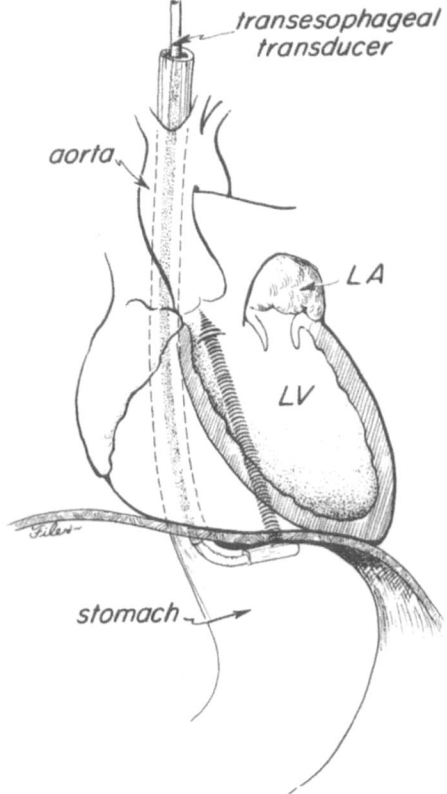

Fig. 3. Diagram of transesophagel echocardiographic probe position to direct the Doppler ultrasound beam parallel to flow across the aortic valve. LA = left atrium, LV = left ventricle. Reprinted with permission from the American Journal of Cardiology, 1993; 71: 853–857

with $r = 0.91$, $y = 1.01x + 0.2$ (Figs. 4A, 4B, 5). Stoddard et al. also confirmed close correlations of transesophagel Doppler estimates of cardiac output at the aortic valve site with thermodilution calculations using either pulsed or continuous-wave Doppler [11]. This method was further refined by Darmon et al. who used direct measurement of the aortic valve orifice, which may be triangular-shaped (Fig. 6), along with continuous-wave Doppler from the transgastric window [12]. They demonstrated a high yield of available data using this approach in 62 of 63

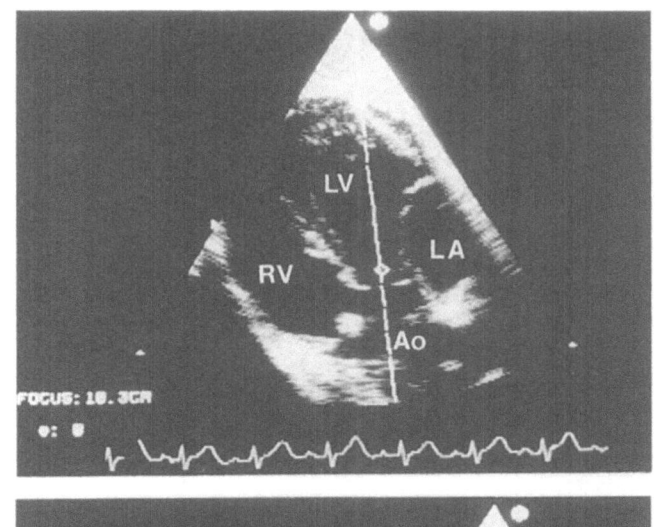

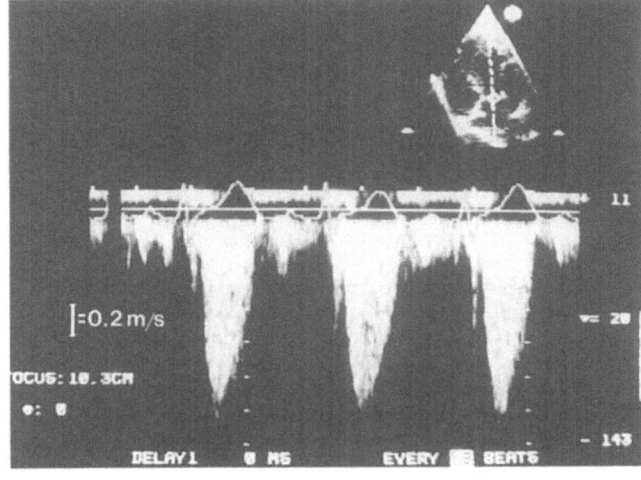

Fig. 4. A Echocardiographic image from transgastric view of the left ventricular outflow tract, aortic valve and aortic root with the continuous wave Doppler cursor. Ao = aorta, LA = left atrium, LV = left ventricle, RV = right ventricle. **B** Transgastric continuous wave Doppler spectral display of blood flow across the aortic valve. Reprinted with permission from the American Journal of Cardiology, 1993; 71 : 853–857

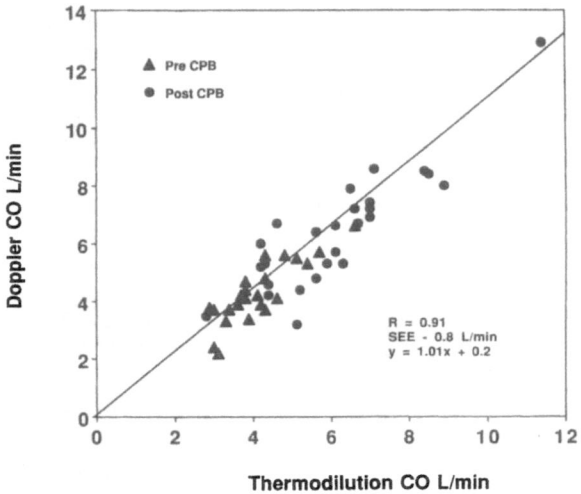

Fig. 5. Results of correlation of transgastric continuous wave Doppler cardiac output determinations with simultaneous thermodilution cardiac output measurements. CPB = cardiopulmonary bypass, CO = cardiac output. Reprinted with permission from the American Journal of Cardiology, 1993; 71 : 853–857

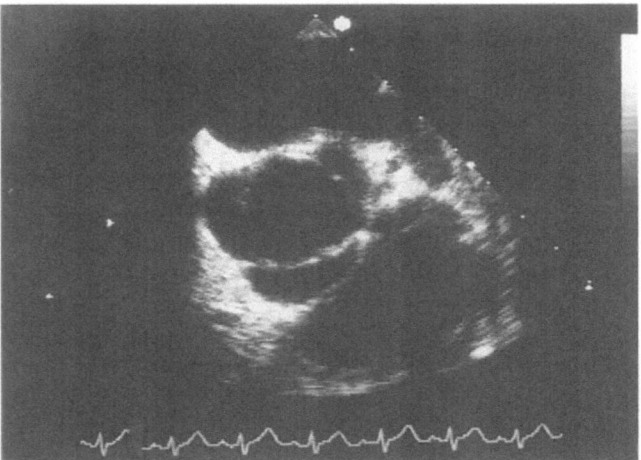

Fig. 6. Transesophageal echocardiographic image of aortic valve orifice in mid-systole, demonstrating triangular shape

patients in whom many had studies before and after cardiac surgery, reporting a total of 109 studies. They observed a very close correlation with thermodilution measures of cardiac output; $r = 0.94$, SEE = 0.4 L/min, $y = 0.94 x + 0.19$. These data combine to demonstrate that the aortic site is the site of first choice for TEE determination of cardiac output. In patients where this method cannot be applied because of aortic stenosis, aortic regurgitation, or left ventricular outflow tract obstruction, the pulmonary artery or mitral valve sites may be employed.

Novel Echocardiographic Approaches to Assess Ventricular Function

Pressure-Area and Pressure-Volume Relations

Although ejection phase indices, such as ejection fraction or cardiac output, have widespread clinical use to describe LV function, these measures are limited by their dependence on loading conditions. Suga and Sugwawa described originally a model to assess LV performance using the pressure-volume relationships that are relatively independent of loading conditions [13]. They demonstrated that the slope of the LV end-systolic pressure-volume relationship, also known as end-systolic elastance (E_{es}) is predominantly linear over a wide range of pressures and volumes and that the slope of this relationship varies with alterations in contractile state. Applications of this model to clinical situations have been limited because of the need for collection of simultaneous LV volume and pressure data while load is altered acutely.

A relatively recent advance has been echocardiographic automated border detection which uses the radiofrequency ultrasound backscatter data to determine the blood-tissue interface within a tomographic image and calculate and display cross-sectional area on-line [14, 15]. Appleyard and Glantz have previously demonstrated that changes in two-dimensional cross-sectional area accurately describe changes in LV volume in a canine sonomicrometry model over a wide range of hemodynamic derangements [16]. We have extended this observation to the use echocardiographic automated border detection (Sonos 1500, Hewlett-Packard, Andover, MA) to show that changes in mid-ventricular cross-sectional area can be used as a surrogate for changes in volume [17]. This has been demonstrated in an intact animal model where measures of stroke area (end-diastolic area – end-systolic area) correlated linearly with changes in stroke volume, measured simultaneously by an aortic electromagnetic flow probe, while preload was acutely altered by inferior vena caval occlusion: $r = 0.93$, SEE = 5%, $n = 7$ dogs (540 beats) [18]. This relationship was also confirmed in humans, in a study of patients undergoing coronary artery bypass surgery (Figs. 7–9) [19]. Measures of mid-ventricular cross-sectional area using TEE were significantly correlated with changes in stroke volume measured by an aortic electromagnetic flow probe during transient inferior vena caval occlusion: group mean $r = 0.94 \pm 0.03$, SEE = 0.33 ± 0.12 cm^2 before bypass, and group mean $r = 0.92 \pm 0.05$, SEE = 0.59 ± 0.81 cm^2 after bypass. Although no reliable method exists to convert mid-ventricular cross-sectional area to volume, these studies combine to demonstrate that changes in cross-sectional area are linearly related to changes in LV volume within physiological ranges and that area may be used as a surrogate for LV volume in the assessment of pressure-volume relations.

Automated measures of cross-sectional area can be used to construct pressure-area loops in a manner similar to pressure-volume loops. We showed that the end-systolic elastance solved from pressure-area loops (E'_{es}) as the slope of the maximum pressure/area points of a family of pressure area loops varied with predictable alterations in contractile state in a canine model of inotropic modulation (Fig. 10) [20]. LV contractility increased with dobutamine ($n = 7$);

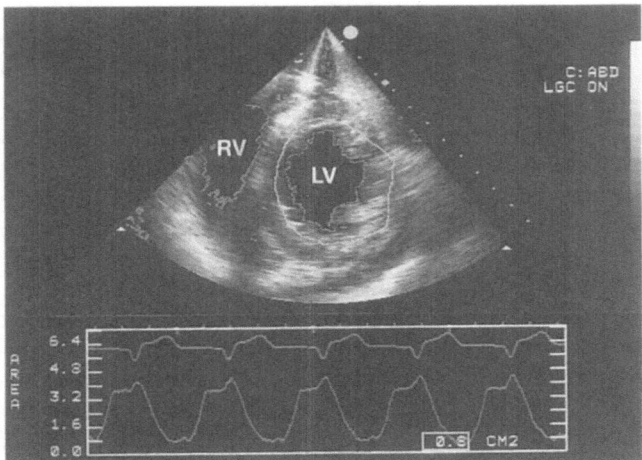

Fig. 7. Transesophageal echocardiographic image at midventricular short-axis plane demonstrating automated border detection measures of left ventricular (LV) cavity area. RV = right ventricle. Reprinted with permission from the American Journal of Cardiology, 1993; 72: 721–727

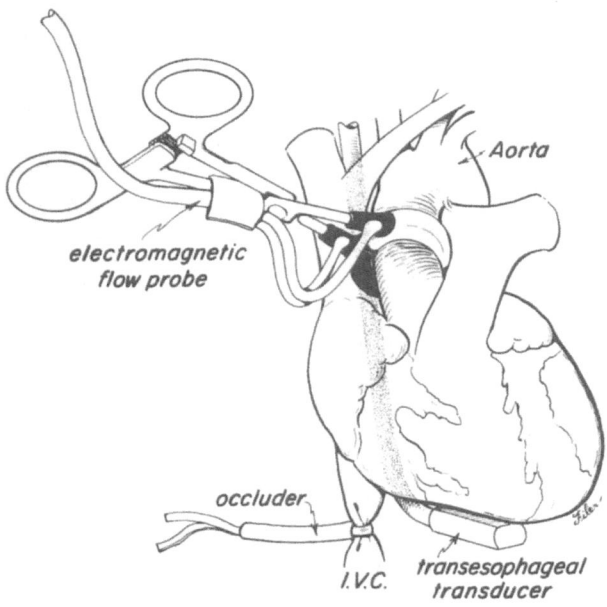

Fig. 8. Diagram of experimental instrumentation in patients undergoing coronary artery bypass surgery. IVC = inferior vena cava. Reprinted with permission from the American Journal of Cardiology, 1993; 72:721–727

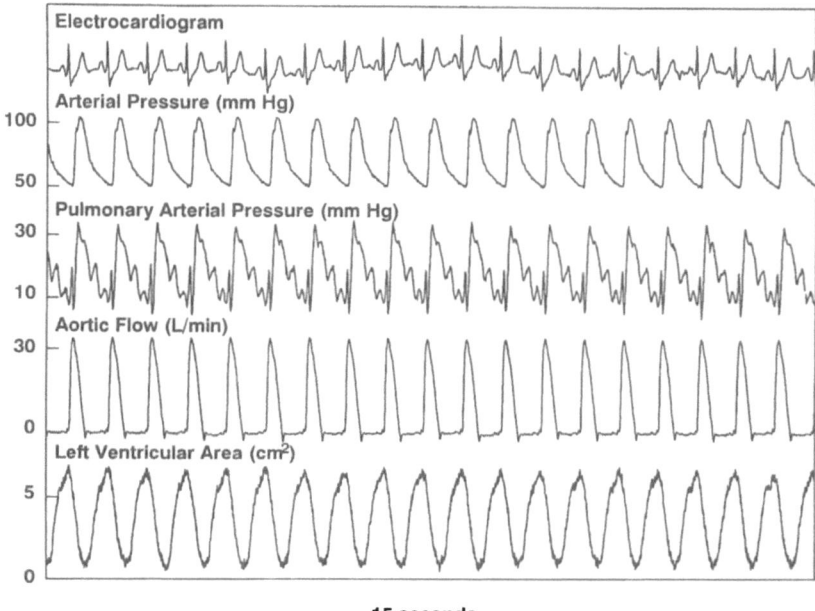

15 seconds

Fig. 9. Examples of simultaneous waveform data with left ventricular area acquired with transesophageal in a patient undergoing coronary artery bypass surgery. Reprinted with permission from the American Journal of Cardiology 1993; 72:721–727

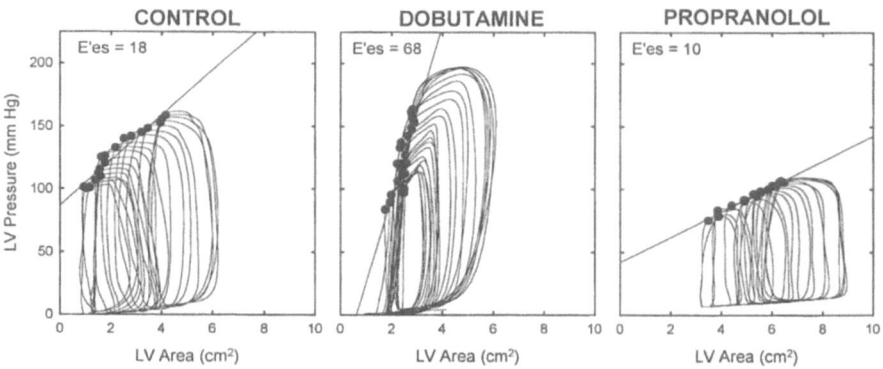

Fig. 10. Examples of pressure-area loops in an open chest canine model with contractile state altered by inotropic modulation. Left ventricular short-axis cross-sectional area was acquired with echocardiographic automated border detection and pressure was acquired with a high fidelity catheter during inferior vena caval occlusion. The slope of the end-systolic pressure-area relation predictably increased with dobutamine and decreased with propranolol. Reprinted with permission from the American College of Cardiology, Journal of the American College of Cardiology, 1994; 23:242–252

E'_{es}: 30 ± 11 to 67 ± 24 mmHg/cm^2, and decreased with propranolol (n = 5); E'_{es}: 20 ± 4 to 13 ± 4 mmHg/cm^2 (both p , < 0.02 vs. control).

A more recent modification of this automated border detection technology is an automated volume algorithm that calculated volume from a longitudinal tomographic LV image [21, 22]. Two different automated algorithms are possible, an area-length method which uses (8 area^2)/3 π length, and a modified Simpson's rule algorithm which sums the volume calculated form 20 equally spaced circular disks (Fig. 11). The Simpson's rule automated border detection LV volume method has been recently evaluated in an animal model using the conductance catheter as a reference standard for LV volume [22, 23]. Relative changes in steady state volume were closely correlated throughout the cardiac cycle, and changes in end-diastolic volume and end-systolic volume were linearly related during acute alterations in preload induced by inferior vena caval occlusion (Fig. 12). However, the automated echocardiographic method had a tendency to underestimate LV absolute volume. This on-line LV volume method was also evaluated for the application of pressure-volume loops in this model. Although absolute values of E_{es} differed when using echocardiographic automated border detection versus the conductance catheter, similar changes in these measures were demonstrated during alterations in contractile state induced by pharmacological inotropic modulation (Fig. 12). The use of this TEE method to estimate LV volume on line in patients has promise, but our initial experience was that it could only be applied to approximately 82% of attempted TEE studies using the longitudinal two-chamber view and 67% of studies using the apical four-chamber view, due to technical limitations [24].

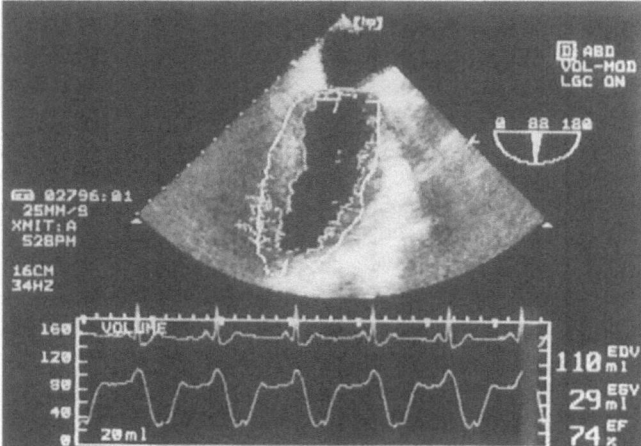

Fig. 11. An example of a transesophageal echocardiographic two-chamber view from a longitudinal plane in a patient with normal ventricular function. Echocardiographic automated border detection calculates left ventricular volume using modified Simpson's rule. Reprinted with permission from the American Heart Journal, 1994; 128:389–396

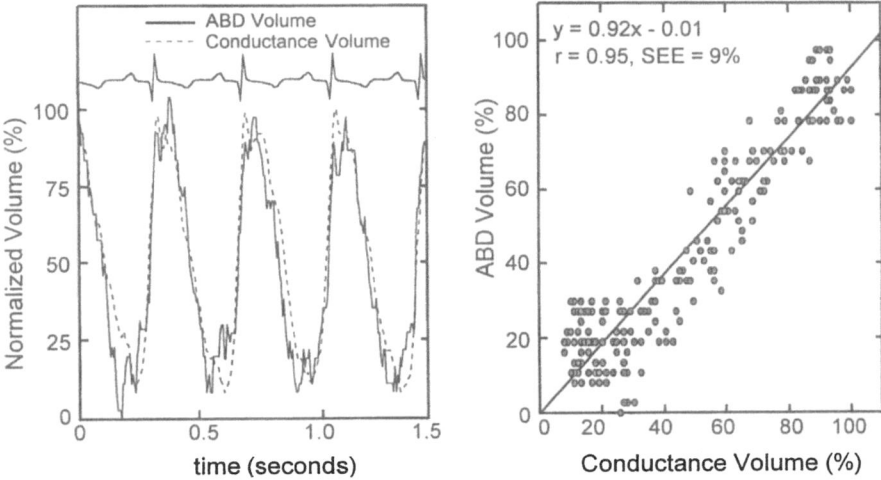

Fig. 12. An example of simultaneous echocardiographic automated border detection (ABD) and conductance catheter volume signals during steady state conditions in an animal model. Relative values are closely related throughout the cardiac cycle. Reprinted with permission from the American Heart Journal 1996; 131:544–552

Echocardiographic automated border detection measures of short axis cross-sectional area could be applied to over 90% of attempted studies using TEE in humans [25, 26]. The utility of pressure-area relations to assess LV performance in humans was shown in a study of the effects of cardiopulmonary bypass on LV contractility in patients undergoing coronary artery bypass surgery [26]. Thirteen patients had measurement of LV pressure and LV cross-sectional area using TEE during inferior vena caval occlusions both before and after bypass. In 7 patients with complete data sets, significant decreases in E'_{es}, maximal elastance and preload recruitable stroke work occurred (Fig. 14) [27]. These observations were consistent with the transient stunning effects of cardiopulmonary bypass that has been described elsewhere [28]. The advantage of this method was that consistent changes in contractility were measured by pressure-area relations where measures of cardiac output and fractional area change were variable in the same patients.

Substitution of Arterial Pressure for Left Ventricular Pressure

A relatively less invasive means of assessing LV contractility using pressure-area relations without having to catheterize the left ventricle was studied using femoral arterial pressure as a surrogate for LV ejection pressure. In a series of 13 patients studied before and after cardiopulmonary bypass, simultaneously acquired LV pressure-area loops were compared with femoral arterial pressure-area loops to assess LV performance [29]. The delay in the femoral arterial pressure with re-

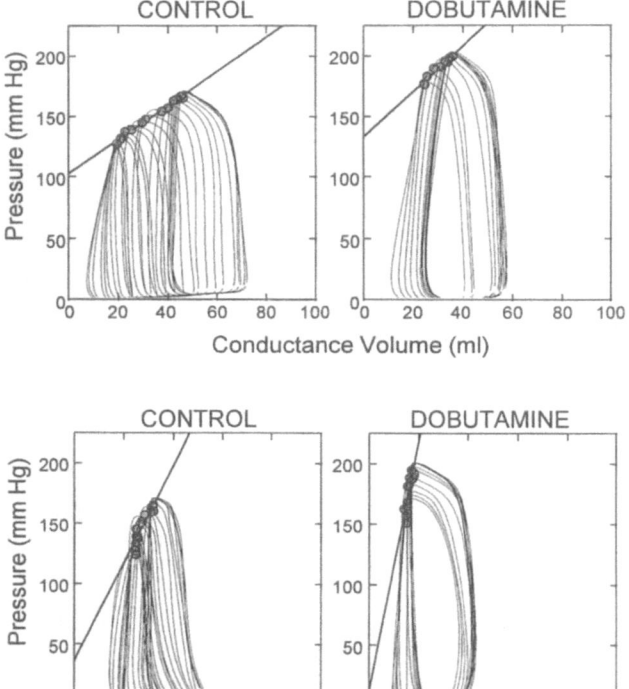

Fig. 13. Examples of simultaneous pressure-volume loops with volume from the conductance catheter (top) and volume from transesophageal echocardiographic automated border detection (ABD) bottom in a canine model. The left panels shows control and the right panels demonstrate increases in the slope of the end-systolic pressure-volume relationship with dobutamine infusion. The end-systolic slopes were comparatively steeper with the echocardiographic technique. Reprinted with permission from the American Heart Journal 1996; 131:544–552

spect to true LV ejection pressure was corrected by aligning minimum arterial pressure with the first occurrence of end-diastolic area (Fig. 15). The same pressure-volume loop analyses were then performed to calculate E'_{es}, and maximal elastance which were similar using both pressure signals (Fig. 16). These data suggest that femoral arterial pressure may be used as a surrogate for LV catheterization when assessing pressure-area relations with echocardiography.

Practical Implementation of Pressure-Area or Pressure-Volume Relations

To assess LV performance by pressure-area or pressure-volume relations using echocardiographic automated border detection, the following are needed: an

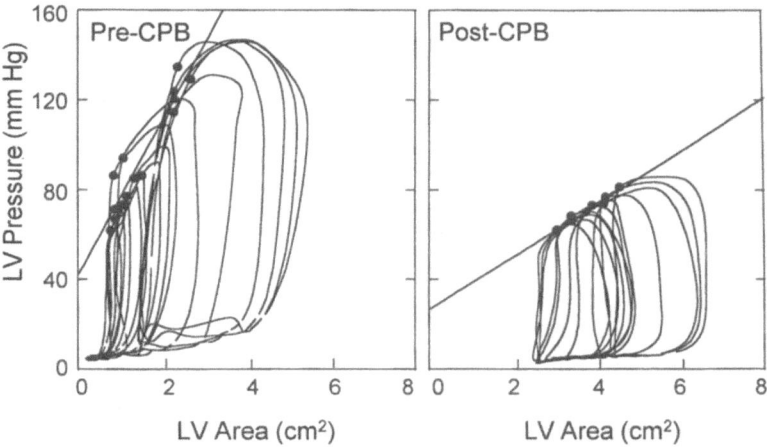

Fig. 14. Pressure-area loops in a patient undergoing coronary artery bypass surgery before and after cardiopulmonary bypass (CPB). The end-systolic pressure-area slope is decreased, consistent with a decrease in left ventricular contractile state immediately after bypass. Reprinted with permission from the American Heart Association, Circulation 1990; 89:180–190

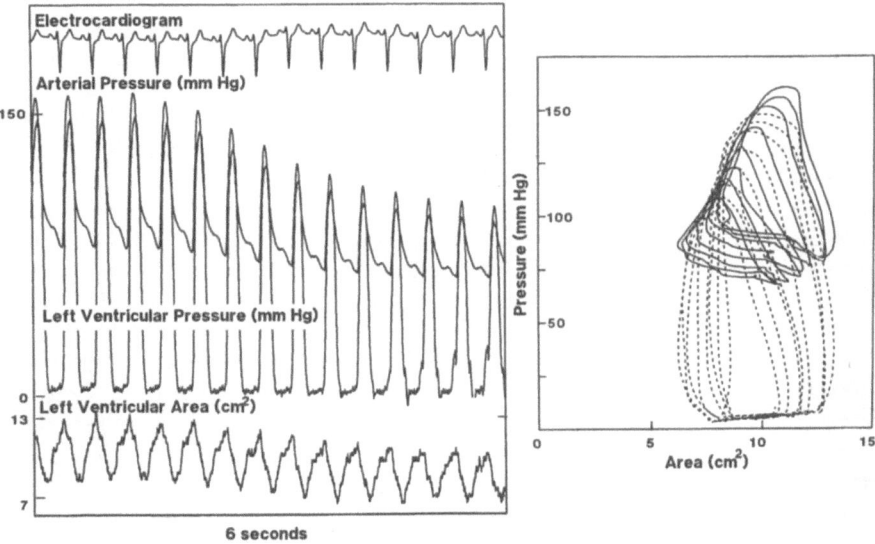

Fig. 15. Simultaneous waveform data (left) and pressure-area loop data (right) from a patient during inferior vena caval occlusion. The left ventricular pressure-area loops are shown as dashed lines and the femoral arterial pressure-area loops appear as solid lines. Reprinted with permission from Anesthesiology 1994; 81:553–562

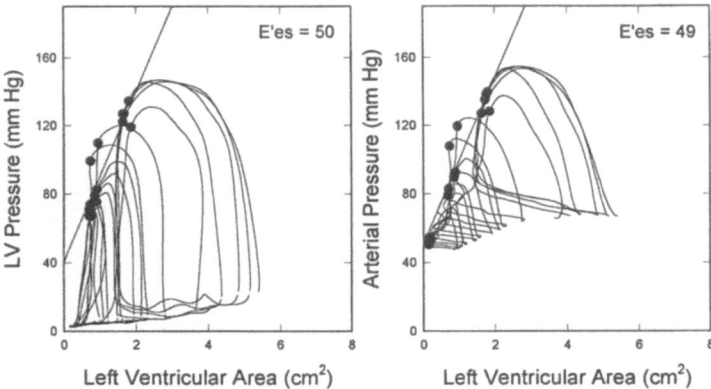

Fig. 16. Examples of similar end-systolic elastance (E'$_{es}$) values from pressure area relations using high fidelity left ventricular pressure (left), and femoral arterial pressure (right) from a patient undergoing cardiac surgery. Reprinted with permission from Anesthesiology 1994; 81: 553–562

interface with the ultrasound system (A. Q. dataport, Hewlett-Packard, Andover, MA), a recording device for simultaneous pressure and area or volume signals, and a pressure-volume loop analysis program. We used an analog-to-digital converter (Model RTS-132, Significat, Hudson, MA) for all of the signals with a sampling rate set at 150 Hz. The multiple physiological signals, such as the electrocardiogram, pressure, electromagnetic flow and echocardiographic area or volume were recorded on a customized computer workstation (Apollo Computer Inc. Model DN3550, Chelmsford, MA) for display, storage and subsequent analysis of data. Other commercially available personal computers for multichannel recording of data may be used. The frame rate of the echocardiographic system was relatively slow at 30 Hz and adjustment of timing was necessary to correctly align pressure and area or volume signals for loop plots. The signal with the highest temporal resolution was the high fidelity pressure catheters used for our studies. Using this as our reference standard, we found an average delay of 13 ± 19 msec in the automated border detection signal for 36 inferior vena caval occlusion runs in a canine model. Time was added to the pressure signal to correctly align end-diastolic pressure (defined as the point immediately before the onset of isovolumic contraction) with the end-diastolic area or volume (defined as the first occurrence of maximal area or volume). Fine tuning of the timing was accomplished by choosing the delay that gave the pressure-volume loop with the most vertical isovolumic portions of the loop (Fig. 17). Pressure-volume loop analysis was performed with a customized computer program (ASYST Software Technologies, Inc., Rochester, NY) to calculate E'$_{es}$, maximal elastance using a time-varying elastance model, and preload recruitable stroke force, described in detail elsewhere. Commercially available programs, such as the CA Recorder and Spectrum (Triton Technologies, San Diego, CA) may perform similar functions [20, 25, 27].

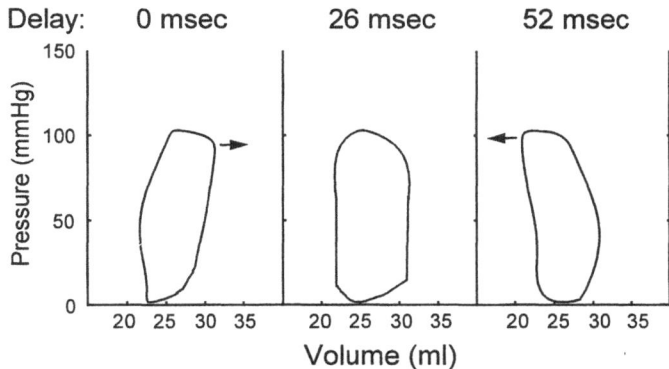

Fig. 17. Examples of automated border detection (ABD) pressure-volume loops plotted with varying delays in the pressure signal. The ABD system has a frame rate of 30 Hz and signals were digitized at 150 Hz. The left panel shows no delay (leans rightward), the middle panel shows 26 ms delay, and the right panel shows 52 msec delay (leans leftward). The 26 msec delay was selected for this run because the isovolumic portions of the loop appear most vertical. Reprinted with permission from Kluwer Academic Press, from New Echocardiographic Techniques for Automated Quantification of Cardiovascular Function 1997

This review demonstrates how TEE may be useful to guide supportive therapy in critically ill patients through the assessment of LV filling and cardiac output. Furthermore, it demonstrates that more recent advances in echocardiography, such as automated border detection, may be used to assess ventricular performance in a relatively load insensitive manner. It is likely that these applications of TEE will continue to evolve along with progressive technological advances, and continue to have an impact on the hemodynamic management of patients who are critically ill.

References

1. Pearson AC, Castello R, Labovitz AJ (1990) Safety and utility of transesophageal echocardiography in the critically ill patient. Am Heart J 119:1083–1089
2. Smith MD, MacPhail B, Harrison MR, Lenhoff SJ, DeMaria AN (1992) Value and limitations of transesophageal echocardiography in determination of left ventricular volumes and ejection fraction. J Am Coll Cardiol 19:1213–1222
3. Clements F, Harpole D, Quill T, Jones R, McCann R (1990) Estimation of left ventricular volume and ejection fraction by two-dimensional transoesophageal echocardiography: Comparison of short-axis imaging and simultaneous radionuclide angiography. Brit J Anaesth 64:331–336
4. Urbanowitz JH, Shaaban MJ, Cohen NH, Cahalan MK, Botvinick EH, Chatterjee K, Schiller NB, Dae MW, Matthay MA (1990) Comparison of transesophageal echocardiographic and scintigraphic estimates of left ventricular end-diastolic volume index and ejection fraction in patients following coronary artery bypass grafting. Anesthesiology 72:607–612
5. Cheung AT, Salvino JS, Weiss SJ, Aukburg SJ, Berlin JA (1994) Echocardiographic and hemodynamic indices of left ventricular preload in patients with normal and abnormal ventricular function. Anesthesiology 81:376–387

6. Nishimura RA, Callahan MJ, Schaff HV, Ilstrup DM, Miller FA, Tajik AJ (1984) Noninvasive measurement of cardiac output by continuous wave Doppler echocardiography: Initial experience and review of the literature. Mayo Clin Proc 59:484–489

7. Stewart WJ, Jiang L, Mich R, Pandian N, Guerrero JL, Weyman AJ (1985) Variable effects of flow rates through the aortic, pulmonary and mitral valves on valve area inflow velocity: Impact on quantitative Doppler flow calculations. J Am Coll Cardiol 6:653–662

8. Muhivdeen IA, Kuecherer HF, Lee E, Cahalan MK, Schiller NB (1991) Intraoperative estimation of cardiac output by transesophageal pulsed Doppler echocardiography. Anesthesiology 74:9–14

9. Gorcsan J, Diana P, Ball BA, Hattler BG (1992) Intraoperative determination of cardiac output by transesophageal continuous wave Doppler. Am Heart J 123:171–176

10. Katz WE, Gasior TA, Quinlan JJ, Gorcsan J (1993) Transgastric continuous-wave Doppler to determine cardiac output. Am J Cardiol 71:853–857

11. Stoddard MF, Prince CR, Ammish N, Goad JL, Vogel RL (1993) Pulsed Doppler transesophageal echocardiographic determination of cardiac output in human beings: Comparison with thermodilution technique. Am Heart J 126:956–962

12. Darmon PL, Hillel Z, Mogtader A, Mindich B, Thys D (1994) Cardiac output by transesophageal echocardiography using continuous-wave Doppler across the aortic valve. Anesthesiology 80:796–805

13. Suga H, Sagawa K, Shoukas (1973) Load independence of the instantaneous pressure-volume ratio of the canine left ventricle and effects of epinephrine and heart rate on the ratio. Circ Res 32:314–322

14. Perez JE, Waggoner AD, Barzilai B, Melton HE, Miller JG, Sobel BE (1992) On-line assessment of ventricular function by automatic boundary detection and ultrasonic backscatter imaging. J Am Coll Cardiol 19:313–320

15. Vandenberg BF, Rath LS, Stuhlmuller P, Melton HE, Skorton D (1992) Estimation of left ventricular cavity area with an on-line semiautomated echocardiographic edge detection system. Circulation 86:159–166

16. Appleyard RF, Glantz SA (1990) Two-dimensions describe left ventricular volume change during hemodynamic transients. Am J Physiol 258:H277–H284

17. Gorcsan J, Morita S, Mandarino WA, Deneault LG, Kawai A, Kormos RL, Griffith BP, Pinsky MR (1993) Two-dimensional echocardiographic automated border detection accurately reflects changes in left ventricular volume. J Am Soc Echocardiogr 6:482–489

18. Gorcsan J, Lazar JM, Romand J, Pinsky MR (1993) On-line estimation of stroke volume by means of echocardiographic automated border detection in the canine left ventricle. Am Heart J 125:1316–1323

19. Gorcsan J, Gasior TA, Mandarino WA, Deneault LG, Hattler BG, Pinsky MR (1993) On-line estimation of changes in left ventricular stroke volume by transesophageal echocardiographic automated border detection in patients undergoing coronary artery bypass grafting. Am J Cardiol 72:721–727

20. Gorcsan J, Romand JA, Mandarino WA, Deneault LG, Pinsky MR (1994) Assessment of left ventricular performance by on-line pressure-area relations using echocardiographic automated border detection. J Am Coll Cardiol 23:242–252

21. Morrisey RL, Siu SC, Guerrero JL, Newell JB, Weyman AE, Picard MH (1994) Automated assessment of ventricular volume and function by echocardiography: Validation of automated border detection. J Am Soc Echocardiogr 7:107–115

22. Gorcsan J, Denault A, Mandarino WA, Pinsky MR (1996) Left ventricular pressure-volume relations using transesophageal echocardiographic automated border detection: Comparison with conductance catheter technique. Am Heart J 131:544–552

23. Baan J, Van Der Velde ET (1988) Sensitivity of left ventricular end-systolic pressure-volume relation to type of loading intervention in dogs. Circ Res 62:1247–1258

24. Katz W, Gasior TA, Reddy SBC, Gorcsan J (1994) Utility and limitations of biplane transesophageal echocardiographic automated border detection for estimation of left ventricular stroke volume and cardiac output. Am Heart J 128:389–396

25. Gorcsan J, Gasior TA, Mandarino WA, Deneault LG, Hattler BG, Pinsky MR (1990) Assessment of the immediate effects of cardiopulmonary bypass on left ventricular performance by on-line pressure-area relations. Circulation 89:180–190
26. Stoddard MF, Keedy DL, Longaker RA (1994) Two-dimensional transesophageal echocardiographic characterization of ventricular filling in real time by acoustic quantification: Comparison with pulsed-Doppler echocardiography. J Am Soc Echocardiogr 7:116–131
27. Glower DD, Spratt, JA, Snow ND, Kabas JS, Davis JW, Olsen CO, Tyson GS, Sabiston DC, Rankin JS (1985) Linearity of the Frank-Starling relationship in the intact heart: the concept of preload recruitable stroke work. Circulation 5:994–1009
28. Breissblatt WM, Stein KL, Wolfe CJ, et al (1990) Acute myocardial dysfunction and recovery: A common occurrence after coronary bypass surgery. J Am Coll Cardiol 15:1261–1269
29. Gorcsan J, Denault A, Gasior TA, Mandarino WA, Kancel MJ, Deneault LG, Hattler BG, Pinsky MR (1994) Rapid estimation of left ventricular contractility from end-systolic relations using echocardiographic automated border detection and femoral arterial pressure. Anesthesiology 81:553–562

Goals of Resuscitation

Physiology of VO_2/DO_2

J.-L. Vincent and P. van der Linden

Introduction

Cellular energy is supplied in the form of high energy phosphate compounds, such as ATP, by metabolic reactions involving the oxidation of hydrocarbons. The concentration of ATP in most cells is maintained by the mitochondrial electron transport systems. Under normal conditions the amount of oxygen present in the mitochondria greatly exceeds that required to maintain oxidative phosphorylation. However when oxygen delivery falls, less efficient anaerobic metabolism takes over, leading to lactate production and acidosis. Cellular processes fail as energy supplies fall, and organ system function deteriorates. Oxygen is thus essential for the normal activity and survival of tissues.

In physiologic conditions, the delivery of oxygen from the environment to the tissues involves several stages whereby oxygen is transported through the lungs, carried in the blood, and unloaded in the tissues. Oxygen demand is determined by the metabolic rate of the particular tissue and is regulated by control of ventilation and of blood flow or cardiac output. This system exhibits great flexibility enabling it to adapt to increases of 15–20 times in oxygen demand.

An understanding of the relationship between oxygen delivery and uptake in normal tissues is therefore fundamental to our understanding of the effects of hypoxia on our patients, the development of organ dysfunction, and the whole concept of life support. Possible alterations to this relationship in the critically ill are discussed in later chapters but let us focus on the physiologic condition.

Oxygen Delivery

Oxygen delivery (DO_2) can be defined as the rate of oxygen transport to the peripheral tissues. It can be calculated as the product of cardiac output (CO) and arterial oxygen content (CaO_2)

$$DO_2 = CO \times CaO_2 \tag{1}$$

CaO_2 is in turn determined by the hemoglobin (Hb) value, the arterial oxygen saturation (SaO_2), and a constant value representing the amount of oxygen bound to 1 g of hemoglobin (neglecting the small amount of oxygen dissolved in blood).

$$DO_2 = CO \times Hb \times SaO_2 \times 1.39 \times 10 \tag{2}$$

For a normal CO of 3 L/min $\cdot$ m^2, a Hb of 12 g/dL, and a SaO$_2$ of 98% one therefore reaches a DO$_2$ value of about 500 mL/min $\cdot$ m^2.

Oxygen Uptake

Oxygen uptake (VO$_2$) can be defined as the total oxygen required by all the aerobic metabolic processes in the body. It can be determined either from the Fick equation or from the analysis of expired gases.

Using the Fick equation it can be calculated as the product of CO and the arteriovenous oxygen difference

$$\begin{aligned} VO_2 &= CO \times (CaO_2 - CvO_2) \\ &= CO \times Hb \times (SaO_2 - SvO_2) \times 13.9 \end{aligned} \tag{3}$$

where CvO$_2$ represents the venous oxygen content and SvO$_2$ the venous oxygen saturation.

Using indirect calorimetry for the analysis of expired gases to calculate VO$_2$ involves the use of cumbersome metabolic carts or mass spectroscopy techniques and the equation

$$VO_2 = (VI \times FIO_2) - (VE \times FEO_2) \tag{4}$$

where VI and VE are the volumes of the inspired and expired gases respectively, and FIO$_2$ and FEO$_2$ are the oxygen fractions of the inspired and expired gases respectively. In practice most devices only measure VE and calculate VI using the Haldane transformation. This makes the method sensitive to errors in the measurement of FIO$_2$ or FEO$_2$, and it has other practical difficulties, but it avoids the risk of mathematical coupling that may occur in comparing VO$_2$ and DO$_2$ when both are calculated using the thermodilution CO. Despite practical problems there is a strong correlation between Fick-derived VO$_2$ values and those obtained by indirect calorimetry [1, 2].

Oxygen Extraction

The ratio of oxygen demand to delivery is the oxygen extraction ratio (O$_2$ER).

$$\begin{aligned} O_2ER &= VO_2/DO_2 \\ &= (CaO_2 - CvO_2)/CaO_2 \\ &= [(Hb \times C \times SaO_2) - (Hb \times C \times SvO_2)]/(Hb \times C \times SaO_2) \\ &= (SaO_2 - SvO_2)/SaO_2 \end{aligned} \tag{5}$$

Oxygen extraction is therefore independent of the hemoglobin level. With an SvO_2 of 75% the O_2ER for normal metabolic needs is about 25%.

VO_2/DO_2 Relationship

The three components of oxygen transport are hemoglobin, oxygen saturation, and cardiac output (equation 2). A reduction in Hb or SaO_2 can be compensated for by an increase in CO, thus maintaining DO_2. On the contrary if CO falls, hemoglobin and SaO_2 are unable to compensate and a drop in CO is therefore a greater threat. If DO_2 falls however, VO_2 is maintained by an increase in tissue oxygen extraction occurring at the microcirculatory level. Terminal arterioles dilate decreasing the intercapillary distance and allowing greater oxygen extraction [3, 4]. However a point is reached, the $DO_{2\,crit}$, when O_2ER reaches 65–70% (O_2ER_{crit}) and further increases are unable to maintain VO_2. VO_2 thus begins to fall and becomes supply dependent (Fig. 1). Tissues become hypoxic, anaerobic metabolism becomes prominent and blood lactate levels rise [5, 6].

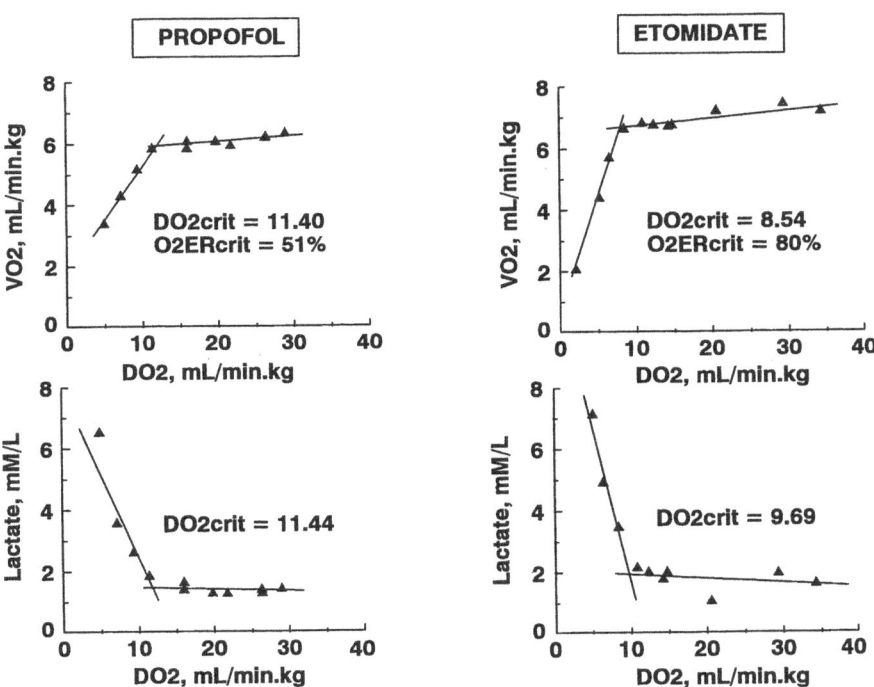

Fig. 1. The physiologic VO_2/DO_2 relationship during acute bleeding in one dog anesthetized with propofol (*left panel*), and one dog with etomidate (*right panel*). Note that the $DO_{2\,crit}$ is identical when calculated from VO_2 or from lactate levels

Experimental Studies. Experimentally, one can investigate the VO_2/DO_2 relationship by adjusting the three components of oxygen delivery, basically employing Barcroft's classification of hypoxia [7].

Anoxic (Hypoxemic) Hypoxia. Achieved by reducing arterial oxygenation to very low levels. If compensatory rises in cardiac output can occur, hypoxia only occurs when PaO_2 reaches levels below 30 mmHg.

Anemic Hypoxia. Lowered Hb decreases the oxygen carrying capacity of the blood. Acute reductions in hemoglobin without a reduction in blood volume result in circulatory disturbances which affect DO_2, although a reduction in hematocrit to as low as 20% can be tolerated by increasing CO [8]. The critical hemoglobin level at which VO_2 becomes DO_2 dependent is around 4 g/dL [9]. Chronic anemia is generally well tolerated by compensatory rises in CO, capillary recruitment, lowered blood viscosity, and a shift in the hemoglobin oxygen dissociation curve to the right.

Circulatory Hypoxia. Essentially this is a reduction in CO and can be divided into several categories: hypovolemic, cardiogenic, or obstructive.

Various experimental models have been used to assess the relationship between DO_2 and VO_2, including hemorrhage, tamponade, and balloon filling of the inferior vena cava. In the experimentally controlled environment, the transition between supply dependency and independency is sharp and well defined and graphically represented by straight lines. Laboratory studies of both whole animals [10–12] and isolated tissues [3, 13, 14] consistently demonstrate this biphasic relationship. The DO_{2crit} varies according to the model used to study it. In hemorrhagic and tamponade models values between 6–10 ml/kg/min have been observed [12, 15, 16]. In a model using balloon inflation in the inferior vena cava, De Backer et al. observed a much higher value of 18.4 ml/kg/min [11]. They suggested that this could, in part, be due to the selective reduction in blood flow in the inferior vena cava with this model, as compared to a global reduction in the hemorrhagic and tamponade models. The DO_{2crit} almost certainly varies between species and according to metabolic requirements, which could also account for some of the different values obtained. Rats have much higher metabolic demands and thus a higher DO_{2crit} (22–23 ml/kg/min) [17, 18] than dogs [12, 19]. However, despite some differences in the DO_{2crit}, many tissues appear to reach oxygen supply dependency at the same critical oxygen extraction in the range of 60–65%.

Clinical Studies. Clinical investigation of this relationship is more difficult as reducing oxygen supply below a critical level is almost certainly detrimental to the tissues. However results from Shibutani [20] and Komatsu [21] in patients undergoing elective cardiac surgery support the biphasic relationship. They made no specific interventions to alter DO_2 but took single measurements from each patient and pooled the results. Using these measures they determined a DO_{2crit} of

8 ml/kg/min with a critical oxygen extraction (O$_2$ER$_{crit}$) of about 30%. The pooled data could however obscure differences between individual patients, and the effects of anesthetic agents on oxygen extraction could also influence these results [15]. Ronco et al. [22] studied values from individual terminal patients after life support systems had been discontinued. They also found the typical biphasic relationship, but with a DO$_{2\,crit}$ value of 4.5 ± 1.3 ml/kg/min, and an O$_2$ER$_{crit}$ consistent with that of animal models. Their lower value of DO$_{2\,crit}$ may be related to the type of patient with different metabolic rates than the elective surgical patient.

Other groups have demonstrated the effects of temporarily increasing DO$_2$ with fluid administration, blood transfusion, or inotropic agents, in patients with raised or normal blood lactate levels. These studies showed no significant rise in VO$_2$ in patients with normal blood lactate levels, but in those with raised lactates, and therefore supply dependency, VO$_2$ levels rose with DO$_2$ [23, 24].

The limited clinical evidence thus certainly supports the experimental data, although it is likely that the exact values for the critical point at which oxygen uptake becomes supply dependent are very person-dependent.

Clinical Assessment

Clinically one can identify the DO$_{2\,crit}$ by looking at the level of DO$_2$ at which VO$_2$ begins to fall, or at which the blood lactate levels begin to rise. A rise in the veno-arterial difference in PCO$_2$ (VAPCO$_2$) has also been shown to occur at the level of DO$_{2\,crit}$ [25]. However it is the relationship between DO$_2$ and VO$_2$ which is most important clinically to determine the adequacy of tissue oxygenation. Direct assessment of this relationship is difficult as both parameters involve complex calculations, and the figures obtained are difficult to interpret with clinical meaning as the exact oxygen requirements of the patient are unknown. Mathematical coupling of data could also occur if the thermodilution cardiac output is used to calculate both values.

The relationship between CO and O$_2$ER [26, 27] may be of more value for the clinician, involving much simpler formulae. The two parameters are obtained independently thus avoiding any potential problems of mathematical coupling of data. By plotting a range of physiological values obtained during exercise in healthy individuals, one can compare patient values with a line of reference. Curvilinear isopleths of VO$_2$ can be drawn on the diagram and VO$_2$/DO$_2$ dependency noted by temporarily increasing DO$_2$. Dobutamine is particularly convenient for this purpose as it increases DO$_2$ while having no effect on Hb levels, a component which is not included in this diagram. If VO$_2$ remains constant and therefore independent of DO$_2$, the data points will move parallel to the VO$_2$ isopleths as compensatory changes in O$_2$ER occur (Fig. 2). However if dependency exists, non-parallel movement will occur. This is thus a simple method to assess and monitor patient condition, although it is not sufficient to base decisions on patient management solely on these measurements.

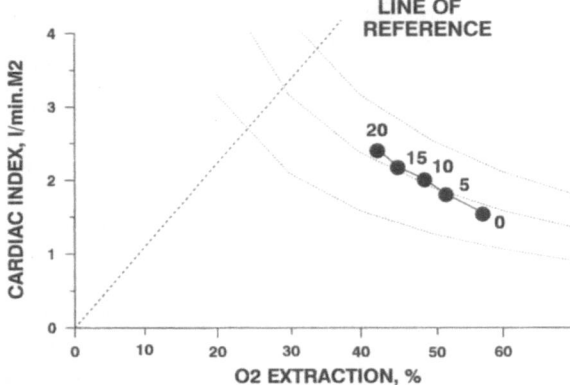

Fig. 2. Effects of a dobutamine infusion in a patient after aortic valve replacement. The numbers on the figure refer to the doses of dobutamine in mcg/kg·min. Note the lack of any significant increase in VO_2, despite the potentially thermogenic effects of dobutamine

Practical Implications

The maintenance of adequate oxygen delivery is of vital importance to the continuing function of organ systems. Once the $DO_{2\,crit}$ has been reached and tissue perfusion is threatened, organ survival is at risk. From a practical point of view, the phase of VO_2/DO_2 dependency represents the onset of shock. Re-establishment of VO_2/DO_2 independency therefore reflects the successful treatment of shock. This can be achieved by either increasing oxygen delivery, reducing oxygen demand, or a combination of both.

Increase DO_2. Referring to equation 2, one can see that DO_2 can be increased by increasing oxygen saturation, hemoglobin concentration, or cardiac output. Respiratory support should be offered to maintain SaO_2 greater than 90%, but remembering potential problems of barotrauma (with high levels of positive end-expiratory pressure) and oxygen toxicity (with high FiO_2). An optimal hemoglobin level is difficult to define as increased viscosity can negatively influence oxygen extraction capabilities. Transfusion is thus not advised for hemoglobin levels greater than 10 g/dl or hematocrits of greater than 30%. Adequate fluid administration is vital to increase cardiac output, but if this alone is not sufficient, inotropic agents should be employed. There is considerable current interest in the influence of these agents on regional blood flow and their effects on oxygen extraction, and we must await further results before any definite recommendation can be made for the use of one agent over another. However, dobutamine is currently considered the safest and most reliable to increase blood flow to the tissues.

Decrease VO_2. This is the alternative approach and is frequently employed in the ICU. Methods to reduce pain, anxiety, and muscular work, are all used in an attempt to reduce oxygen demand and improve tissue oxygenation. However the use of sedative agents, analgesics, and anesthetic agents may reduce oxygen extraction capabilities and thus potentially be detrimental [15, 28]. Mechanical ventilation is often employed to reduce VO_2 by resting respiratory muscles and decreasing respiratory workload. Cooling has been advocated as a means of reducing oxygen demand but lowering body temperature below normal also has its problems. While hypothermia may protect the injured brain, even mild reductions in core temperature may favor bleeding [33], delay healing, and predispose to infection [34]. Fever itself may be an adequate response. Experiments have shown that in infected poikilothermic animals if the febrile response is prevented, mortality increases [29]. Anti-pyretic treatments may thus be more therapeutic for the physician than for the patient.

Increase O_2ER. Improving the microcirculation may increase oxygen availability to the cells for the same global DO_2 (i.e., the same arterial oxygen content and the same CO). Experimentally under physiologic conditions, it seems the microvascular blood flow is optimally tuned and it is not possible to improve it [30, 31]. In pathophysiologic conditions, however, it may be possible to influence oxygen extraction [32].

As has been shown both clinically and experimentally, the decrease of DO_2 to a value known as $DO_{2\,crit}$, leads to the consequent occurrence of VO_2/DO_2 dependency that effectively constitutes shock. All attempts must be made to prevent this situation developing. Clinical observation and hemodynamic parameters such as cardiac index and SvO_2, must be combined with measures of tissue perfusion such as blood lactate and gastric pH (pHi) or PCO_2 ($PgCO_2$) to continually monitor the critically ill patient. The CI/O_2ER diagram may be useful in assessing more complex cases. Most interventions to prevent or correct VO_2/DO_2 dependency must aim at increasing DO_2 as reducing VO_2 is usually insufficient, and is more complex as the methods used often adversely affect DO_2 and oxygen extraction.

References

1. De Backer D, Moraine JJ, Berré J, Kahn RJ, Vincent JL (1994) Effects of dobutamine on oxygen consumption in septic patients: Direct vs indirect determinations. Am Rev Respir Crit Care Med 150:95–100
2. Takala J, Keinänen O, Väisänen P (1989) Measurement of gas exchange in intensive care: Laboratory and clinical validation of a new device. Crit Care Med 17:1041–1047
3. Kvietys PR, Granger DN (1982) Relationship between intestinal blood flow and oxygen uptake. Am J Physiol 242:G202–G209
4. Lindbom L, Tuma RF, Arfors KE (1980) Influence of oxygen on perfused capillary density and capillary red cell velocity in rabbit skeletal muscle. Microvasc Research 19:197–208
5. Cain SM, Adams RP (1965) Appearance of excess lactate in anesthetized dogs during anemic and hypoxic hypoxia. Am J Physiol 209:604–608
6. Heusser F, Fahey JT, Lister G (1987) Effect of hemoglobin concentration on critical cardiac output and oxygen transport. Am J Physiol 253:H527–H532
7. Barcroft J (1920) Physiological effects of insufficient oxygen supply. Nature 106:125–129
8. Levine E, Rosen A, Sehgal L (1992) Physiologic effects of acute anemia: Implication for a reduced transfusion trigger. Transfusion 30:11–16
9. Van Woerkens EC, Trouwborst A, Van Lanschot JJ (1992) Profound hemodilution: What is the critical level of hemodilution at which oxygen delivery-dependent oxygen consumption starts in an anesthetized human? Anesth Analg 75:818–821

10. Fahey JT, Lister G (1987) Postnatal changes in critical cardiac output and oxygen transport in conscious lambs. Am J Physiol 22:H100–H106
11. De Backer D, Roman A, Van der Linden P, Armistead C, Schiltz G, Vincent JL (1992) The effects of balloon filling into the inferior vena cava on the VO_2/DO_2 relationship. J Crit Care 7:167–173
12. Cain SM (1977) Oxygen delivery and uptake in dogs during anemic and hypoxic hypoxia. J Appl Physiol 42:228–234
13. Samsel RW, Cherqui D, Pietrabissa A, Sanders WM, Edmond JC, Schumacker PT (1991) The limits of oxygen extraction in the isolated liver. J Appl Physiol 70:186–193
14. Schlichtig R, Kramer DJ, Boston R, Pinsky MR (1991) Renal O_2 consumption during progressive hemorrhage. J Appl Physiol 70:1957–1962
15. Van der Linden P, Gilbert E, Engelman E, Schmartz D, Vincent JL (1991) Effects of anesthetic agents on systemic critical O_2 delivery. J Appl Physiol 71:83–93
16. Zhang H, Spapen H, Benlabed M, Vincent JL (1993) Systemic oxygen extraction can be improved during repeated episodes of cardiac tamponade. J Crit Care 8:93–99
17. Cain SM, Bradley WE (1983) Critical O_2 transport values at lowered body temperatures in rats. J Appl Physiol 55:1713–1717
18. Adams RP, Dieleman LA, Cain SM (1982) A critical value for O_2 transport in the rat. J Appl Physiol 53:660–664
19. Nelson DP, Beyer C, Samsel RW, Wood LDH, Schumacker PT (1987) Pathological supply dependence of O_2 uptake during bacteremia in dogs. J Appl Physiol 63:1487–1492
20. Shibutani K, Komatsu T, Kubai K, Sarchala V, Kumar V, Bizarri DV (1983) Critical level of oxygen delivery in anesthetized man. Crit Care Med 11:640–643
21. Komatsu T, Shibutani K, Okamoto K, Kumar V, Kubal K, Sanchala V, Lees DE (1987) Critical level of oxygen delivery after cardiopulmonary bypass. Crit Care Med 15:194–197
22. Ronco JJ, Fenwick JC, Tweeddale MG, Wiggs BR, Phang PT, Cooper DJ, Cunningham KF, Russell JA, Walley KR (1993) Identification of the critical oxygen delivery for anaerobic metabolism in critically ill septic and nonseptic humans. JAMA 270:1724–1730
23. Kaufman BS, Rackow EC, Falk JL (1984) The relationship between oxygen delivery and consumption during fluid resuscitation of hypovolemic and septic shock. Chest 85:336–340
24. Vincent JL, Roman A, DeBacker D, Kahn RJ (1990) Oxygen uptake/supply dependency: Effects of short-term dobutamine infusion. Am Rev Respir Dis 142:2–8
25. Zhang H, Vincent JL (1993) Arteriovenous differences in PCO_2 and pH are good indicators of critical hypoperfusion. Am Rev Respir Dis 148:867–871
26. Silance PG, Simon C, Vincent JL (1994) The relation between cardiac index and oxygen extraction in acutely ill patients. Chest 105:1190–1197
27. Vincent JL (1996) Determination of O_2 delivery and consumption vs cardiac index vs oxygen extraction ratio. Crit Care Clin 12:995–1006
28. Berton CC, Schnitzler B, Thill B (1996) Reduction in oxygen demand, normalization of oxygen delivery and oxygen extraction. Réan Urg 5:302–312
29. Bernheim HA, Kluger MJ (1976) Fever: Effect of drug-induced antipyresis on survival. Science 193:237–239
30. Zhang H, Spapen H, Vincent JL (1994) The effects of dobutamine and norepinephrine on oxygen availability in tamponade-induced stagnant hypoxia. Crit Care Med 22:299–305
31. Zhang H, Nguyen DN, Spapen H, Moock M, Maciel F, Vincent JL (1995) Sodium nitroprusside does not influence tissue oxygen extraction capabilities during a critical reduction in oxygen delivery. Cardiovasc Res 30:240–245
32. Zhang H, Spapen H, Manikis P, Rogiers P, Vincent JL (1995) Tirilazad mesylate (U74006F) improves systemic and splanchnic oxygen extraction capabilities following endotoxic shock. Am J Physiol 268:H1847–H1855
33. Schmied H, Kurz A, Sessler DI, Kozek S, Reiter A (1996) Mild hypothermia increases blood loss and transfusion requirements during total hip arthroplasty. Lancet 347:289–292
34. Kurz A, Sessler DI, Lenhardt R (1996) Perioperative normothermia to reduce the incidence of surgical-wound infection and shorten hospitalization. Study of wound infection and temperature. N Engl J Med 334:1209–1215

Pathophysiology of VO_2/DO_2 in Sepsis

B. Vallet

Introduction

The high molar demand for oxygen (O_2) compared to other metabolic substrates implies that tissues deplete blood of O_2 much sooner than of these other substrates. Under normal resting conditions, tissue O_2 demand rather than tissue O_2 supply (DO_2) determines the rate of O_2 uptake (VO_2). When blood carries less than the normal amount of O_2 or when blood flow is reduced, DO_2 is reduced and compensatory adjustments occur in an attempt to satisfy the O_2 requirements of peripheral tissues. As DO_2 is gradually reduced, O_2 consumption (VO_2) is maintained by increases in the O_2 extraction ratio ($ERO_2 = VO_2/DO_2$), until a critical point at which VO_2 falls with further declines in DO_2. At this critical point, tissues shift toward a chemically reduced state with elaboration of reduced substrate forms such as lactate. It has been proposed that increased ERO_2 is a consequence of regulation of the circulation and the result of the simultaneous activation of both central and local factors. Central factor induces a regional redistribution of blood flow among tissues via sympathetic vasoconstrictor tone while local factor or autoregulation induces an increase in the density of perfused capillaries within tissues via metabolic vasodilator tone. Local autoregulatory processes include local release and action of vasodilating substances. An inability to regulate blood flow distribution, between and within tissues, could result in hyperperfusion of some tissue beds at the expense of other hypoperfused areas resulting in O_2 extraction defect as seen in sepsis.

Matching of DO_2 to VO_2

Interregional Matching of DO_2 to O_2 Demand

Redistribution of whole body DO_2 among organs may promote macrovascular O_2 regulation by reducing perfusion of organs that are normally overperfused relative to need. Thus diversion of unnecessary flow from organs such as the kidneys and splanchnic viscera to the heart and brain during critically low whole body DO_2 could enhance VO_2 of the whole organism [1]. The question of blood flow redistribution among organs in response to declining whole body DO_2 is closely related to the question of whether all organs become supply dependent simultaneously, or in a hierarchical fashion. Under normal circumstances, blood flow to each organ is matched to prevailing needs such that each organ receives a given fraction of the whole body DO_2. However, when the whole body DO_2 is compromised, it is redistributed so that some organs receive a progressively smaller fraction of whole body DO_2, while others receive progressively more. Laboratory animal demonstrations generally support that all organs become O_2 supply-dependent at the same whole body DO_2 value (for a review see Ref. [2]). For example, during progressive hemorrhage the intestine appears to become O_2 supply-dependent at about the same systemic O_2 delivery as the whole body (9.7 ± 2.7 ml·min^{-1}·kg^{-1} vs 7.9 ± 1.9 ml·min^{-1}·kg^{-1} respectively) [3, 4]. Likewise, Ward et al. [5] demonstrated that the whole body O_2 delivery at which the resting diaphragm VO_2 becomes supply limited is similar to that for nondiaphragmatic tissue. In the isolated canine hindlimb, it has been found VO_2 becoming supply-limited at a systemic O_2 delivery of ~ 6 ml·min^{-1}·kg^{-1} during hemorrhage when whole body critical DO_2 was 6 to 8 ml·min^{-1}·kg^{-1} [6, 7].

Schlichtig et al. [1] mathematically demonstrated that redistribution of whole body DO_2 among organs is a determinant of whole body critical DO_2, i.e. that redistribution of whole body DO_2 among organs enhances the ability of the whole animal to maintain VO_2 supply independent. Supporting this finding Cain [8] previously demonstrated that a vigorous constrictor tone was necessary during whole body hypoxia for improving efficiency in extracting O_2, presumably by redistribution of flow. After O_2 delivery was lowered during hypoxic hypoxia ($FiO_2 = 9\%$) in control anesthetized and paralyzed dogs, O_2 extraction ratio increased from 54% at 10 min of hypoxia to 87% at the end of hypoxia, just before death. Survival time in this group was 70 ± 30 min. In another group of dogs treated with phenoxybenzamine, a potent α-blocker, O_2 extraction did not increase (46% vs 43%) with time and was significantly less than in the unblocked group. Survival time in this group was only 35 ± 16 min. These results proved that a vigorous vasoconstrictor sympathetic tone during hypoxia conserved oxygenation and increased survival time by promoting greater extraction by the tissues. Presumably, the sympathetic tone maintains arteriolar blood flow to metabolically active tissues while reducing blood flow to nonactive ones [9]. Thereby, an increase in sympathetically mediated vasoconstrictor tone prevents the "vascular steal" of blood flow away from regions with high metabolic demand.

Local Tissue Matching of DO_2 to O_2 Demand

However, even if arteriolar blood flow goes to the correct tissues in proportion to their needs, there is no guarantee that the downstream capillaries receive this blood in an amount proportional to the needs of their tissues. According to the metabolic theory of microvascular regulation, metabolic vasodilation in tissues with relatively high metabolic rates competes with sympathetic vasoconstrictor tone, thereby affecting a balance between local tissue O_2 supply and demand. Basically, the proponents of the direct PO_2 hypothesis suggest that interstitial PO_2, through its proposed direct effect on vascular smooth muscle tone, is the necessary link between parenchymal metabolism and microvascular tone. Hence, any condition leading to a decreased interstitial PO_2 will elicit a vascular dilation and therefore tissue oxygenation will be returned to normal. On the other hand, excessive tissue oxygenation causes a vasoconstriction and consequent fall of interstitial PO_2 toward normal.

Granger et al. [10] have identified a useful dichotomy in blood vessels controlling peripheral microcirculatory flow: flow controlling vessels and distribution vessels. Total regional flow is determined by large vessels (medium-sized arterioles) where the majority of the arteriovenous pressure gradient is dissipated. By contrast, local distribution of flow is determined downstream, by precapillary sphincters in tissues that have them, or by similarly sized precapillary arterioles in all tissues. It has been argued that these vascular regions are separately controlled. The distribution vessels are primarily under local control, responding to buildup of vasodilator metabolites, and largely refractory to sympathetic control. Upstream flow controlling vessels are mainly controlled by sympathetic and other regional control systems, although ultimately they are also subject to metabolic feedback (for a review see Ref. [11]).

According to this, Paul Schumacker and his group [12, 13] determined whether cardiovascular reflex responses to hypovolemia contribute to local O_2 extraction efficacy during progressive reductions in blood flow. They first examined the role of sympathetically mediated vasoconstriction on the critical level of O_2 extraction in dog hindlimb during progressive reduction in O_2 delivery [12]. They used two different approaches to limit sympathetic contributions. In a first group, delivery to the limb was locally reduced while sympathetic tone was minimized by using volume administration to maintain cardiac output. In a second group, α-adrenergic efferent activity was blocked with phenoxybenzamine. Both methods produced a significant impairment in critical O_2 extraction by hindlimb. By contrast, when sympathetic activity was stimulated by blood removal, hindlimb VO_2 was preserved to a higher O_2 extraction ratio. In another study, the same group using the same study design [13] investigated the contribution of the autonomic nervous system in intestinal O_2 extraction. In the intestine, the critical O_2 extraction ratio was significantly poorer in the normovolemic group ($45 \pm 11\%$) than in either α-intact-hypovolemic group ($69 \pm 3\%$) or α-blocked-hypovolemic group ($62 \pm 9\%$). Although phenoxybenzamine treatment markedly reduced gut vascular resistance, it did not alter O_2 extraction ability.

For the authors, these observations suggested
1) that relative roles of humoral and neural mechanisms in controlling the microvascular adjustment to lowered QO_2 may differ among tissues (humoral mechanisms – vasopressine or renin – may contribute to intestinal vasoconstriction); and
2) that a functional difference exists between the vessels controlling microvascular distribution of capillary blood flow and those responsible for intestinal vascular resistance.

The authors referred to the functional distinction between flow- and distribution-controlling vessels proposed by Granger et al. [10], stating that it is possible that sympathetic nerve activity alone may not be sufficient to achieve high O_2 extraction.

Therefore, although it appears to be true for the whole body that a vigorous constrictor tone is necessary during hypoxia for improving efficiency in extracting O_2, it does not hold at the level of organ systems. In support of this, Cain and Chapler [14] infusing norepinephrine intraarterially into canine hindlimb demonstrated that O_2 uptake was able to be maintained by increased O_2 extraction despite a threefold increase in vascular resistance and a 30% decrease in blood flow. This provided another indication that increased vasoconstrictor tone does not interfere with greater O_2 extraction at the level of an organ. Cain and Chapler suggested that to achieve greater O_2 extraction precapillary vessels (distribution-controlling vessels) must be relaxed and capillary surface area enlarged. They noticed that despite continuous infusion of norepinephrine, resistance decreased by approximately 40%, consistent with a local metabolic regulation-mediated relaxation phenomenon. Central and humoral vasoconstrictor responses were thought to be overridden by local chemical control of microvascular tone.

O_2-Sensing Structures and Their Localization

In parallel to global control systems there exist local mechanisms which regulate the matching of O_2 demand and O_2 supply within an individual organ. The nature of the O_2-sensitive structures acting at the local tissue level is not completely understood. There is evidence that parenchymal cells, under conditions of hypoxia, release increased amounts of metabolites such as adenosine, lactate, hydrogen ions and potassium ions, which accumulate in the tissue. These metabolites induce relaxation of the vascular smooth muscle resulting in an increased blood flow in the hypoxic area [15]. This mechanism, however, implies that the cells must suffer from a certain degree of hypoxia before the organ blood flow will be affected. Therefore, another principle of control could be located in arterial vessels themselves, allowing a more rapid response to changes of blood O_2 tension without involvement of parenchymal cells. This implies that blood vessels are directly affected if the O_2 content or tension of the blood is reduced, either as a result of hypoxemia or owing to an augmented extraction of O_2.

Endothelial cells which are in direct contact with the flowing blood have a number of properties which predestinate them as effective functional O_2 sensors [16]. The endothelium lining the entire circulatory system is a highly specialized tissue involved in immune responses, vascular cell growth, and in the regulation of the level of hemostatic, inflammatory, and vasoactive agents in the blood. The endothelium releases autacoids (tissue hormones) which decisively affect vascular tone and platelet function [17]. Many endothelium-derived relaxing autacoids have been described and characterized, among them prostacyclin (PGI_2), the potent vasodilator compound endothelium-derived relaxing factor [EDRF, which is believed to be nitric oxide (NO) or a related compound], and a putative endothelium-dependent hyperpolarizing factor (EDHF). EDRF/NO stimulates soluble guanylate cyclase in vascular smooth muscle directly and induces vasodilation by cyclic GMP-dependent mechanisms; PGI_2 elicits an increase of cellular cyclic AMP by a receptor dependent stimulation of adenylate cyclase; EDHF (and to some extent EDRF and PGI_2) induce hyperpolarization through opening of potassium channels, inhibiting calcium influx and mediating vasodilation.

The release of these autacoids is not only stimulated by receptor-dependent stimuli but also by a number of physical stimuli, and it was hypothesized that endothelial cells may also respond specifically to changes in O_2 tension. Indeed, altough synthesis of these autacoids is dependent on molecular O_2, investigators suggested that progressive hypoxia significantly augmented production of EDRF/NO [18], PGI_2 [19] and/or activated ATP-sensitive K^+ channels possibly via increased EDHF release [20–22]. Moreover, it has been demonstrated that endothelial cells are involved in tissue O_2 extraction ability [23]. An endothelial O_2 sensor in the vascular wall would enable the vasculature to respond rapidly to decreases in arterial PO_2 without need from previous accumulation, with the potential risk of hypoxia-induced parenchymal cell damage. Such an hypoxic signal would be particularly effective in conduit arteries which are not reached by tissue metabolites for the balance of the vasomotor tone in these vessels and for the adjustment of global tissue perfusion.

VO₂ to DO₂ Dependency

Whole Body O₂ Extraction is Impaired During Sepsis

A decreased ability to extract O_2 has been reported in patients and in animal models of sepsis. When anesthetized dogs are injected with either live bacteria or endotoxin (lipopolysaccharide, LPS) and hemorrhaged in steps to lower DO_2, critical DO_2 is raised and ERO_2 is lowered in the whole body [4, 24]. The mathematical model of no blood flow distribution described above [1] suggests that only minor disturbance of blood flow redistribution can produce a significant change in the value of whole body critical DO_2. The blood flow among organs is altered during bacteremia or endotoxemia [25, 26] suggesting that bacterial infection might cause regional changes in vascular tone. Nelson et al. [24] hypothesized that during sepsis maldistribution of blood flow among organs relative to organ O_2 demand could produce an abnormal O_2 supply dependency for the whole body by preferentially forcing some tissues into supply limitation while other tissues were relatively hyperperfused. They tested this hypothesis by comparing a control group of dogs and a group receiving a continuous infusion of live *Pseudomonas aeruginosa*. Their results demonstrated that infusion of live bacteria was associated with an increased whole body critical DO_2 threshold and a reduced critical O_2 extraction ratio.

In a further study, Nelson et al. [4] tested whether endotoxin administration, and not only live bacteria, also reduces the efficacy of systemic extraction in dogs. They found that treatment with *E. coli* endotoxin doubled the minimum systemic DO_2 needed to maintain VO_2 in dogs. This type of situation resembles that of the phenoxybenzamine-treated animals in the study from Cain [8] that was previously discussed.

Evidence of regional hypoperfusion resulting from dysregulation of vascular tone in arterial and venous vessels has been reported in sepsis. Dissimilar effects may occur among different vascular beds, resulting in abnormalities with respect to the distribution of capillary blood flow and blood volume [27]. For example, in non-resuscitated endotoxemic shock models, a vasodilatory response was noted in the hepatic circulation [28] whereas an intense vasoconstriction was seen in the gut circulation. Moreover, large differences among vascular beds have been noted regarding the effects of endotoxemia on the responsiveness of isolated blood vessels [29], although convincing evidence exists today that a general effect of endotoxin infusion *in vivo* is a loss of contractile responsiveness in *ex vivo* vascular tissue.

Vascular Reactivity is Impaired During Sepsis

Numerous studies have presented results of impaired contractile responses to α-adrenergic agonists in vessels from endotoxemic animals [29–32]. Umans et al. [29] confirmed and extended these findings by demonstrating impaired contractions in response to angiotensin II and serotonin. This generalized contractile defect suggested for the authors basic alterations in calcium mobilization or in the contractile apparatus within vascular smooth muscle. NO synthase (NOS) inhibitors largely restore the contractile responses to agonists. Importantly, it has been demonstrated that this effect of NOS inhibitors was maintained in vessels whose endothelium have been removed, suggesting that *in vivo* LPS administration leads to the expression of a NO synthase (inducible NOS isoform) within vascular smooth muscle cells [29, 32] increasing the activity of guanylate cyclase and impairing contractile responses. These changes correspond to the pathophysiologic features of clinical and experimental sepsis and may account for the profound vasodilation and the limited response to the normal endogenous stimuli that regulate blood flow distribution among organs.

Also, Parker et al. [33] and Umans et al. [29] have demonstrated attenuated acetylcholine-induced endothelium-dependent relaxation *in vitro* following canine endotoxemia and hypothesized that this defect was due to impaired release of EDRF/NO by the endothelial constitutive NOS isoform. Alternatively, the induction of smooth muscle NOS, leading to the enhanced basal activation of guanylate cyclase, might limit further relaxation in response to the acetylcholine-stimulated release of EDRF/NO.

However, the hypothesis that the vascular defect during sepsis is due entirely to excessive NO synthesis appears too simplistic since inhibition of NO synthase using the nonspecific inhibitor L-nitroarginine methyl ester (L-NAME) *in vivo* failed to restore a normal O_2 extraction ability during endotoxemia [34]. Administration of that compound during endotoxemia produced a partial restoration of systemic blood pressure, but cardiac output decreased significantly even though left atrial pressures were maintained. It is conceivable that an inhibitor that acts selectively on the inducible isoform of NO synthase might be of benefit, since physiological NO synthesis by the constitutive isoform in endothelial cells would be preserved. However, the observation that the nonspecific inhibitor L-NAME does not significantly impair critical O_2 extraction in non septic animals suggests that endothelial NO synthesis is not essential for the vascular regulation that determines tissue O_2 extraction at low levels of O_2 delivery [34, 35]. Moreover, recent work has questioned the specificity of individual NO synthase inhibitors [36-38] as well as the usefulness of NO synthase inhibitors [39] in septic shock [40]. Further studies are required to fully clarify the cellular mechanisms underlying the vascular dysfunction that occurs in sepsis.

Regional O_2 Extraction is Impaired During Sepsis

Clearly, we also have to consider that the blood vessels described in previous studies are conduit arteries and are not directly responsible for either vascular resistance or blood flow distribution. However, recent studies in the isolated perfused rabbit heart [41], autoperfused rat cremaster[42], and rat mesenteric microvascular segment [43] suggest that similar mechanisms may be operative in the microvasculature. Using intravital microscopy on extensor digitorum longus muscle in rats made septic by caecal ligation and puncture (CLP), Lam et al. [44] found that sepsis was associated with a 36% reduction in tissue perfused capillary density. The spatial distribution of perfused capillaries was also more heterogeneous, and the mean intercapillary distance increased by 30%. They concluded that sepsis affects the ability of the skeletal muscle microcirculation to distribute red blood cells flux and consequentely O_2 appropriately. Moreover, when using laser Doppler flowmetry to assess the functional hyperemic response of the muscle before and after a period of maximal twitch designed to increase O_2 demand, the authors observed after contraction that the relative increase in red blood cell flux was less in CLP rats. They further concluded that sepsis affects the ability of microcirculation to respond to increases in O_2 need.

An impaired reactivity to catecholamines associated with a direct inhibitory effect of LPS on endothelial NO biosynthesis might result in a defective blood flow distribution and inappropriate focal vasodilation/vasoconstriction. Moreover, these EDRF/NO-related perfusion abnormalities may be enhanced or complicated by other mechanisms affecting vascular reactivity such as activation of ATP-sensitive K^+ channels in vascular smooth muscle [45].

In view of such abnormalities, Nelson et al. [4] suggested that sepsis could cause a maldistribution of blood flow not only among organs but also within organ systems. They tested the hypothesis that abnormal O_2 supply dependence seen at the whole-body level also existed within organ systems by measuring the local O_2 extraction efficacy in an autoperfused loop of small intestine. The intestine was chosen for study because it normally exhibits a high rate of VO_2 compared with other tissues. The authors observed a pathological O_2 supply dependency in their analysis of the VO_2-DO_2 relation of endotoxemic dog intestine, suggesting that endotoxemia impairs O_2 extraction at the organ level. This impairment was associated with an ablated reactive hyperemia in six of seven animals, and Nelson et al. [4] suggested that the defect in efficacy of O_2 extraction is due to microvascular injury and/or appearance of greater heterogeneity of microvascular distribution of DO_2 with respect to O_2 demand in endotoxin-treated animals. The authors stated that if microvascular smooth muscle responsiveness to catecholamines is altered, the effective regulation of local blood flow in relation to local perivascular metabolic activity will be disordered, leading to onset of O_2 supply dependence along some capillaries, whereas others are excessively perfused.

In another study, Samsel et al. [6] examined the isolated hindlimb to determine if an O_2 extraction defect similar to that seen in the intestine arises in skeletal muscle. After giving endotoxin, they measured systemic and hindlimb O_2 extraction as systemic DO_2 was reduced by withdrawal of blood. They found that the hindlimb, unlike the intestine, extracted O_2 normally after endotoxin administration, suggesting that the tissue response to endotoxin is not uniform. Of interest, they found that endotoxin did not ablate reactive hyperemia after brief arterial occlusions in the hindlimb. In contrast, in two separate studies, Bredle et al. [7, 46] observed that a mild O_2 extraction defect was produced in dog hindlimb by endotoxin. However, the increase in critical O_2 delivery in these studies was smaller than that seen earlier for the whole body or the gut and it was concluded that muscle is not a major contributor to the impaired O_2 extraction in endotoxemia.

In the absence of proof that a disruption in blood flow distribution occurs within organ during sepsis and that this disruption is linked to decreased O_2 extraction ability, we attempted to answer that question by generating surface tissue PO_2 ($PtiO_2$) measurements from skeletal muscle and gut mucosa and serosa during endotoxemia, before and after volume resuscitation [47]. Distribution of $PtiO_2$ histograms may be used to characterize the relationship between capillary O_2 delivery and cellular O_2 requirements and to reflect changes in microvascular control [48]. Under normal physiological conditions, relationship of capillary perfusion to cellular O_2 demand is well matched and the $PtiO_2$ histogram has a shape approximating a Gaussian distribution. When the microcirculation is disturbed. the histogram becomes irregular with a dispersion of values. In our study, skeletal muscle exhibited preserved O_2 extraction ability. Its VO_2 remained unchanged and ERO_2 reached 78% by the end of LPS infusion suggesting that muscle microcirculation was probably not severely disturbed. Consistent with this interpretation, the tissue PO_2 histograms in muscle maintained a near-Gaussian distribution supporting the finding of Gutierrez et al. [49], that skeletal muscle microcirculatory heterogeneity did not increase during endotoxin-induced sepsis. In the gut, VO_2 and intramucosal pH (pHi) significantly decreased, and although intestinal DO_2 returned to baseline with volume resuscitation, VO_2 and pHi never recovered. The failure of gut VO_2 to rebound with resuscitation is consistent with earlier LPS dog studies [50] but is in sharp contrast to non-LPS models of gut ischemia, including studies of systemic hypoxic hypoxia [51] or ischemic hypoxia [52, 53]. In these non-LPS models, gut VO_2, as well as pHi, returned to baseline with resuscitation despite a more severe period of decreased DO_2 than in our study. This suggested that the physiology of shock associated with LPS has features such as inflammatory mediators that are non present in non-LPS hypoxia or ischemia that cause a sustained disturbance in gut VO$_2$. This may be related to cell death, microcirculatory supply limitation, or both. The tissue PO$_2$ distribution suggested that, during endotoxemia, tissue hypoxia persisted in the mucosa despite resuscitation, and that increased blood flow within the gut wall was heterogeneously redistributed from the mucosa to the muscularis. Therefore, after LPS infusion, blood flow-controlling sites in the gut microcirculation appeared to be inadequate to maintain mucosal perfusion and oxygenation, and unable to prevent the preferential onset of supply dependency in the gut despite more than adequate blood flow following fluid infusion.

In support of changes in reactive properties of vascular tissue, Drazenovic et al. [54] showed that gut adjustments in perfused capillary surface density, in response to changes in DO$_2$, were impaired after LPS administration. Whithworth et al. [55] showed that the vascular tone between intestinal little arterioles was imbalanced in an hyperdynamic model of sepsis in rats. Third-order arterioles, which terminate as central villous arterioles, were more constricted than first or second-order arterioles, leading specifically to compromised mucosal blood flow. Therefore, local tissue hypoperfusion during endotoxemia could result from a failure of vascular tissue to respond normally to metabolic vasodilatory stimuli and to match the local O$_2$ supply to demand. Even in the setting of systemic vasodilation, an inappropriate focal vasoconstriction could occur as a potential mechanism for focal tissue hypoxia.

Conclusion

Several authors have suggested that an among-organ defect in blood flow distribution may account for impaired whole body O$_2$ regulation. The first, Cain [8] observed, in a hypoxic hypoxia model, that O$_2$ extraction ratio and whole body VO$_2$ were considerably lower at the point of circulatory crisis in dogs treated with phenoxybenzamine than in control dogs, suggesting that whole body O$_2$ utilization is more efficient when vasoconstrictor tone is intact than during α-adrenergic blockade. Schumacker and Cain [56] hypothesized later that a within-organ defect in blood flow related to an abnormal vascular reactivity may account for impaired organ O$_2$ regulation.

If specific classes of microvessels must constrict or relax to achieve efficient O$_2$ extraction during limitation of DO$_2$, then impaired vascular reactivity might produce pathological supply limitation. In this regard, infusion of lipopolysaccharide produces an O$_2$ extraction impairment.

In sepsis, the inflammatory response profoundly alters the homeostatic circulatory process of the body. The proposed mechanisms operative in this response and some of the putative mediators induce decreased adrenergic receptor sensitivity and abnormal microvascular events. These events involve microemboli of formed cellular elements, endothelial swelling, and release of vasoconstricting or vasodilating substances. This has been referred as a malignant intravascular inflammation that alters vasomotor tone and the distibution of blood flow among and within organs [9]. As endotoxin elicits release of endogenous vasodilators (EDRF/NO, PGI_2, EDHF) and/or constrictors (endothelin, platelet activating factor, thromboxane A_2), it may

1) undermine the systemic compensatory vasoconstriction that normally occurs when blood flow is reduced, and
2) compromise the local autoregulatory processes, thereby limiting tissue extraction responses to decreased O_2 supply.

References

1. Schlichtig R, Kramer DJ, Pinsky MR (1991) Flow redistribution during progressive hemorrhage is a determinant of critical O_2 delivery. J Appl Physiol 70:169–178
2. Schlichtig R (1993) O_2 uptake, critical O_2 delivery, and tissue wellness. In: Pinsky MR, Dhainaut JF (eds) Pathophysiologic foundations of critical care. Williams and Wilkins, Baltimore, pp 119–139
3. Nelson DP, King CE, Dodd SL, Schumacker PT, Cain SM (1987) Systemic and intestinal limits of O_2 extraction in the dog. J Appl Physiol 63:387–394
4. Nelson DP, Samsel RW, Wood LDH, Schumacker PT (1988) Pathological supply dependence of systemic and intestinal O_2 uptake during endotoxemia. J Appl Physiol 64:2410–2419
5. Ward ME, Chang H, Erice F, Hussain SNA (1994) Systemic and diaphragmatic oxygen delivery-consumption relationships during hemorrhage. J Appl Physiol 77:653–659
6. Samsel RW, Nelson DP, Sanders WM, Wood LDH, Schumacker PT (1988) Effect of endotoxin on systemic and skeletal muscle O_2 extraction. J Appl Physiol 65:1377–1382
7. Bredle DL, Samsel RW, Schumacker PT, Cain SM (1989) Critical O_2 delivery to skeletal muscle at high and low PO_2 in endotoxemic dogs. J Appl Physiol 66:2553–2558
8. Cain SM (1978) Effects of time and vasoconstrictor tone on O_2 extraction during hypoxic hypoxia. J Appl Physiol 45:219–278
9. Pinsky MR (1995) Regional blood flow distribution. In: Pinsky MR, Dhainaut JF, Artigas A (eds) The splanchnic circulation: no longer a silent partner. Springer-Verlag. Berlin, pp 1–13
10. Granger HJ, Goodman AH, Cook Billy H (1975) Metabolic models of microcirculatory regulation. Federation Proc 34:2025–2030
11. Samsel RW, Schumacker PT (1992) Pathologic supply dependence of oxygen utilization. In: Principles of critical care medicine. Williams and Wilkins, Baltimore, pp 667–678
12. Maginiss LA, Connolly H, Samsel RW, Schumacker PT (1994) Adrenergic vasoconstriction augments tissue O_2 extraction during reductions in O_2 delivery. J Appl Physiol 76:1454–1461
13. Samsel RW, Schumacker PT (1994) Systemic hemorrhage augments local O_2 extraction. J Appl Physiol 77:2291–2298
14. Cain SM, Chapter CK (1981) Effects of norepinephrine and alpha-block on O_2 uptake and blood flow in dog hindlimb. J Appl Physiol 51:1245–1250
15. Skinner NS, Costin JC (1968) Tissue metabolites and regulation of local blood flow. Fed Proc 27:1426–1429
16. Pohl U (1990) Endothelial cells as a part of a vascular oxygen-sensing system: hypoxia-induced release of autacoids. Experientia 46:1175–1179
17. Vanhoutte PM (1989) Endothelium and control of vascular function. State of the art lecture. Hypertension 13:658–667
18. Pohl U, Busse R (1989) Hypoxia stimulates release of endothelium-derived relaxant factor. Am J Physiol 956:H1595–1600
19. Michiels C, Arnould T, Dieu M, Remacle J (1993) Stimulation of prostaglandin synthesis by human endothelial cells exposed to hypoxia. Am J Physiol 264:C866–C874
20. Standen NB, Quayle JM, Davies NW, Brayden JE, Huang Y, Nelson MT (1989) Hyperpolarizing vasodilators activate ATP-sensitive K^+ channels in arterial smooth muscle. Science Wash DC 245:177–180

21. Daut J, Maier-Rudolph W, Von Beckerath N, Mehrke G, Günther K, Goedel-Meinen L (1990) Hypoxic dilation of coronary arteries is mediated by ATP-sensitive potassium channels. Science Wash DC 247:1341–1344

22. Vallet B, Curtis SE, Guery B, Mangalaboyi J, Menager P, Cain SM, Chopin C, Dupuis BA (1995) ATP-sensitive K$^+$ channel blockade impairs oxygen extraction during progressive ischemia in pig hindlimb. J Appl Physiol 79:2035–2042

23. Curtis SE, Vallet B, Winn MJ, Caufield JB, Cain SM (1995) Ablation of the vascular endothelium causes an oxygen extraction defect in canine skeletal muscle. J Appl Physiol 79:1352–1360

24. Nelson DP, Bever C, Samsel RW, Wood L, Schumacker PT (1987) Pathological supply dependence of O$_2$ uptake during bacteremia in dogs. J Appl Physiol 63:1487–1492

25. Van Lambalgen AA, Bronsveld W, Van den Bos GC, Thijs KG (1984) Distribution of cardiac output, oxygen consumption and lactate production in canine endotoxic shock. Cardiovasc Res 18:195–201

26. Breslow MJ, Miller CF, Parker SD, Walman AT, Traystman RJ (1987) Effect of vasopressors on organ blood flow during endotoxin shock in pigs. Am J Physiol 252:H291–300

27. Carrol G, Synder J (1982) Hyperdynamic severe intravascular sepsis depends on fluid administration in cyonomolgus monkey. AmJ Physiol 243:R131–141

28. Garrisson RN, Ratcliffe DJ, Fry DE (1980) Hepatocellular function and nutrient blood flow in experimental peritonitis. Surgery 92:713–719

29. Umans JG, Wylam ME, Samsel RW, Edwards J, Schumacker PT (1993) Effects of endotoxin *in vivo* on endothelial and smooth-muscle function in rabbit and rat aorta. Am Rev Repir Dis 148:1638–1645

30. Wakabayashi I, Hatake K, Kakishita E, Nagai K (1987) Diminution of contractile response of the aorta from endotoxin-injected rats. Eur J Pharmacol 141:117–122

31. Mc Kenna TM (1988) Enhanced vascular effects of cyclic GMP in septic rat aorta. Am J Physiol 23:R436–R442

32. Julou-Schaeffer G, Gray GA, Fleming I, Schott C, Parratt JR, Stoclet JC (1990) Loss of vascular responsiveness induced by endotoxin involves L-arginine pathway. Am J Physiol 259:H1038–H1043

33. Parker JL, Keller RS, DeFily DV, Laughlin MH, Novotny MJ, Adams HR (1991) Coronary vascular smooth muscle function in *E. coli* endotoxemia in dogs. Am J Physiol 260:H832–H842

34. Schumacker PT, Kazaglis J, Connolly HV, Samsel RW, O'Connor MF, Umans JG (1995) Systemic and gut oxygen extraction during endotoxemia: role of nitric oxide synthesis. Am J Respir Crit Care Med 151:107–115

35. Vallet B, Curtis SE, Winn MJ, King CE, Chapler CK, Cain SM (1994) Hypoxic vasodilation does not require nitric oxide (EDRF/NO) synthesis. J Appl Physiol 76:1256–1261

36. Peterson DA, Peteron DC, Archer S, Weir EK (1992) The nonspecificity of specific nitric oxide synthase inhibitors. Biochem Biophys Res Commun 187:797–801

37. Winn MJ, Asante NK, Ku DD (1993) Vasomotor responses of canine arterial rings to N^G-monomethyl-L-arginine and N$^\omega$-nitro L-arginine methyl ester. J Pharmacol Exp Ther 264:265–270

38. Winn MJ, Vallet B, Asante NK, Curtis SE, Cain SM (1993) Effects of N^G-substituted arginines on coronary vascular function after endotoxin. J Appl Physiol 75:424–431

39. Wright CE, Rees DD, Moncada S (1992) Protective and pathological roles of nitric oxide in endotoxin shock. Cardiovasc Res 26:48–57

40. Cobb JP, Natanson C, Quezado ZMN, Hoffman WD, Koev CA, Banks S, Correa R, Levi R, Elin RJ, Hosseini JM, Danner RL (1995) Differential hemodynamic effects of L-NMMA in endotoxemic and normal dogs. Am J Physiol 268:H1634–H1642

41. Smith RE, Palmer RMJ, Moncada S (1991) Coronary vasodilation induced by endotoxin in the rabbit isolated perfused heart is nitric oxide-dependent and inhibited by dexamethasone. Br J Pharmacol 140:5–6

42. Lübbe AS, Garrison RN, Cryer HM, Alsip NL, Harris PD (1992) EDRF as a possible mediator of sepsis-induced arteriolar dilation in skeletal muscle. Am J Physiol 262:H880–H887

43. Schneider F, Schott C, Stoclet JC, Julou-Schaeffer G (1992) L-arginine induces relaxation of small mesenteric arteries from endotoxin-treated rats. Eur J Pharmacol 211:269–272

44. Lam C, Tyml K, Martin C, Sibbald W (1994) Microvascular perfusion is impaired in a rat model of normotensive sepsis. J Clin Invest 94:2077–2083
45. Landry DW, Oliver JA (1992) The ATP-sensitive K$^+$ channel mediates hypotension in endotoxemia and hypoxic lactic acidosis in dog. J Clin Invest 89:2071–2074
46. Bredle DL, Cain SM (1991) Systemic and muscle oxygen uptake/delivery after dopexamine infusion in endotoxic dogs. Crit Care Med 19:198–204
47. Vallet B, Lund N, Curtis SE, Kelly DR, Cain SM (1994) Gut and muscle tissue PO$_2$ in endotoxemic dogs during shock and resuscitation. J Appl Physiol 76:793–800
48. Thorborg P, Malmqvist LA, Lund N (1988) Surface oxygen pressure distributions in rabbit skeletal muscle: dependence on arterial PO$_2$. Microcirc Endothel Lymphatics 4:169–192
49. Gutierrez G, Lund N, Palizas F (1991) Rabbit skeletal muscle PO$_2$ during hypodynamic sepsis. Chest 99:224–229
50. Curtis SE, Cain SM (1992) Regional and systemic oxygen delivery/uptake relations and lactate flux in hyperdynamic, endotoxin-treated dogs. Am Rev Respir Dis 145:348–354
51. Dodd SL, King CE, Cain SM (1987) Responses of innervated and denervated gut to whole-body hypoxia. J Appl Physiol 62:651–657
52. Curtis SE, Cain SM (1992b) Systemic and regional O$_2$ delivery and uptake in bled dogs given hypertonic saline, whole blood, or dextran. Am J Physiol 262:H778–H786
53. Montgomery A, Hartmann M, Jonsson K, Haglund UH (1989) Intramucosal pH measurement for detecting gastrointestinal ischemia in porcine hemorrhagic shock. Circ Shock 29:319–327
54. Drazenovic R, Samsel RW, Wylam ME, Doerschuk CM, Schumacker PT (1992) Regulation of perfused capillary density in canine intestinal mucosa during endotoxemia. J Appl Physiol 72:259–265
55. Whithworth PW, Cryer HM, Garrison RN, Baumgarten TE, Harris PD (1989) Hypoperfusion of the intestinal microcirculation without decreased cardiac output during live *Escherichia coli* sepsis in rats. Circ Shock 27:111–122
56. Schumacker PT, Cain SM (1987) The concept of a critical oxygen delivery. Intensive Care Med 13:223–229

Metabolic Targets in Acute Resuscitation

S. Beloucif, Nathalie Kermarrec, and D. Payen

The metabolic targets in acute resuscitation are to correct two separate but frequently intricated syndromes:
1) a "forward failure" (hypoperfusion), with an acute circulatory failure characterized by systemic hypotension, cyanosis, oliguria and possible signs of decreased cerebral and splanchnic perfusion;
2) a "backward failure" (congestion), with acute pulmonary edema or congestive hepatomegaly and jugular venous distension.

Some patients present with an association of both syndromes, which indicates a pejorative prognostic value. The therapeutic interventions should be aimed at obtaining an adequate peripheral oxygen delivery and peripheral tissular oxygenation, and suppress the signs of vascular engorgement. When needed, myocardial contractility should be restored or improved, without deleterious effect on cardiac rate or rhythm, and ideally with a reduction of myocardial oxygen consumption.

If it is difficult in clinical practice to reach all this goals, a better knowledge of the pathophysiologic mechanisms involved may help determine which specific therapeutic intervention needs to be established for a given condition. In the last decade, several authors have proposed that therapeutic optimization strategies aimed at normalizing or maximalizing metabolic end-points such as oxygen delivery should be beneficial [1, 2]. However, several theoretical and methodological biases have been later evidenced, leading to a relative disappointment of this approach. Therefore, this short review will:
1) analyze the consequences for the organism of hypoperfusion/congestion states;
2) present the discussions at the origin of the controversy regarding the interest of improving oxygen delivery with regards to outcome; and
3) propose a simplified algorithm for the hemodynamic management of critically ill patients.

Consequences of Circulatory Dysfunction

When right ventricular (RV) dysfunction predominates, signs of backward failure will mainly induce renal or hepatic dysfunction, with marked biological abnormalities, specially if renal and hepatic arterial blood flows are reduced because of a systemic hypoperfusion. Besides usual symptomatic treatment (forced diuresis or continuous hemofiltration), improvement of systemic hemodynamics is essential to increase cardiac output and arterial pressure, while relieving the signs of venous congestion, thus participating in the correction of organ perfusion pressure. In the case of an acute hepatic dysfunction, these latter considerations are of paramount importance in the absence of an available symptomatic supportive therapy improving hepatic function. The conjunction of a hepatic venous congestion and a decreased arterial inflow pressure can rapidly increase hepatic transaminases, coagulation times and lactate production as a consequence of centrilobular hepatic necrosis [3]. Although continuous hemofiltration might be a way to control deleterious increases in venous pressures, treatment is aimed at improving organ perfusion. In a patient with massive RV dysfunction and massive increases in hepatic transaminases, inhaled nitric oxide was reported to increase both mixed venous and hepatic venous oxygen saturations, with a normalization of biological signs of hepatic failure [4].

Left ventricular (LV) failure elevates left atrial and pulmonary artery occlusion pressures, and may lead to pulmonary edema and pleural effusions. Such a pulmonary congestion secondary to LV failure may aggravate a pulmonary hypertension in patients with border-line RV function, worsen pulmonary gas exchange, and cause an additional load for the right ventricle. This pulmonary vascular engorgement might also be potentiated by an impairment of the alveolo-interstitial membrane if an acute lung injury is present, requiring added specific therapeutic interventions like titration of optimal PEEP level and prevention of baro/volo trauma.

For the organism, acute circulatory failure is accompanied by a compensatory hyperstimulation of the sympathetic system in order to maintain systemic vascular resistance and arterial blood pressure. However, this additional load for the heart may further impair cardiac performance [5, 6]. Considering the liver and the kidney, forward failure with shock induces a splanchnic or renal ischemia with decreased arterial flow that amplifies the decreased regional perfusion pressure secondary to the venous congestion. If overall organ perfusion is not improved by the optimization of loading conditions, the administration of inotropic/vasoactive agents might restore blood pressure by improving forward flow. In cases of severe and persistent systemic hypotension despite therapy, the perfusion of coronary and systemic vascular beds can be compromised. In these cases, the utilization of vasopressors can be discussed in order to treat this refractory hypotension and try to counteract a vicious circle of severe cardiac dysfunction with hypotension, aggravating the cardiac performance *via* secondary coronary and systemic ischemia.

The relationship between DO_2 and VO_2 has been the subject of many studies and have fueled numerous controversies. The normal adaptative response to a decreased DO_2 is an enhanced O_2 extraction by the organism, thus maintaining VO_2 constant over a wide range of DO_2 values, i.e. a O_2 supply-independency is observed. In cases of extreme decreases in DO_2 below a "critical DO_2" level, maximal O_2 extraction capacities will be reached, and VO_2 will decrease. However, in critically ill patients (suffering from sepsis, trauma, ARDS, or following a high-risk surgery...) the normal O_2 supply-independency failed to be initially observed, and changes in DO_2 were described to be associated with corresponding changes in VO_2. Accordingly, in this situation, O_2 extraction fails to increase to maintain a relatively stable VO_2. As a consequence of this mismatching, an anaerobic metabolism and lactic acid production will be observed [7, 8].

Based on these considerations, several authors in the the last decade [1, 9] have proposed that aggressive therapies in critically ill patients aimed at "restoring" elevated DO_2 would lead to a return to a more physiologic relationship of O_2 supply-independency. Indirect evidences that would support this approach were that ARDS survivors had higher DO_2 and VO_2 values than non-survivors [10, 11], and that deliberate increases in DO_2 towards "supra-normal" values in high-risk surgical patients have been proposed to be associated with a decreased mortality [1, 2]. These high DO_2 values were obtained with large volumes of fluid loading, blood transfusions, and inotropic support, mainly using dobutamine.

However, these initially promising results failed to be confirmed by several prospective studies [12–14], and several major methodologic biases of the O_2 supply-dependency studies were evidenced. Accordingly, since VO_2 was calculated from cardiac output data obtained by the Swan-Ganz catheter, the correlation between DO_2 and VO_2 might have been forced by a mathematical coupling of shared measurement error [15]. Accordingly, the majority of authors studying calculated VO_2s observed a O_2 supply-dependency, whereas studies of measured VO_2s by analysis of respiratory gases generally did not [16]. Phang et al. even showed that calculated VO_2 were dependent on DO_2, whereas measured VO_2 (by calorimetry) in the same patients was independent on DO_2 [17]. Finally, data originating from the same group demonstrated that critical DO_2 and critical extraction ratios of septic and non-septic patients did not differ [18].

Finally, Gattinoni et al. in an impressive study concerning more than 700 patients from 56 Italian intensive care units failed to evidence any benefit of therapeutic optimisation strategies aimed at obtaining supra-normal values of cardiac index or normal SvO_2 values compared to a control group whose target was to reach a normal cardiac output [19]. They thus questionned the efficacy of obtaining supranormal DO_2 values since although several previous studies [12, 13] failed to observe any difference in mortality between treated and control groups, a secondary, *a posteriori* analysis showed that the patients achieving the higher supra-normal hemodynamic values had a better survival. However, Gattinoni et al. pointed out that *"this approach is misleading, since it confounds what is to be proved (i.e., that increasing hemodynamic values to supranormal levels improves survival) with what has been observed (i.e., that patients with a high cardiac index survive at a higher rate than patients with a low cardiac index)"* [19].

If this approach considering global oxygenation parameters is inaccurate or disapointing, it has been suggested that the consequences of ischemia/reduced flow states could be more readily assessed in the splanchnic circulation, since this organ is extremely sensitive to hypoperfusion. This regional circulation is particularly and early affected despite an initially "normal" or increased cardiac output. pHi has been valued as a warning parameter associated with a defavorable outcome [20–22]. The rationale of this appproach is that the mesenteric circulation being extremely sensitive to hypoperfusion, local anaerobic metabolism will develop at an early stage, with increased intramural PCO_2 at the mucosa level. Since CO_2 is very diffusible, it will equilibrate with local gastric CO_2 tension, becoming accessible to a measurement using a modified gastric tonometer. pHi is calculated according to this local PCO_2 value and Henderson-Hasselbach equation. When this measurement is performed under strict methodological conditions, a decrease in pHi would be closely correlated with reduced tissular PO_2, reduced mesenteric VO_2, and increased mesenteric lactate flux [23]. Accordingly, increased lactate level is, like pHi, frequent during mesenteric ischemia. Friedman et al. [24], studied the interest of a therapy guided by the combined measurement of pHi and lactate level. They observed that if these two variables are good indexes of severe sepsis, their value as prognostic indicators was improved when considered in association.

In fact, such measurements targeted at the regional level need further investigations with regards to the value of their correction in determining outcome. They however might be proven superior to globally-based evaluations such as DO_2–VO_2 relationships. While the interest of these more recent techniques become solid facts, easily used at the bedside, one could reasonnably assume that the therapeutic optimisation strategies to be proposed should be "taylored" for a given individual patient. This approach should consider the patient's individual status and the pathophysiologic mechanisms involved in the observed hemodynamic alteration. This should then help determine which specific therapeutic intervention needs to be established in this particuliar patient. The last part of this review will propose a simplified algorithm for the hemodynamic management of critically ill patients.

A Simplified Algorithm for Hemodynamic Management in Critically Ill Patients

Classically, the hemodynamic management of such patients can rely on simultaneous measurements of pulmonary artery occlusion pressure (PAOP) and cardiac index (CI), leading to four different situations:
1) a normal low PAOP-normal CT situation;
2) a decreased CI (usually defined as < 2.2 L/min/m²) associated with a low PAOP (usually defined as < 18 mmHg), that would indicate the existence of a hypovolemia;
3) a "normal" CI with an elevated PAOP would indicate the presence of pulmonary congestion, even if PAOP is not always a reliable indicator of preload; and
4) the association of a decreased CI with an elevated PAOP that would indicate the existence of a cardiogenic shock with congestion and low-cardiac output syndrome.

In addition to this classical format, we propose a clinical decision making based on ventricular function and mean systemic arterial pressure. Ventricular function is considered rather than CI since CI is not a regulated variable: rather than considering a value of CI as being "normal", "low", or "high", one should consider a given CI value as being "adapted" or not to peripheral oxygen requirements.

The simultaneous consideration of CI values, indexes of cardiac performance such as echographic ejection fraction (EF), and SvO_2 (an overall indicator of the peripheral extraction of oxygen by the organism that can help ensure that CI is adapted to the peripheral needs of the organism) allows to separate ventricular function as "adequate", "poor" (with for eg. EF < 35%, CI < 2.2 L/min/m², and SvO_2 < 55%), or "dynamic" (with for eg. EF > 65%, CI > 5 L/min/m², and SvO_2 > 80%). Figure 1 describes such a format during which several theoretical hemodynamic situations can be considered [25].

Systemic Hypertension with a Low CI

In this case, arterial vasodilators are usually considered in order to reduce afterload, thus lowering arterial pressure while simultaneously correcting the decreased CI. This frequent hemodynamic profile is however sometimes the consequence of a hypovolemia. Before prescribing an arterial vasodilator, one should therefore eliminate this diagnosis, and fluid loading in such patients will result in a normalization of blood pressure with a marked increase in CI.

The early detection and treatment of an associated hypovolemia is essential, specially when more aggressive therapies using inotropic or vasoactive drugs are considered. Volume replacement is especially important when cardiac performance is altered since marked decreases in cardiac output can be observed when cardiac filling pressures are not elevated. This condition can be suspected when hypoperfusion develops in a patient with normal ventricular function, or after inappropriate diuretic therapy or excessive use of vasodilators. When myocardial function is impaired, hypovolemia can be recognized when signs of congestion of the pulmonary vascular bed are modest or absent, with a low PAOP (classically

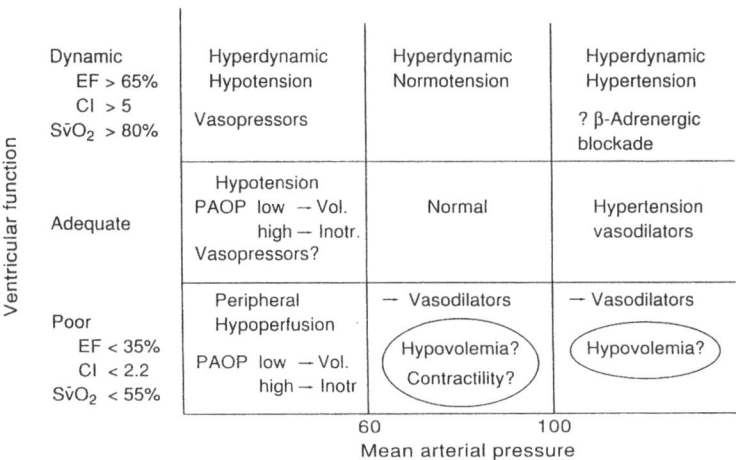

Fig. 1. A simplified algorithm for the hemodynamic management of critically ill patients. (From [25] with permission)

< 15 mmHg). This diagnosis is confirmed if rapid infusions of 50–100 ml of fluid under control of PAOP and CI values correct the hemodynamic alteration. However, if PAOP markedly rises without a corresponding increase in CI, then additional therapies are warranted in this failing heart to increase CI.

If the diagnosis of hypovolemia was not considered, the administration of an arterial vasodilator, even like intravenous nicardipine, a less potent and more easy-to-use vasodilator than sodium nitroprusside, might be poorly tolerated, with important decrease in arterial pressure without simultaneous improvement in stroke volume. However, in the absence of a hypovolemia, arterial vasodilators are very effective in this case of systemic hypertension with a low CI, both considering the peripheral circulation (since CI will increase) and the heart (since myocardial oxygen consumption will be normalized).

Systemic Hypertension with a High or Normal CI

Before prescribing a vasodilator, an etiology must be sought, such as pain, inadequate sedation or shivering. Etiologic treatment of this form of hypertension must always be considered, rather than simply symptomatically lowering arterial pressure at a time when the organism would have a high oxygen consumption.

Hypotension Associated with a Low CI

The hemodynamic strategy will be better optimized considering the evolution of preload (assessed by echocardiography or PAOP) and CI. The existence of a low PAOP reflects a small left ventricular filling pressure (hypovolemic state) and should be treated with fluid loading. When PAOP is markedly increased (typically > 18 mmHg), a cardiogenic component should be suspected and an inotropic treatment such as dobutamine is usually indicated. In addition to control of heart rate, the aims of treatment should thus be directed towards establishing an adequate preload, then improving contractility if needed [26].

Dobutamine is a synthetic catecholamine with predominant β_1-adrenergic agonist properties and slight α-adrenergic effects, that are partially clinically offset by a peripheral β_2 vasodilating action. Thus, the net effect of dobutamine is an enhanced inotropic effect *via* stimulation of the cardiac β_1-adrenergic receptors. Dobutamine has usually minimum effects on heart rate and rhythm, without deleterious increases in arterial blood pressure. This hemodynamic response explains its usual beneficial effects on the balance between myocardial oxygen consumption and myocardial oxygen supply (coronary blood flow).

Hypotension with a Normal CI

The rationale for therapeutic intervention is usually similar than in the previous case since it might be difficult to assess the "normality" of CI. SvO_2 monitoring is helpful in identifying patients with a non adapted CI. Systemic oxygen delivery should therefore be increased in such cases with a similar reasoning (i.e. fluid loading when PAOP is low or inotropes when PAOP is high).

Low CI at a Normal Systemic Blood Pressure

Although measurement of PAOP will help appreciate the presence of a hypovolemia or of an impaired contractility, the existence of a maintained blood pressure in these cases allows to reduce afterload selectively with lesser (but not absent) concerns regarding associated hypovolemia. If the low output syndrome is associated to normal-elevated PAOP, the prescription of inotropic drugs with some arterial vasodilating properties such as dobutamine is of interest.

Hyperdynamic Hypotension (Systemic Hypotension at a High CI)

This hemodynamic profile is frequently observed in the resuscitated stage of hyperdynamic septic shock. Besides the concern for general organ perfusion the existence of a severe hypotension is of pejorative prognosis as the gradient for coronary perfusion is decreased. The therapeutic optimisation strategy in this case is to increase systemic blood pressure to adequate levels and improve peripheral perfusion, while avoiding a deleterious increased load to the heart. When vasopressors are considered, estimation of ventricular function is mandatory since the addition of a pure α agonist such as phenylephrine might be poorly tolerated when baseline cardiac function is impaired. In such cases, norepinephrine or epinephrine, which have combined α and β effects on the peripheral vasculature are more appropriate since the inotropic effect induced by the stimulation of the cardiac β receptors will help overcome a potentially deleterious effect on the cardiac function during a stimulation of the vascular α receptors increasing LV afterload. The doses used should be carefully titrated to maintain coronary perfusion pressure without deleterious effects on cardiac output, since administration of high doses bear the risk of an excessive peripheral vasoconstriction that can adversely affect organ perfusion while increasing cardiac work and perpetuate a myocardial ischemia.

Hyperdynamic Normotension

In this situation, blood pressure is in the normal range, and CI is increased. Hemodynamic manipulations should be limited in such patients. The appropriate therapeutic attitude might then consist in subsequent frequent hemodynamic evaluations, since these patients can spontaneously return to a normal state (normal CI at a normal blood pressure) and have no need for agressive therapies. If a hyperdynamic hypertension develops (for example as the effects of anesthetic drugs become less marked), analgesic agents, sympatholytic agents, or vasodilators would be efficient. Finally, if the patient's condition evolves towards a situation of hyperdynamic hypotension, vasoconstrictive agents will be necessary.

Conclusion

The care of the complicated patient requires recognition of the parameters involved in the observed disturbances while keeping in consideration the particular past medical condition of the patient. Treatment should be directed towards improving the peripheral circulation while simultaneously maintaining the heart function since these two elements need to be considered in terms of pathophysiologic and therapeutic consequences.

Acknowledgement: The authors wish to express their sincere appreciation to Dr. Jean-Louis Teboul for his help during the preparation of this manuscript.

References

1. Shoemaker WC, Appel PL, Kram HB, Waxman K, Lee TS (1988) Prospective trial of supranormal values of survivors as therapeutic goals in high-risk surgical patients. Chest 94:1176–1186
2. Boyd O, Grounds RM, Bennet ED (1993) A randomized clinical trial of the effect of deliberate perioperative increase of oxygen delivery on mortality in high-risk surgical patients. JAMA 270:2699–2707
3. Birgens HS, Hendricksen J, Poulsen H (1978) The shock liver: Clinical and biological findings in patients with centrilobular liver necrosis following cardiogenic shock. Acta Med Scand 204:417–723
4. Gatecel C, Mebazaa A, Kong R, Guinard N, Kermarrec N, Matéo J, Payen D (1995) Inhaled nitric oxide improves hepatic tissue oxygenation in right ventricular failure: value of hepatic venous oxygen monitoring. Anesthesiology 82:588–590
5. Mason DT (1978) Afterload reduction and cardiac performance. Am J Med 65:106–125
6. Ross J (1976) Afterload mismatch and preload reserve. Prog Cardiovasc Dis 18:255–270
7. Cain SM (1977) Oxygen delivery and uptake in dogs during anemic and hypoxic hypoxia. J Appl Physiol 42:228–234
8. Danek SJ, Lynch JP, Weg JG, Dantzker DR (1980) The dependence of oxygen uptake on oxygen delivery in the adult respiratory distress syndrome. Am Rev Respir Dis 122:387–395
9. Hayes MA, Yau EHS, Timmins AC, Hinds CJ, Watson D (1993) Response of critically ill patients to treatment aimed at achieving supranormal oxygen delivery and consumption. Chest 103:886–895
10. Russel JA, Ronco JJ, Lockhat D, Belzberg A, Kiess M, Dodek PM (1990) Oxygen delivery and consumption and ventricular preload are greater in survivors than in nonsurvivors of the adult respiratory distress syndrome. Am Rev Respir Dis 141:659–665
11. Hankeln KB, Gronemeyer R, Held A, Böhmert F (1991) Use of continuous noninvasive measurement of oxygen consumption in patients with adult respiratory distress syndrome following shock of various etiologies. Crit Care Med 19:642–649
12. Tuchschmidt J, Fried J, Astiz M, Rackow E (1992) Elevation in cardiac output and oxygen delivery improves outcome in septic shock. Chest 102:216–220
13. Yu M, Levy MM, Smith P, Takiguchi SA, Miyasaki A, Myers SA (1993) Effect of maximalizing oxygen delivery on morbidity and mortality rates in critically ill patients: A prospective, randomized, controlled study. Crit Care Med 21:830–838

14. Hayes MA, Timmins AC, Yau EHS, Palazzo M, Hinds CJ, Watson D (1994) Elevation of systemic oxygen delivery in the treatment of critically ill patients. N Engl J Med 330: 1717–1722
15. Stratton H, Feustel P, Newell J (1987) Regression of calculated variables in the presence of shared measurement error. J Appl Physiol 62:2083–2093
16. Annat G, Viale JP, Percival C, Froment M, Motin J (1986) Oxygen delivery and uptake in the adult respiratory distress syndrome. Am Rev Respir Dis 133:999–1001
17. Phang TP, Cunningham KF, Ronco JJ, Wiggs BR, Russel JA (1994) Mathematical coupling explains dependence of oxygen consumption on oxygen delivery in ARDS. Am J Respir Crit Care Med 150:318–323
18. Ronco J, Fenwick J, Tweeddale (1993) Identification of the critical oxygen delivery for anaerobic metabolism in critically ill septic and nonseptic humans. JAMA 270:1724–1730
19. Gattinoni L, Brazzi L, Pelosi P, Latini R, Tognoni G, Pesenti A, Fumagalli R (1995) A trial of goal-oriented hemodynamic therapy in critically ill patients. N Engl J Med 333:1025–1032
20. Gys T, Hubens A, Neels H (1988) The prognostic value of gastric intramural pH in surgical intensive care patients. Crit Care Med 16:1222–1224
21. Gutierrez G, Bismar H, Dantzker DR, Silva N (1992) Comparison of gastric intramucosal pH with measures of oxygen transport and consumption in critically ill patients. Crit Care Med 20:451–457
22. Marik PE (1993) Gastric intramucosal pH. A better predictor of multiorgan dysfunction syndrome and death than oxygen-derived variables in patients with sepsis. Chest 104: 225–229
23. Vallet B, Lund N, Curtis SE, Kelly DR, Cain SM (1994) Gut and muscle tissue PO_2 in endotoxemic dogs during shock and resuscitation. J Appl Physiol 76:793–800
24. Friedman G, Berlot G, Kahn RJ, Vincent JL (1995) Combined measurements of blood lactate concentrations and gastric intramucosal pH in patients with severe sepsis. Crit Care Med 23:1184–1193
25. Beloucif S, Payen D (1996) Hemodynamic management. In: Postoperative management of the cardiac surgical patient. In: Williams JP (ed) Churchill Livingstone, New York, pp 123–143
26. Moreno-Cabral C, Mitchell R, Miller C (1988) Manual of postoperative management in adult cardiac surgery. Williams & Wilkins, Baltimore, pp 102–136

Cardiovascular Support
by Hemodynamic Subsets

Hemorrhagic Shock:
From Physiology to Molecular Biology

L. A. Omert and T. R. Billiar

Hemorrhagic shock (HS) is accompanied by a unique set of cardiovascular derangements that are well-described in standard physiology texts. The molecular basis for the physiologic and inflammatory changes during HS, however, has not been fully clarified, and research in this area is ongoing. It has been shown that many of the events which follow HS in the resuscitation and post-resuscitation phases characterize the inflammatory response. This complex series of molecular events includes cytokine upregulation, nitric oxide synthase and stress protein induction, and adhesion molecule production, to name only a few. Some of these events appear to occur due to changes in gene expression with consequent appearance of new cell phenotypes. The phenotypic alterations may vary with the severity of HS as well as with the presence or absence of resuscitation. The link between the physiology of HS and the subsequent elicitation of the inflammatory response is an area of continuing research and experimentation.

Physiology of Hemorrhagic Shock

HS is caused by a diminution of circulating blood volume which results in impaired oxygen delivery ($\dot{D}O_2$) to the tissues. As $\dot{D}O_2$ decreases, oxygen consumption ($\dot{V}O_2$) also decreases in a linear fashion (Fig. 1). The end organ responses to HS are due to the degree of reduction in perfusion, $\dot{D}O_2$, and $\dot{V}O_2$ as well as to the effects of attempts to normalize these parameters by resuscitation.

HS should not be confused with traumatic shock (TS) which combines HS with soft-tissue injury and/or fractures. The additional insult of TS extends beyond hypovolemia and is responsible for a synergistic activation of mediator cascades resulting in a profound inflammatory response. The lower threshold for mediator activation is due to the underlying physiology of TS with respect to tissue perfusion. Stated another way, HS alone will result in impaired oxygen delivery. In a traumatized animal, however, an equivalent diminution of tissue perfusion will occur with a much lesser degree of hemorrhage [1].

Defined stages of HS have been described and are important in studying the molecular changes that occur [2]. *Compensated shock* is the term applied to the physiologic state wherein adrenosympathetic reflexes are activated and maintain the circulation so that the patient or animal can recover. These reflexes include the baroreceptor and chemoreceptor responses, stimulation of the renin-angio-

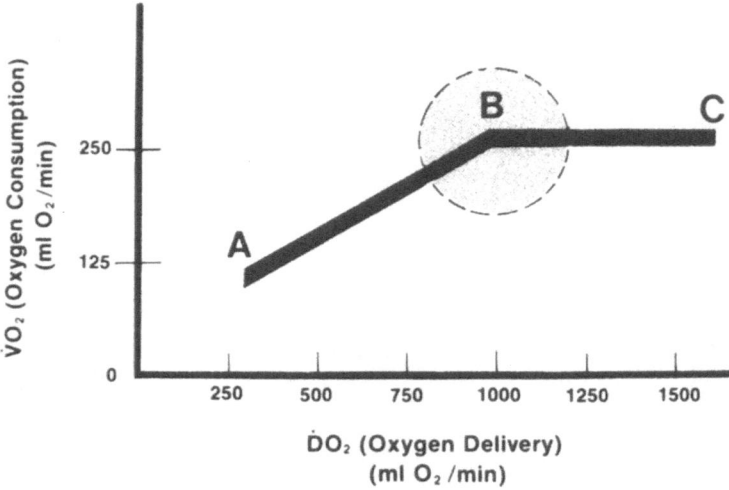

Fig. 1. Dependence of $\dot{V}O_2$ on $\dot{D}O_2$. As $\dot{D}O_2$ decreases, $\dot{V}O_2$ decreases in a linear fashion. (From: Omert, LA (1996) Hemodynamics Management in Critical Care Report, Mosby-Year Book, Inc., Vol 1 (3)

tensin-aldosterone axis, and increased production of ACTH, cortisol, growth hormone, glucagon, and antidiuretic hormone. Local autoregulation insures the maintenance of cerebral and coronary perfusion in the face of global vasoconstriction.

As shock progresses, compensatory mechanisms fail and vascular collapse associated with vasodilation, vascular leak, and depressed cardiac output ensues (Fig. 2). Additonally, liver function becomes depressed, and pulmonary edema may develop with subsequent impairment of oxygenation. Persistent hypoperfusion results in a global increase in microvascular permeability, intravascular thrombosis, and cell death. This phase of *decompensated shock* is characterized by a 30–60% mortality rate [3]. Finally, a threshold exists beyond which so much

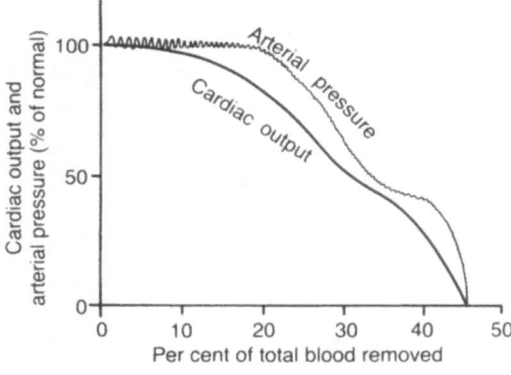

Fig. 2. Effect of hemorrhage on cardiac output and blood pressure. (From [2] with permission)

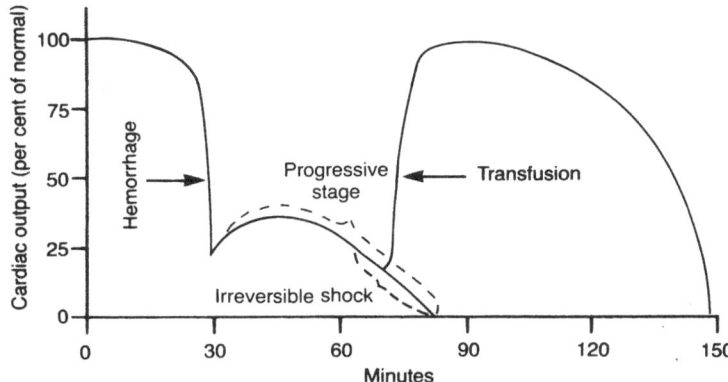

Fig. 3. Failure of transfusion to prevent death in irreversible shock. (From [2] with permission)

cellular necrosis has occurred that recovery is impossible even though cardiac output can be transiently supported. This is the stage of *irreversible shock*, which is characterized by acidosis, vasomotor unresponsiveness, capillary leak, depletion of high energy phosphates, and death of the organisms (Fig. 3).

Hemorrhagic Shock in the Trauma Patient

Hemorrhage is the most common cause of shock in the trauma patient and it is necessary to both recognize and treat this condition expeditiously. The aforementioned physiologic categories have been reiterated as 5 classes of shock in order to facilitate clinical managements [4] (Table 1).

Table 1. Estimated fluid and blood losses[a] based on patient's initial presentation

	Class I	Class II	Class III	Class IV
Blood Loss (mL)	Up to 750	750–1500	1500–2000	> 2000
Blood Loss (%BV)	Up to 15%	15–30%	30–40%	> 40%
Pulse Rate	< 100	> 100	> 120	> 140
Blood Pressure	Normal	Normal	Decreased	Decreased
Pulse Pressure (mmHg)	Normal or increased	Decreased	Decreased	Decreased
Respiratory Rate	14–20	20–30	30–40	> 35
Urine Output (mL/hr)	> 30	20–30	5–15	Negligible
CNS/Mental Status	Slightly anxious	Mildly anxious	Anxious and confused	Confused and lethargic
Fluid Replacement (3:1 Rule)	Crystalloid	Crystalloid	Crystalloid and blood	Crystalloid and blood

[a] For a 70-kg male

Class I hemorrhage is the state in which loss of up to 15% of intravascular volume occurs. A mild tachycardia is usually the only clinical sign that accompanies this state. Blood replacement is not necessary for most patients.

In Class II hemorrhage, 15–30% of blood volume has been lost, or between 750–1500 ml. Tachycardia is always present in patients with normal hearts, and they may be anxious and tachypneic as well. Decreased pulse pressure can be noted by the careful examiner. The systolic component of blood pressure is usually maintained in Class II hemorrhage, but the diastolic will be elevated due to circulating catecholamines. Replacement of blood loss with crystalloid will generally be sufficient to restore normal physiology.

Loss of 30–40% (2000 ml) of blood places the patient in Class III hemorrhage. In addition to the previous clinical findings, the systolic blood pressure will be decreased and urine output will diminish reflecting the global hypoperfusion. Most of these patients will require blood transfusion.

Finally, Class IV hemorrhage, or loss of > 40% blood volume, is an acutely life-threatening situation. The patient is usually unresponsive and the diastolic blood pressure will be unobtainable. Airway protection and blood and crystalloid infusion should be expeditiously provided along with attempts to minimize ongoing blood loss.

It has become increasingly evident in both humans and animals that the ability to recover from HS depends on its duration and severity. Obviously, some degrees of blood loss are so great that resuscitation is futile. If a patient is successfully resuscitated, however, the ensuing clinical course is not automatically a smooth path toward discharge. Instead, the patient will often remain critically ill for days to months, experiencing the complications of a condition which has come to be known as the systemic inflammatory response syndrome (SIRS). SIRS is characterized by multiple organ system dysfunction and repeated septic episodes and carries with it a mortality rate of up to 60% [5].

Why hemorrhagic shock, a non-infectious process, leads to SIRS is a question which still cannot be definitively answered. However, exploration of the molecular mechanisms underlying HS may provide some of the answers.

Molecular Responses in Hemorrhagic Shock

It is becoming increasingly evident that the different stages of HS may be accompanied by changes in gene expression and cell phenotype which results in their unique physiologic and metabolic characteristics. Additionally, changes in gene expression may be facilitated by resuscitation following shock and may occur in the post-resuscitation phase as well.

Cytokines

Much of the data regarding cytokine production in HS is conflicting and reflects the problem that local upregulation of mRNA transcripts may not be reflected in circulating blood levels. In 1990, Chaudry et al. demonstrated that macrophages harvested from hemorrhaged mice showed decreased production of TNF, IL-1 and IL-6, but that blockade of prostaglandin production prevented this depression of macrophage function [6]. Supernatants obtained from Kuppfer cells, however, showed a consistent increase in these three cytokines at both two and 24 hours post-shock [7]. Experiments by Zapata-Sirvent published in 1992 illustrated that the shock-induced increases in TNF production persisted for 48 hours in their model of HS which examined splenic leukocytes obtained from animals subjected to two episodes of blood loss [8]. Serum from human patients admitted to the hospital in HS was also found to contain increased levels of IL-1 and TNF [9]. Studies from deMaria et al. showed that the hemorrhage-induced increase in TNF that occurs in normal mice is not found in endotoxin-resistant (C3H/HeJ) mice or mice pretreated with anti-TNF antibody [10]. Additionally, Rhee demonstrated that the shock-induced increase in TNF did not persist with resuscitation [11].

In the mid 1990's, more attention was devoted to elucidating the molecular basis for hemorrhagic shock. In 1994, the Chaudry group found that an upregulation of mouse peritoneal macrophage mRNA transcripts of IL-1, IL-6, TNF and TGF-beta occurs at one hour following HS [12]. A year later, Schwartz and colleagues illustrated a similar increase in IL-1 and TNF in mRNA from pulmonary macrophages [13]. This response was inhibited by DMTU, a low molecular weight antioxidant which scavenges hydrogen peroxide, hydroxyl radicals and hypochlorous acid in vitro. The authors speculated that oxygen radicals generated during resuscitation activate the transcriptional factor NF-kB which binds to enhancer sequences in the gene promoter region to upregulate cytokine production.

The role resuscitation plays in cytokine modulation in hemorrhagic shock is another area which remains poorly understood. Jiang and colleagues elegantly demonstrated that TNF levels increased in portal and systemic blood of hemorrhaged rats at 1 hour post-shock and peaked at 120 minutes after resuscitation [14]. Our laboratory has utilized a rat model of hemorrhagic shock which illustrates the effects of shock alone versus shock with resuscitation. Male Sprague Dawley rats were anesthetized and cannulae placed in their jugular vein and carotid artery. They were then subjected to an initial bleed of 2.25 ml/100 g over 15 minutes. Blood was continuously withdrawn to maintain mean arterial pressure (MAP) at 40 mmHg. The point at which blood could no longer be removed, but had to be returned in order to maintain the MAP at 40 mmHg, was each animal's unique physiologic compensation endpoint. In general, this occurred at 63 minutes following the initial hemorrhage. We prolonged the shock state to specified endpoints by reinfusing small aliquots of blood to maintain MAP at 40 mmHg and then sacrificed the animals. For example, the point at which 35% of shed blood was returned marked a time point representing decompensated shock, while 70% blood return was well into the irreversible shock state. Additionally, we used these endpoints as times at which the animal was resuscitated with all of its remaining shed blood and two times that amount as a crystalloid infusion. We have shown that while mRNA levels for IL-6 increase in the liver and

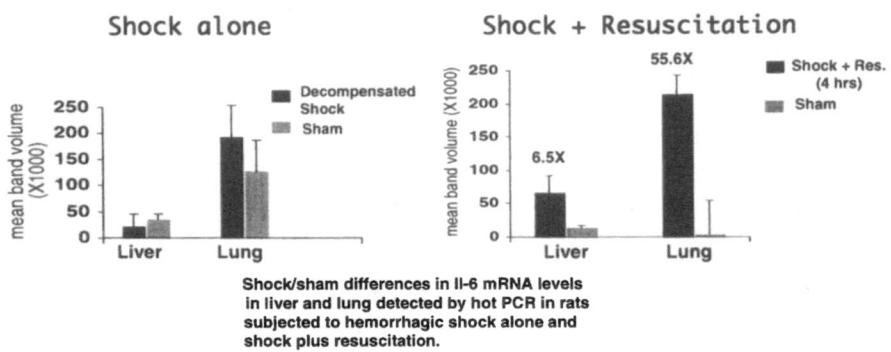

Shock/sham differences in Il-6 mRNA levels
in liver and lung detected by hot PCR in rats
subjected to hemorrhagic shock alone and
shock plus resuscitation.

Fig. 4. Unpublished data (Omert LA, Billiar TR, presented at the Nineteenth Annual Conference on Shock, 1996)

lungs of shocked rats as demonstrated by semi-quantitative RT-PCR, this increase is not significantly greater than in animals who undergo anesthesia and vascular cannulation alone. When the animals are resuscitated, however, a much more pronounced increase in IL-6 occurs which is six times greater than sham in the liver and 55 times greater in the lung [15] (Fig. 4).

Stress Proteins

Another molecular response to HS includes the expression of heat shock protein and metallothionein. The heat shock response is a primitive reflex designed to protect a cell from environmental stress. The proteins expressed in the response bind to injured structural proteins to facilitate their repair. Heat shock protein expression is initially beneficial but has the eventual untoward effect of rendering the cell susceptible to subsequent apoptosis, or programmed cell death, when it is subjected to a second noxious stimulus. One may speculate that this is a reason why patients who have survived severe hemorrhagic shock later succumb to multiple organ failure that appears to have been triggered by a non-lethal insult such as nosocomial pneumonia or vascular catheter infection. Our laboratory has shown that mRNA for heat shock protein 72 (HSP-72), an inducible member of the heat shock group, increased during HS, but this increase was not significantly greater than that evidenced by sham animals undergoing anesthesia and cannulation. However, resuscitation of the animals in decompensated shock resulted in a strong increase of HSP-72 over sham [16].

Metallothionein is another stress protein that has been found to be upregulated in HS. Like HSP-72, metallothionein is potentially protective in HS with respect to its role in reducing oxidative injury. Induction of metallothionein mRNA occurs later than HSP 72 and is significantly greater than sham induction only in severe resuscitated HS [16].

Nitric Oxide

Although nitric oxide (NO) is short-lived in the circulation, it is both ubiquitous and functionally diverse. Originally called endothelium-derived relaxing factor due to its effect on vasomotor tone and regulation of blood pressure, NO is now known to be synthesized solely from L-arginine by one of the isoforms of NO synthase. Due to its extremely lipophilic nature, it freely diffuses across cell membranes to exert its multiple effects. The role that NO plays in HS is still being clarified, but some interesting findings have emerged. In 1993, Peitzman's group found that nitrate/nitrite levels, the endproducts of NO, are significantly lower in trauma patients than in normal controls [17]. Levels rise if the trauma patient becomes septic, but are still relatively suppressed. It was initially postulated by some investigators that the cytokine-inducible isoform of NO synthase, Type II NOS, would be elevated in decompensated HS [18]. This would provide a rational explanation for the vasomotor instability seen in this stage. Our group has found, however, that NOS II induction occurs only in the late stages irreversible HS [19]. Shocked rats did not demonstrate any increase in NOS mRNA or protein over sham animals until 5 hours of shock was reached (irreversible phase) and also did not exhibit any pressor response to N^G-monomethyl-L-arginine, an inhibitor of all NOS isoforms.

Clearly, molecular events underlie the physiologic changes which occur during HS. The stimuli for these events include ischemia, hypoxia, generation of oxygen radicals and probably numerous other factors yet to be elucidated. The addition of resuscitation to the shocked animal or patient is necessary for survival in many cases, but, in turn, may generate an inflammatory cascade with it's own adverse sequelae.

It is increasingly evident that hemorrhage, metabolic stress and inflammation are linked; the catalysts responsible for facilitating this complex interaction are yet to be understood.

References

1. Rady MY, Kirkman E, Cranley J, et al (1993) A comparison of the effects of skeletal muscle injury and somatic afferent nerve stimulation on the response to hemorrhage in anesthetized pigs. J Trauma 35:756–761
2. Guyton AC (1991) Textbook of Medical Physiology. 8th ed. WB Saunders, Philadelphia
3. Kelly E, Billiar T, Peitzman A (1996) Current problems in surgery: Hemorrhagic shock. Mosby Year-Book
4. ATLS Instructors Manual (1993) 5th ed. American College of Surgeons, Chicago
5. Civetta JM, Taylor RW, Kirby RR (1988) Critical Care. JB Lippincott, Philadelphia
6. Ertel W, Morrison MH, Ayala A, Chaudry IH (1990) Blockade of prostaglandin production increases cachectin synthesis and prevents depression of macrophage functions after hemorrhagic shock. Annals of Surgery
7. Ertel W, Morrison MH, Ayala A, Chaudry IH (1991) Eicosanoids regulate tumor necrosis factor synthesis after hemorrhage in vitro and in vivo. J of Trauma 31 (5):609–616
8. Zapata-Sirvent RL, Hansbrough JF, Cox MC, Carter WH (1992) Immunologic alterations in a murine model of hemorrhagic shock. Critical Care Medicine 20 (4):508–517

9. Roumen RMH, Hendriks R, van der Ven-Jongekrijg J, et al (1993) Cytokine patterns in patients after major vascular surgery, hemorrhagic shock, and severe blunt trauma. Annals of Surgery 218 (6):769–776
10. DeMaria EJ, Pellicane JV, Lee RB (1993) Hemorrhagic shock in endotoxin-resistant mice: Improved survival unrelated to deficient production of tumor necrosis factor. J of Trauma 35 (5):720–725
11. Rhee P, Waxman K, Clark L, et al (1993) Tumor necrosis factor and monocytes are released during hemorrhagic shock. Resuscitation 25:249–255
12. Zhu XL, Ayala A, Zellweger R, et al (1994) Peritoneal macrophages show increased cytokine gene expression following haemorrhagic shock. Immunology 83:378–383
13. Schwartz MD, Repine JE, Abraham E (1995) Xanthine oxidase-derived oxygen radicals increase lung cytokine expression in mice subjected to hemorrhagic shock. Am J Respir Cell Mol Biol 12:434–440
14. Jiang J, Bahrami S, Leichtfried et al (1995) Kinetics of endotoxin and tumor necrosis factor appearance in portal and systemic circulation after hemorrhagic shock in rats. Annals of Surgery 221 (1):100–106
15. Omert, LA, Hierholzer C, Peitzman A, Billiar TR (1996) The role of reperfusion in IL-6 and ICAM-1 expression in hemorrhagic shock. Presented at the Nineteenth Annual Conference on Shock, Grand Traverse Village, Michigan, June 2–5
16. Kelly E, Morgan N, Woo ES, et al (in press) Metallothionein and HSP–72 are induced in the liver by hemorrhagic shock and resuscitation but not by shock alone
17. Jacob TD, Ochoa JB, Peitzman AB, et al (1993) Nitric oxide production is inhibited in trauma patients. J of Trauma 35 (4):590–597
18. Thiemermann C, Szabo C, Mitchell JA, et al (1993) Vascular hyporeactivity to vasoconstrictor agents and hemodynamic decompensation in hemorrhagic shock is mediated by nitric oxide. Proc Natl Acad Sci USA 90:267–271
19. Kelly E, Shah NS, Morgan N, et al (in press) Physiologic and molecular characterization of the role of nitric oxide in hemorrhagic shock: Evidence that Type II nitric oxide synthase does not regulate vascular decompensation

Cardiogenic Shock

A. Boujoukos

Introduction

Cardiogenic shock is defined by poor systemic perfusion despite adequate volume due to a low cardiac output so that basal metabolic needs of a patient can not be met. Hemodynamically, a low cardiac index (CI) of $< 1.8–2.1$ l/min/m^2 is coupled with an elevated arteriovenous oxygen difference and a low mixed venous oxygen saturation. The clinical presentation of cardiogenic shock is variable depending on the acuity of onset and the ability of the body to compensate for the progressive decline in cardiac output. In previously healthy patients, an abrupt loss of left ventricular (LV) function following an extensive myocardial infarction (MI) often results in diaphoresis, tachycardia, frank or relative hypotension and cool, clammy, vasoconstricted extremities. Confusion, oliguria, lactic acidosis and evidence of respiratory muscle fatigue manifest as sequellae of end organ hypoperfusion. Systemic hypotension fuels the ventricular failure further by reducing coronary perfusion and increasing the ischemic insult to already hypoperfused myocardium. Less dramatic initial presentations are often evident in patients in whom the deterioration in cardiac output is more insidious. Fatigue, anorexia, progressive tachycardia, a drop in blood pressure from baseline, and oliguria with rising blood urea nitrogen and creatinine may be seen well in advance of the frank hypotension. A state of compensated low output with normal systemic blood pressure can often be maintained chronically though the lack of cardiovascular reserve may quickly, with minimal insult, precipitate a state where perfusion and oxygen delivery do not meet the body's needs leading to a state of overt shock.

General Therapeutic Principles

The management of patients with the acute onset of cardiogenic shock centers around rapid stabilization of the hemodynamics to prevent ischemic organ and tissue injury along with prompt assessment of the etiology. Adequate oxygen delivery and perfusion are addressed by
- assuring adequate preload,
- maintaining sinus rhythm,
- preventing hypoxemia,

- utilizing inotropes, and
- titrating vasopressors judiciously to maintain critical organ perfusion.

Volume loading in low output states is to assure that preload is optimized and to exclude a component of relative volume depletion. For patients in shock, a pulmonary artery occlusion pressure (Ppao) of 15–18 mmHg should be an initial target unless there are substantial derangements of gas exchange. Ventricles with a significant component of diastolic dysfunction and which appear underfilled echocardiographically despite Ppao ot 15 mmHg should be volume loaded further. Continued improvement in cardiac output, urine output, capillary refill and other markers of perfusion with crystalloid challenges, in the absence of pulmonary edema, is perhaps the best marker of the appropriateness of continued volume therapy.

The electrocardiogram allows for the diagnosis of rhythm disturbances and aids in the evaluation of ischemia. Loss of atrial contraction because of either atrial fibrillation or junctional rhythms may lead to shock in the setting of severe diastolic dysfunction or right ventricular (RV) failure. Conversion of atrial fibrillation to sinus rhythm should be an immediate goal in these patients. Immediate electric cardioversion is appropriate though often an intravenous antiarrhythmic is required to maintain the patient early on. In patients with chronic atrial fibrillation, conversion is generally not possible. Rate control with digoxin, for patients with systolic failure or calcium blockers/β blockers, for patients with diastolic failure should be a priority to allow for a longer diastolic ventricular filling time. Accelerated junctional rhythms are problematic from a management and hemodynamic standpoint but fortunately are usually self limited. Slow junctional rhythms should be managed with a trial of catechol infusions to bring out the sinus rhythm or atrial pacing may be required.

Inotropes/Pressors. A variety of catechol and phosphodiesterase inhibitor inotropes are used in the setting of cardiogenic shock to maintain perfusion of vital organs. The selection of inotropes is a clinical judgment based on the physiology of the individual patient. If the systolic blood pressure (SBP) is < 80 mmHg, catechols with vasopressor properties such as dopamine or norepinephrine are first line drugs.

Two points should be noted with regard to pressor titration. First, it is important to titrate these drugs to a well functioning arterial pressure tracing. Peripheral vasoconstriction can cause a radial arterial pressure recordings to be substantially dampened leading to inappropriate upward titration of vasopressors at the expense of elevated afterload and increased myocardial work. A femoral arterial catheterization site may demonstrate substantially higher central pressures.

Additionally, since a hypotensive patient is at high risk of death from both the current episode of shock as well as the complications of the shock such as stroke, renal failure, extension of a myocardial infarction and mesenteric ischemia, pressers should be titrated up aggressively to achieve an adequate perfusion pressure and prevent organ damage. Generally, a mean arterial blood pressure (MAP) goal > 65 mmHg and SBP > 85 mmHg are sought. The management of hypotension requires titration of the first pressor, such as dopamine, up rapidly so that within 15–20 minutes, a dose of 15 µg/kg/min has been reached. With ongoing MAP < 65 mmHg, the prompt addition and titration of norepinephrine, beginning at 0.02 µg/kg/min, should be undertaken along with simultaneous consideration of intraaortic balloon counterpulsation (IABP) placement.

Inotropic Support

Dopamine has inotropic and chronotropic effects throughout its dose range. Pressor effects are evident starting in the 5–10 µg/kg/min range. Supraventricular arrhythmias are common with dopamine. Norepinephrine is comparatively a more potent pressor and, at doses of 0.05–2 µg/kg/min, often effectively treats hypotension that is refractory to dopamine.

Epinephrine is a potent inotrope, chronotrope and pressor. Is seldom used in the setting of active coronary disease since myocardial oxygen consumption increases substantially. However in the absence of active ischemia it can be effectively titrated, beginning at low doses of 0.05 µg/kg/min, to provide effective inotropic and blood pressure support.

Dobutamine, a β_1 selective agent, increases inotropy, increases CI, augments coronary artery flow, reduces ventricular filling pressures, and causes systemic vasodilation. It is the mainstay of therapy in patients without profound hypotension (SBP > 80 mmHg). It is also appropriate used to augment inotropy in situations where the blood pressure is being effectively being supported with a vasopressor or IABP. Atrial arrhythmias and exacerbations of sinus tachycardia limit its upward titration in some patients.

The phosphodiesterase inhibitors amrinone and milrinone may be valuable adjuncts, especially in the settings of reversible pulmonary hypertension and RV failure. The inotropic properties appear to be minimal compared with their vasodilator actions although postischemic myocardium may be more responsive to the β_1 effects [1]. The pulmonary vasodilator properties may be valuable in some postcardiotomy settings where pulmonary hypertension precipitates RV failure. However, because they are potent vasodilators, the use of these drugs is limited in the setting of severe hypotension. As a rule, vasodilators such as phosphodiesterase inhibitors and nitroprusside should be considered only after the hypotension is well controlled. The possible utility of combinations of vasopressors and vasodilators to manage cardiogenic shock is unpredictable and requires individual assessment in each patient.

Triiododothyronine (T_3) has been used as a support of the failing heart in the myxedema cardiogenic shock and in the postcardiotomy setting [2]. Support for the latter comes from animal models indicating that active T_3 levels are reduced due to cardiopulmonary bypass and that triiododothyronine significantly enhances the recovery of ischemic myocardium during the reperfusion period [3, 4]. A prospective, randomized, placebo controlled trial in 142 high-risk patients undergoing coronary artery bypass grafting (CABG) demonstrated that triiododothyronine did in fact produce higher stroke volume and CI (2.88 ± 0.73 l/min/

m^2 vs 2.61 ± 0.60 l/min/m^2) although morbidity, mortality (4.9%) and other inotrope use was not measurably different [5].

When limitations of oxygen delivery are at such a critical state such, it is appropriate to reduce excessive metabolic demands by treating fever and preventing shivering. In patients with moderate to severe cardiogenic shock, early institution of controlled mechanical ventilation and sedation can reduce oxygen consumption substantially. Finally, mechanical support of the patient with IABP, extracorporeal membrane oxygenation (ECMO), or a ventricular assist device (VAD) may be appropriate in specific settings where more conservative therapy has failed and where the possibility of recovery or transplantation exists.

Specific Diagnostic and Management Strategies

The final common physiologic pathways leading to cardiogenic shock are impaired ventricular ejection and/or impaired ventricular filling. In a patient with new onset of pressor dependent hypotension, a pulmonary artery (PA) catheter is critical in confirming the cardiogenic etiology of the shock. A CI < 1.8 l/min/m^2 along with Ppao > 15 mmHg is consistent with the diagnosis. Although there are multiple potential etiologies, the history, exam, hemodynamic profile, electrocardiogram, chest radiograph, arterial blood gas and echocardiogram should allow for the establishment of a diagnosis (Table 1). It is critical to pursue the diagnosis during the process of aggressive resuscitation since, in many case, therapy must be tailored to the specific diagnosis.

The history and setting may suggest a pulmonary embolism. Hypotension, low output and RV failure manifests usually with > 50% of the pulmonary arterial tree occluded by emboli [6]. Pulmonary pressures are usually above normal but not remarkably so perhaps because of the resultant RV failure. An arterial blood gas and chest radiograph may reveal hypoxemia and CO_2 retention in the face of a high minute ventilation (> 15 l/min) and a clear radiograph which suggests a massive pulmonary embolism. Although definitive data is not available, thrombolytic therapy is associated with a more rapid recovery of RV function and should be considered once the diagnosis has been confirmed by ventilation-perfusion scan or angiogram [7].

High intrathoracic pressures associated with tension pneumothorax or excessive PEEP, either applied or auto-PEEP, need to be excluded since hemodynamically they can masquerade as a low output, high central venous pressure (CVP) cardiogenic shock state. A radiograph excludes the former and transiently removing the patient's endotracheal tube from the ventilator circuit will expose the latter.

Acute drug induced cardiogenic shock, such as seen with protamine reactions and poisoning with calcium channel blockers or β-blockers, are generally evident by history. The catastrophic pulmonary vasocontrictive reactions occur immediately following protamine administration and quickly precipitate RV failure and shock in the absence of rapid catechol support [8]. Once suspected, both β-blocker and calcium channel blocker poisonings should be treated with glucagon

Table 1. Causes of cardiogenic shock

Acute myocardial infarction
- LV pump failure
- RV pump failure
- Acute papillary muscle rupture
- Ventricular septal rupture
- Free wall rupture

Postcardiotomy cardiogenic shock

Myocardial contusion

Myocarditis

End-stage cardiomyopathy
- Dilated
- Restrictive
- Hypertrophic
- Aortic insufficiency
- Mitral regurgitation

Obstruction to flow
- Aortic stenosis
- Mitral stenosis
- Myxoma
- Pulmonary embolism

Impaired ventricular filling
- Tamponade
- Tension pneumothorax
- PEEP

Cardiac rejection

Arrhythmias

Myxedema

Drug toxicity
- Protamine
- β-blockers
- Calcium Channel blockers

which increases chronotropy and myocardial contractility independent of adrenergic receptors by increasing myocardial cyclic AMP [9, 10]. A 5–10 mg bolus of glucagon can be followed by an infusion of 1–20 mg/hr and should be used along with a catechol or possibly phosphodiesterase inhibitor infusion [11].

The echocardiogram provides extremely valuable diagnostic and management data in the setting of cardiogenic shock. The diagnoses of myxoma, ventricular septal rupture, free wall rupture, and severe valvular disease require consideration of definitive surgical intervention or balloon valvuloplasty. New wall motion abnormalities suggest an ischemic etiology. In patients with acute cardiogenic shock and CVPs of 16–20 mmHg, distinguishing RV failure from tamponade is most effectively done echocardiographically. In a medical setting, a transthoracic echo is generally acceptable in diagnosing a pericardial effusion which can be managed with percutaneous drainage. In the postcardiotomy setting, a transesophageal is often required to exclude the possibility of localized mediastinal clot compressing the RV or either atrium. Reexploration is generally required for management.

Shock primarily due to RV infarction is seen in 10% of patients with inferior wall MIs [12]. Both aggressive volume challenges to prevent RV underfilling and inotropic support are known to be important in improving LV filling and CI [13]. Central venous pressures of 15–18 mmHg are empiric targets though the optimal CVP will vary from patient to patient and will also vary depending upon the level of inotropic support. Maintaining atrial-ventricular sequential contraction is critical to maintain RV output and A–V sequential pacing should be instituted if junctional rhythms or heart block become manifest. Intraaortic balloon counterpulsation has been shown to improve RV function in the setting of MI and may be useful adjunct [14]. Additionally, since the relative risk of in-hospital death has been shown to be 7.7 times higher for RV infarctions than for inferior wall infarcts alone, aggressive attempts at early reperfusion have been suggested [12, 15].

In the postcardiotomy setting, RV failure due to air embolism or other ischemic insults can be particularly difficult to manage. The pericardium, and sometimes the chest itself, cannot be closed without precipitating major hypotension, therefore the normal ventricular interdependence seen in medical RV failure is less applicable. Overdistention of the RV with volume may precipitates severe tricuspid regurgitation. Inotropic support is the mainstay along with reduction of pulmonary resistance with vasodilators if tolerated. Mechanical assist with an RVAD for 2–7 days may be necessary to allow for recovery.

The diagnosis of cardiogenic shock associated with acute MI is made by history, myocardial enzyme detection, electrocardiogram with right sided leads and the echocardiogram. Although supportive strategies are initially appropriate, there is some evidence and the bulk of opinion suggestive that early reperfusion therapy should be undertaken.

Mechanical Support

Intraaortic balloon counterpulsation has been used since the late 60's to increase coronary and systemic perfusion by augmenting diastolic pressure and to reduce the LV afterload in multiple settings of cardiac failure. In patients with cardiogenic shock, the IABP has proven to be efficacious in increasing cardiac output, peripheral perfusion, mean and diastolic arterial pressure, coronary blood flow, stroke volume (SV), RV and LV ejection fraction and reducing myocardial oxygen extraction, LV end-systolic and diastolic volumes, and pulmonary blood volume [14, 16–19]. The indications for IABP in patients with cardiogenic shock are pump failure, papillary muscle rupture and ventricular septal rupture. Other shock settings where IABP is of value include postcardiotomy cardiogenic shock, mitral regurgitation, bridge to transplantation, and transplant rejection. Significant aortic insufficiency, aortic dissection or severe atherosclerotic disease of the aorta are the major absolute contraindications to IABP.

The IABP is reported to be a useful tool for stabilizing the hemodynamics in 40–90% of patients with cardiogenic shock. Despite the improved physiologic parameters, the in-hospital mortality with IABP support alone is quite substantial. The in-hospital mortality rate in post-MI patients studied by Scheidt (n = 87), Mueller (n = 10), Bardet (n = 18), and Dunkman (n = 25) were 83%, 90%, 83% and 84% respectively [16–19]. In 21 post MI cardiogenic shock patients reported by DeWood, IABP was associated with only a 52% in-hospital mortality [20]. However, the average pre-IABP CI in this group was 1.93 l/min/m² compared with 1.22–1.5 l/min/m² seen in the reports with 80–90% mortality rates [17–19]. Even in DeWood's less compromised population, an additional 19% of the group died within 12 months of progressive pump failure. In summary, the IABP may be a valuable adjunct in stabilizing a patient in shock post MI but a subsequent supportive strategy alone likely confers no survival benefit.

A VAD is a mechanical pump that augments or replaces the output of a failing ventricle. Successful univentricular and biventricular support has allowed for myocardial recovery and survival in several settings of intractable cardiogenic shock. The development and use of VADs has emerged from 2 primary clinical environments. Short-term VADs have been used as an extension of cardiopulmonary bypass (CPB) to allow for myocardial recovery over several days in the setting of postcardiotomy cardiogenic shock. Second, the development of long-term VADs has evolved to allow for bridging unstable end-stage cardiomyopathy patients to transplant and consideration of partially implantable VAD support as an alternative to transplantation [21].

Failure to wean from CPB because of severe LV or RV failure occurs in 0.5–1% of patients following coronary artery or valvular heart surgery. The etiology of postcardiotomy cardiogenic shock includes MI, coronary air embolus, coronary spasm, ventricular distention, inadequate myocardial protection and incomplete revascularization. If inotropes and IABP fail to allow for separation from CPB in a heart with preserved preoperative function, a VAD may be indicated. For this purpose, centrifugal pumps made by Medtronic and Sarns and pneumatically driven devices by ABIOMED and Thoratec have served as effective VADs in postcardiotomy patients and short term bridge to transplant since 1980 [22, 23]. In contrast to implantable devices which can only serve as LVADs, each of these devices is capable of providing biventricular as well as univentricular support. The Medtronic pump can additionally be coupled with an oxygenator to provide venoarterial ECMO as a bridge to recovery in patients with concomitant pulmonary failure. An additional investigational device, the Hemopump, functions only as an LVAD. This 21F percutaneously placed turbine pump traverses the aortic valve and, utilizing the principle of an Archimedes screw, pulls blood from the LV cavity and ejects into the aorta [24]. Mechanical support with these devices provides flows of 3.5–5.5 l/min and generally lasts for 3–7 days which is considered by most to be an adequate period to allow for myocardial recovery.

The outcome of postcardiotomy cardiogenic shock patients supported with various VADs are relatively consistent. Fifty percent of patients are weaned from support, 25% die in the hospital subsequently and 25% are discharged home. Of patients discharged, 86% are NYHA class I or II and survival at 2 years is 82% [25]. Certain subgroups derive less benefit from postcardiotomy cardiogenic shock including patients who undergo cardiac arrest in the operating room prior to VAD support (7% hospital survival), are >70 years of age (13% survival), or are on CPB >6 hours (17% survival) [25–27]. Since postcardiotomy cardiogenic shock patients are unable to support themselves hemodynamically off of CPB, a 25% survival to home with recovered cardiac function likely represents a true mortality benefit.

In patients with end stage heart failure awaiting heart transplantation, the onset of shock may be insidious. Inotrope dependent candidates may deteriorate clinically and require an IABP confining them to bedrest until transplant. Ventricular assist devices can resolve the shock state, improve survival to transplantation and allow ambulation and rehabilitation in preparation for transplantation [28]. The Heartmate, Novacor, and Thoratec VADs have been used as a long term bridge to transplant since the mid 1980s. The Heartmate and Novacor are partially implantable devices use solely for long term support of the LV. The Thoratec is the only long-term assist device which provides biventricular support. At rest, these devices provide outputs of 4.5–6 l/min and may produce in excess of 8 l/min during exercise [29]. A survival benefit through the bridge and transplantation period has not been demonstrated in a controlled setting and likely it will be difficult to do given the 80–90% 1 year survival achieved with current heart transplantation. Potentially, VADs may be shown to improve the survival of transplant recipients overall by reversing organ failure, allowing reconditioning and optimizing nutrition prior to surgery.

Mechanical VADs as bridges to myocardial recovery have been undertaken in patients with myocarditis, cardiac allograft rejection and acute MI [24, 26]. The numbers are small for acute MI patients supported with VADs to recovery rather than transplant. In the 96 patients reported in registry data, only 26% were weaned and 11% were discharged from the hospital. The average support duration was 5.4 days, with the longest support with ultimate discharge being 23 days [27]. The 30 day survival for 17 patients with acute MI in the Hemopump study was 41% [24]. Since this study was undertaken in the reperfusion era, it is possible that the improvement in survival additionally reflects a more aggressive revascularization algorithm.

Reperfusion Therapy

The acute onset of cardiogenic shock is by far most commonly seen in the setting of a myocardial infarction. Autopsy series of patients who have died with pump failure in this setting suggest that the vast majority have lost an average of 40% of the myocardium as a result of the infarction and subsequent infarct extension due to the persisting hypotension and coronary hypoperfusion [30, 31]. Papillary muscle rupture and acute ventricular septal rupture are further mechanical complications responsible for cardiogenic shock in the days following the MI. Recent thrombolytic trials have placed the incidence of post-MI cardiogenic shock at 4–7% [32–35]. Of these, 20% present with shock and 80% develop shock subsequently [32, 34]. The mortality in patients managed with supportive strategies alone utilizing inotropes, vasopressors and IABP and those with unsuccessful attempts al restoring coronary perfusion is 68–93% [19, 33, 36–40].

Because of the poor outcome of cardiogenic shock in the setting of acute MI, reperfusion strategies using thrombolytics, percutaneous transluminal coronary angioplasty (PTCA) and emergent CABG have been examined. This seems particularly important since in-hospital and long-term survival of patients with cardiogenic shock is most closely related to the patency of the infarct related artery [41]. In 200 patients, the in-hospital mortality for those with a patent infarct related artery was 33% compared with 75% if the infarct related artery was closed and 84% if the patency of the infarct related artery was unknown. Although thrombolytics have been shown in multiple trials to decrease mortality in acute MI, GISSI-1 is the only randomized, prospective controlled trial in which the therapy of cardiogenic shock is addressed [42]. As part of GISSI-1, 280 Killip IV patients received either streptokinase or placebo. No benefit of lytic therapy was demonstrated with the 70% in-hospital mortality in each group [33]. The lack of efficacy of lytic therapy in the setting of shock may be related to less effective clot lysis in the setting of arterial hypotension [43].

The reported experience for early CABG for cardiogenic shock is also uncontrolled. The current approach is to completely revascularize the heart with the first priority being revascularization of the myocardium at most risk, be it the IRA or remote from it. The bulk of the published literature suggests that the in-hospital mortality is in the range of 9–60% with an average around 30% (Table 2). This compares favorably with medical, lytic and PTCA therapy. Furthermore, long-term survival appears to be substantial, particularly in those patients in

Table 2. Reports of CABG for cardiogenic shock (uncontrolled)

Investigators (30 day mort)	n	Med/IABP + CABG n (% mort)	Med/IABP n (% mort)	Notes
Dunkman [19] 1968–71	40	15 (60%)	(25 (84%))	
Dewood [20] 1973–78	40	19 (53%)	21 (42%)	Long-term mortality with CABG 25% if CABG < 16 h after shock onset 72% if CABG > 18 h after shock onset
Phillips [47] 1975–82	26	26 (38%)	—	78 mo survival with CABG − 53%
Subramnian [39] 1976–78	47	34 (50%)	13 (92%)	22 mo survival with CABG − 47%
Laks [45] 1981–86	50	50 (30%)	—	24 mo survival with CABG − 48%
Guyton [44] 1983–86	17	17 (12%)	—	36 mo survival with CABG − 88%
Allen [48] 1986–91	66	66 (9%)	—	
Total =	286	227 (30%)	59 (71%)	

whom early intervention has prevented continued myocardial loss [20, 44, 45]. In the setting of post MI cardiogenic shock due to mechanical disruption, such as with papillary muscle or ventricular septal rupture, the survival with medical therapy is extremely small. With early surgical intervention, reported survival rates are in the range of 50–75% [18].

There is substantial enthusiasm for the use of early PTCA in the setting of acute MI and, as an extension, in the setting of cardiogenic shock. Although several groups have published their experience, no randomized, controlled studies are available yet to answer this question [46]. Nonetheless, there is a common theme in the reported interventional experience (Table 3). In the setting of post MI cardiogenic shock, in the subgroup of patients

a) considered candidates for invasive intervention (often younger, with less organ failure and without refractory shock),
b) who have disease amenable to a trial of PTCA (non-left main and non-multivessel disease) and
c) who undergo successful PTCA on the infarct related vessel.

The in-hospital mortality rate is 20–60% compared with the 70–95% mortality in those with a failed PTCA (Table 1).

Patients with cardiogenic shock deemed suitable for aggressive intervention (i.e. cardiac catheterization) as a group have a lower mortality than those patients treated conservatively (mortality 51% vs 85%) even if not revascularized [38]. Furthermore, even within the group of patients undergoing cardiac catheterization, series have reported equivalent mortalities with subsequent PTCA or medical therapy [18, 38]. Although the obvious biases of these selected reports prevent

Table 3. Reports of PTCA for cardiogenic shock (uncontrolled)

Investigators (30 day mortality)	Overall PTCA n (% mort)	Successful PTCA n (% mort)	Unsuccessful PTCA n (% mort)	
Lee [49] 1982–85	69 (45%)	49 (31%)	20 (80%)	Survival @ 32 mos: – Successful PTCA − 55% – Unsuccessful PTCA − 20%
Hibbard [36] 1982–89	45 (44%)	28 (29%)	17 (71%)	Survival @ 27 mos: – Successful PTCA − 54% – Unsuccessful PTCA − 29%
Gacioch [37] 1985–90	48 (55%)	35 (39%)	13 (93%)	Survival @ 12 mos: – Successful PTCA − 48% – Unsuccessful PTCA − 7%
Eltchaninoff [50] 1986–90	33 (36%)	25 (24%)	8 (75%)	Survival @ 12 mos: – Successful PTCA − 52% – Unsuccessful PTCA − 12%
Hochman [38] 1991–93	48 (65%)	33 (61%)	15 (73%)	
Total =	243 (49%)	170 (37%)	73 (78%)	

generalization to patients with cardiogenic shock as a whole, the data is suggestive that successful PTCA either produces or is a marker of a better outcome than is seen in either patients with unsuccessful PTCA or those treated conservatively. Given the poor prognosis of conservatively treated post MI cardiogenic shock and the broader PTCA and lytic data that suggest that reperfusion strategies improve mortality particularly in sicker patients, it is reasonable to consider early reperfusion a sensible, probably important therapy in this group of patients pending results from randomized trials [46].

Conclusion

Cardiogenic shock continues to carry a high mortality. The goals of management include rapid stabilisation of the hemodynamics, aggressive investigation as to the etiology, and prevention of further myocardial loss. Upon making the diagnosis of ischemic cardiogenic shock, reperfusion therapy should be immediately considered given the understanding we have about this disease and the evidence that reperfusion is beneficial in MI patients overall. For patients who are potential transplant candidates, emergent transplantation and mechanical bridge to transplantation have roles. Soon, the possibility of permanent replacement VADs (destination VAD) may provide options to many other end-stage patients. For viable patients, stabilization followed by early evaluation by a center capable of providing this broad range of invasive interventions may offer the best chance of salvaging more patients with cardiogenic shock.

References

1. Caldarone CA, Krukenkamp IB, Burns PG, Misare BD, Gaudette GR, Levitsky S (1994) Ischemia-dependent efficacy of phosphodiesterase inhibition. Ann Thorac Surg 57:540–545
2. MacKerrow SD, Osborn LA, Levy H, Eaton RP, Economou P (1992) Myxedema-associated cardiogenic shock treated with intravenous triiodothyronine. Ann Intern Med 17: 1014–1015
3. Holland FW, Brown PS, Clark RE (1992) Acute severe postischemic myocardial depression reversed by triiodothyronine. Ann Thorac Surg 54:301–305
4. Kadletz M, Mullen PG, Ding M, Wolfe LG, Wechsler AS (1994) Effect of triiodothyronine on postischemic myocardial function in the isolated heart. Ann Thorac Surg 57:657–662
5. Klemperer JD, Klein I, Gomez M, et al (1995) Thyroid hormone treatment after coronary artery bypass surgery. N Engl J Med 333:1522–1527
6. Thames MD, Alpert JS, Dalen JE (1977) Syncope in patients with pulmonary embolism. JAMA 238:2509–2511
7. Come PC, Kim D, Parker JA, Goldhaber SZ, Braunwald E, Markis JE (1987) Early reversal of right ventricular dysfunction in patients with acute pulmonary embolism after treatment with intravenous tissue plasminogen activator. J Am Coll Cardiol 10:971–978
8. Lowenstein E, Johnston WE, Lappas DG, et al (1983) Catastrophic pulmonary vasoconstriction associated with protamine reversal of heparin. Anesthesiology 59:470–473
9. Koshinski EJ, Malindzak GS (1973) Glucagon and isoproterenol in reversing propanolol toxicity. Arch Intern Med 132:840–843
10. Doyon S, Roberts JR (1993) The use of glucagon in a case of calcium channel blocker overdose. Ann Emerg Med 22:1229–1233

11. Wolf LR, Spadafora MP, Otten EJ (1993) Use of amrinone and glucagon in a case of calcium blocker overdose. Ann Emerg Med 22:1225–1228
12. Zehender M, Kasper W, Kauder E, Schonthaler M, Geibel A, Olschewski M (1993) Right ventricular infarction as an independent predictor of prognosis after acute inferior infarction. N Engl J Med 328:981–988
13. Dell'Italia LJ, Starling MR, Blumhardt R, Lasher JC, O'Rourke RA (1985) Comparative effects of volume loading, dobutamine, and nitroprusside in patients with predominant right ventricular infarction. Circulation 72:1327–1335
14. Weiss AT, Engel S, Gotsman CJ, et al (1984) Regional and global left ventricular function during intra-aortic balloon counterpulsation in patients with acute myocardial infarction shock. Am Heart J 108:249–254
15. Wellens HJJ (1993) Right ventricular infarction (editorial). N Engl J Med 328:1036–1038
16. Mueller H, Ayres SM, Conklin EF, et al (1971) The effects of intra-aortic counterpulsation on cardiac performance and metabolism in shock associated with acute myocardial infarction. J Clin Invest 50:1885–1900
17. Scheidt S, Wilner G, Mueller H, et al (1973) Intra-aortic balloon counterpulsation in cardiogenic shock. N Engl J Med 288, No 19:979–984
18. Bardet J, Masquet C, Kahn JC, et al (1977) Clinical and hemodynamic results of intraaortic balloon counterpulsation and surgery for cardiogenic shock. Am Heart J 93, No 3:280–288
19. Dunkman WB, Leinbach RC, Buckley MJ, et al (1972) Clinical and hemodynamic results of intraaortic balloon pumping and surgery for cardiogenic shock. Circulation 46:465–477
20. DeWood MA, Notske RN, Hensley GR, et al (1980) Intraaortic balloon counterpulsation with and without reperfusion for myocardial infarction. Circulation 61, No 6:1105–1112
21. Frazier OH (1994) Outpatient LVAD: Its time has arrived. Ann Thorac Surg 58:1309–1310
22. Magovern GJ Jr, Wampler RK, Joyce LD, Wareing TH (1993) Circulatory support 1991 symposium; Nonpulsatile circulatory support: techniques of insertion. Ann Thorac Surg 55:266–272
23. Bolman RM III, Cox JL, Marshall W, et al (1989) Circulatory support with a centrifugal pump as a bridge to cardiac transplantation. Ann Thorac Surg 47:108–112
24. Wampler RK, Frazier OH, Lansing AM, et al (1991) Treatment of cardiogenic shock with the Hemopump left ventricular assist device. Ann Thorac Surg 52:506–513
25. Pae WE Jr (1993) Ventricular assist devices and total artificial hearts: a combined registry experience. Ann Thorac Surg 55:295–298
26. Guyton RA, Schonberger JP, Everts PA, et al (1993) Postcardiotomy shock: clinical evaluation of the BVS 5000 biventricular support system. Ann Thorac Surg 56:346–356
27. Aufiero, TX, Miller C (1994) Combined registry for the clinical use of mechanical ventricular assist pumps and the total artificial heart, presented April 1994. ASAIO, San Francisco
28. Frazier OH, Macris MP, Myers TJ, et al (1994) Improved survival after extended bridge to cardiac transplantation. Ann Thorac Surg 57:1416–1422
29. Kormos RL, Borovetz HS, Gasior T, et al (1990) Experience with univentricular support in mortally ill cardiac transplant patients. Ann Thorac Surg 49:261–271
30. Page DL, Caulfield JB, Kastor JA, DeSanctis RW, Sanders CA (1971) Myocardial changes associated with cardiogenic shock. N Engl J Med 285, No 3:133–137
31. Harnarayan C, Bennett MA, Pentecost BL, Brewer DB (1970) Quantitative study of infarcted myocardium in cardiogenic shock. British Heart Journal 32:728–732
32. Holmes DR Jr, Bates ER, Kleinman NS, et al (1995) Contemporary reperfusion therapy for cardiogenic shock: the GUSTO-1 trial experience. J Am Coll Cardiol 26:668–674
33. Gruppo Italiano per lo Studio della Streptochinasi nell'infarcto miocardico (GISSI) (1986) Effectiveness of intravenous thrombolytic treatment in acute myocardial infarction. Lancet i:397–402
34. Gruppo Italiano per lo Studio delta Streptochinasi nell'infarcto miocardico (GISSI) (1990) GISSI-2: A factorial randomised trial of alteplase versus streptokinase and heparin versus no heparin among 12,490 patients with acute myocardial infarction. Lancet 336:65–71
35. Hands ME, Rutherford JD, Muller JE, et al (1989) The in-hospital development of cardiogenic shock after myocardial infarction; incidence, predictors of occurrence, outcome and prognostic factors. J Am Coll Cardiol 14:40–46

36. Hibbard MD, Holmes DR Jr, Baily KR, Reeder GS, Bresnahan JF, Gersh BJ (1992) Percutaneous transluminal angioplasty in patients with cardiogenic shock. J Am Coll Cardiol 19: 639–646

37. Gacioch GM, Ellis SG, Lee L, et al (1992) Cardiogenic shock complicating acute myocardial infarction: the use of coronary angioplasty and the integration of the new support devices into patient management. J Am Coll Cardiol 19: 647–653

38. Hochman JS, Boland J, Sleeper LA, et al (1995) Current spectrum of cardiogenic shock and effect of early revascularization on mortality: results of an international registry. Circulation 91: 873–881

39. Subramian XA, Roberts AJ, Zema MJ, et al (1980) Cardiogenic shock following acute myocardial infarction: late functional results after emergency cardiac surgery. NY State Med Jour, May: 947–951

40. Lee L, Bates ER, Pitt B, Walton JA, Laufer N, O'Neill WW (1988) Percutaneous transluminal coronary angioplasty improves survival in acute myocardial infarction complicated by cardiogenic shock. Circulation 78: 1345–1351

41. Bengtson JR, Kaplan AJ, Pieper KS, et al (1992) Prognosis in cardiogenic shock after acute myocardial infarction in the interventional era. J Am Coll Cardiol 20: 1482–1489

42. Bates ER, Topal EJ (1991) Limitations of thrombolytic therapy for acute myocardial infarction complicated by heart failure and cardiogenic shock. J Am Coll Cardiol 18: 1077–1084

43. Garber PJ, Mathieson AL, Ducas J, Patton JN, Geddes JS, Prewitt RM (1995) Thrombolytic therapy in cardiogenic shock: effect of increased aortic pressure and rapid tPA administration. Can J Cardiol 11 (1): 30–36

44. Guyton RA, Arcidi JM, Langford DA, Morris DC, Liberman HA, Hatcher CR Jr (1987) Emergency coronary bypass for cardiogenic shock. Circulation 76 (V): 22–27

45. Laks H, Rosenkranz E, Buckberg GD (1986) Surgical treatment of cardiogenic shock after myocardial infarction. Circulation 74 (III): 11–16

46. Moscucci M, Bates ER (1995) Cardiogenic shock. Cardiology Clinics 13, No 3: 391–406

47. Phillips SJ, Kongtahworn C, Skinner JR, Zeff RH (1983) Emergency coronary artery reperfusion: a choice therapy for evolving myocardial infarction. J Thorac Cardiovasc Surg 86: 679–688

48. Allen BS, Buckberg GD, Fontan FM, et al (1993) Superiority of controlled surgical reperfusion versus transluminal coronary angioplasty in acute coronary occlusion. J Thorac Cardiovasc Surg 105: 864–884

49. Lee L, Erbel R, Brown TM, Laufer N, Meyer J, O'Neill WW (1991) Multicenter registry of angioplasty therapy of cardiogenic shock: initial and long term survival. J Am Coll Cardiol 17: 599–603

50. Eltchaninoff H, Simpfendorfer C, Franco I, Raymond RE, Casale PN, Whitlow PL (1995) Early and 1-year survival rates in acute myocardial infarction complicated by cardiogenic shock: a retrospective study comparing coronary angioplasty with medical treatment. Am Heart J 130: 459–464

Cardiovascular Support by Hemodynamic Subset: Sepsis

A. Meier-Hellmann and K. Reinhart

Introduction

Multiple organ failure (MOF) is the major cause of death in patients with sepsis [1]. Macro and microcirculatory maldistribution of blood flow to the tissues and hypoxia of certain organs plays an important role in the pathogenesis of sepsis [2, 3]. In addition, there is evidence in the literature for an oxygen extraction deficit. Therefore a supranormal oxygen delivery (DO_2) is considered by many to be essential for adequate tissue oxygenation [4, 5]. Sufficient volume substitution and treatment with catecholamines are usually required to achieve a supranormal oxygen delivery and an adequate systemic perfusion pressure. Despite this, the mortality rate of sepsis and the incidence of MOF remains persistantly high [6]. It is obvious that under the conditions of a supranormal DO_2 tissue hypoxia in various tissues may still occur [2, 4]. Information regarding perfusion and oxygenation in different regions of the body is mandatory for the detection of regional tissue hypoxia.

Renal and gastrointestinal failure are major complications in sepsis [7-9]. Bacterial translocation from the gut is considered by some authors to induce and maintain sepsis [10-12]. Nelson et al. [13] demonstrated that the critical DO_2 of the small intestine in septic sheep was higher than whole body DO_2. Thus, the achievement of critical whole body DO_2 does not exclude oxygen supply dependency in specific tissues [13].

Previous studies have not conclusively demonstrated a reduction of splanchnic perfusion in sepsis. One reason for this may be that different methods were used measure splanchnic perfusion [14]. In septic patients, Dahn et al. [15] demonstrated that splanchnic perfusion increased to the same extent as the cardiac output (CO), although the splanchnic oxygen consumption (VO_2hep) increased to a far greater extent than whole body oxygen consumption (VO_2). In experimental settings [16, 17] it has been reported that redistribution of blood flow and relative improvement of hepatic and small intestine perfusion occurs. In healthy individuals, an infusion of endotoxin doubled splanchnic blood flow [18]. We found that 60% of the cardiac output in septic patients was distributed through the splanchnic region, in comparison to 18-30% in healthy individuals [19, 20].

Little is known about the influence of various catecholamines on regional blood flow and oxygenation [21, 22] and the catecholamines used most often in the clinical setting, e.g. dobutamine, dopamine, norepinephrine, epinephrine, and dopexamine, were typically investigated in patients without sepsis or not in septic shock (Table 1 and 2).

Dobutamine

Many authors suggest that dobutamine due to its beta 1 receptor mediated effects is the catecholamine of choice for increasing myocardial contractility and achieving supranormal CO and DO_2 levels [23–26]. Animal investigations [27] and clinical studies [4, 28] have shown that an increase in DO_2 induced by dobutamine infusion leads to an increased VO_2. Furthermore, it is hypothesized that the beta 2 mediated effects counteract peripheral vasoconstriction and hence improve tissue oxygenation [26]. Under the conditions of an adequate volume replacement, dobutamine increases cardiac output and DO_2 to a greater extent than dopamine [27]. Vincent et al. [28] demonstrated that an infusion of dobutamine at 5 µg/kg/min in adequately volume replaced septic patients increased the DO_2 by

Table 1. Effects of the different catecholamines on the different receptors

	alpha 1	alpha 2	beta 1	beta 2	DA 1	DA 2
Catecholamine						
Dobutamine	+ +	0	+ + +	+ +	0	0
Epinephrine	+ + +	+ + +	+ +	+ + +	0	0
Norepinephrine	+ + +	+ + +	+ +	+	0	0
Dopamine						
0–3 µg/kg/min	0	+	0	0	+ + +	+ +
2–10 µg/kg/min	+	+	+ +	+	+ +	+ +
> 10 µg/kg/min	+ +	+ +	+ +	+	+	+
Dopexamine	0	0	+	+ + +	+ +	+

Table 2. Effects of the different catecholamines on regional blood flow

	Kidney	Brain	Heart	Splanchnic	Muscle	Skin
Catecholamine						
Dobutamine	+	+	+	+	+ +	+
Epinephrine	− / +	+	+	− / +	+ /0	−
Norepinephrine	− / +	+	+	− / +	− /0	0
Dopamine						
0–3 µg/kg/min	+ + +	+	0	+ + +	0	0
2–10 µg/kg/min	+ + / +	+	+	+ / +	0	0
> 10 µg/kg/min	− / +	+	+	− / +	−	−
Dopexamine	+ + +	+	+	+ + +	+	+

29% and VO_2 by 18%. Furthermore, they speculated that dobutamine decreased tissue perfusion maldistribution. To our knowledge it is not clear whether dobutamine selectively influences splanchnic or renal perfusion. Improvement in splanchnic oxygenation is supported by the results of Silverman et al. [29] who found that infusion of dobutamine at 5 µg/kg/min increased a pathologically reduced gastric mucosal pH (pHi). In contrast, blood transfusion did not influence pHi but increased DO_2 to a similar extent. In septic pigs Schneider et al. [30] found that adequate volume substitution alone restored a decreased cardiac output and led to redistribution of blood flow in favour of the splanchnic region. An additional infusion of dobutamine did not influence the distribution of blood flow to the kidneys and the splanchnic region. In patients with congestive heart failure, Leier et al. [31] found that those who received dobutamine at 7.5 µg/kg/min experienced an increase in CO accompanied by a decrease in splanchnic perfusion. In the same study renal perfusion was increased to a lesser extent than CO. Mousdale et al. [32] were able to measure only a minor increase in renal blood flow under dobutamine and dopexamine. However different doses of dopamine induced remarkable increases in renal blood flow.

Hayes et al. [33] demonstrated that there was no difference in global VO_2 between a group of 50 patients treated with dobutamine up to 200 µg/kg/min to achieve three goals (cardiac index above 4.5 l/min/m², DO_2 above 600 ml/min/m², VO_2 above 170 ml/min/m²) established on the basis of previously published recommendations [34–36] and 50 patients who were treated only with an adequate volume filling. Contrary to what might have been expected, the survival in the patients with the dobutamine treatment was lower than in the control group. The authors speculated that the aggressive dobutamine treatment in an attempt to increase VO_2 may have been detrimental in some patients. A benefical effect of dobutamine on gastric mucosal pH (pHi) is demonstrated from Gutierrez et al. [37]; they also found an unchanged VO_2 after treatment with dobutamine but an increase in pHi in septic patients. In conclusion, if dobutamine is used to increase DO_2 there is some evidence of an improvement in tissue oxygenation.

Whether dobutamine selectively influences regional blood flow is unknown. Management of septic shock with dobutamine alone is often not sufficient to restore adequate blood pressure. Whether the combination of dobutamine and norepinephrine is superior to the treatment with dopamine alone has not yet been investigated.

Norepinephrine

Norepinephrine has only moderate $beta_1$ and $beta_2$-mimetic effects. In experimental models it increased splanchnic vascular resistance and decreases splanchnic blood flow [38–40]. Norepinephrine is used in animal studies to induce renal failure [41]. Consequently, norepinephrine is often only used as a last resort if hemodynamic stabilisation is not achieved with other catecholamines [42].

Melchior et al. [43] found that an infusion of 0.5 or 1.0 µg/kg/min norepinephrine did not change whole body VO_2 despite an increased cardiac index (CI) and mean arterial pressure (MAP). They concluded that the beneficial beta mimetic effects of norepinephrine outweigh the possible deleterious effects mediated by alpha receptors. In septic dogs, Bakker et al. [44] demonstrated an increase of right and left ventricular stroke work index with an infusion of norepinephrine ranging from 0.1 to 0.2 µg/kg/min and an increase of DO_2 and VO_2 with an infusion of norepinephrine from 0.5 to 1.0 µg/kg/min. Schneider et al. [30] recommended norepinephrine over dobutamine for the treatment of right heart failure in septic shock since an increase in diastolic blood pressure improves myocardial perfusion. Schreuder et al. [45] reported that a norepinephrine infusion in patients in septic shock increased VO_2 but did not change the DO_2. However it remains unknown how much of the increase in VO_2 was due to an improvement in perfusion pressure which increased simultaneously from 57 mmHg to 75 mmHg. This finding underlines the importance of an adequate perfusion pressure and shows that treatment with norepinephrine is indicated if an adequate perfusion pressure cannot be maintained with volume substitution and dobutamine or dopamine. In 6 patients with septic shock in whom hemodynamic stabilisation by dopamine or dobutamine infusion was not achieved, DO_2 and VO_2 values were inconsistent when they were treated with norepinephrine [46]. In our own investigations [47], the change in catecholamine treatment from dobutamine to norepinephrine in patients with septic shock led to a decrease in DO_2 but VO_2 remained unchanged. The unchanged VO_2 can be explained by an unchanged tissue oxygenation. However, redistribution of blood flow with norepinephrine treatment alone, undetected by the measurement of the global O_2 transport related variables cannot be excluded.

Several authors have demonstrated an increase in urine output in patients with septic shock treated with norepinephrine [48–50]. However it should be emphasized that these patients had markedly decreased blood pressures. In the study from Desjars et al. [48] the infusion of 0.5–1.0 µg/kg/min norepinephrine increased the MAP from 48 mmHg to 62 mmHg. Hesselvik and Brodin [49] reported an increase in MAP from 50 mmHg to 69 mmHg after the infusion of 0.5 µg/kg/min norepinephrine. The principal mechanism of improved renal function in these studies is the increase of perfusion pressure to an adequate level. Redl-Wenzl et al. [51] reported an increase in creatinine clearance after treatment with norepinephrine in 56 patients with septic shock. However, in this study the patients also had an inadequate perfusion pressure of 56 mmHg before treatment with norepinephrine. There is a lack of knowledge about whether treatment with norepinephrine has beneficial effects on the renal function in the presence of an adequate perfusion pressure. Fukuoka et al. [52] reported in septic patients with lactate levels in a normal range that a norepinephrine infusion increased urine output and did not change creatinine clearance, whereas in patients with elevated lactate levels norepinephrine had no effect on urine output but decreased creatinine clearance.

The findings concerning the effects of norepinephrine on splanchnic perfusion are inconsistent. Bersten et al. [53] compared the effects of different catecholamines on regional blood flow in septic and non septic sheep. In the non septic animals there was a redistribution of blood flow measured by microsphere technique to the heart away from brain, kidneys, liver and pancreas with norepinephrine, dobutamine, dopamine, dopexamine or salbutamol treatment. Thus, a deleterious effect of norepinephrine on splanchnic perfusion is demonstrated in these animals. In contrast, in septic animals such a redistribution of regional blood flow was not found. The authors explained these findings by a decreased sensitivity of alpha receptors and a direct sepsis associated vasodilation [54–58].

Schneider et al. [30] infused pigs with E. coli and stabilized the animals initially only by volume substitution. Further treatment with dobutamine or norepinephrine did not influence the distribution of the given volume, measured with radio-labelled erythrocytes. There was a decreased pooling of blood in the legs after norepinephrine infusion. Breslow et al. [59] infused pigs with E. coli and kept the pulmonary capillary wedge pressure within the normal range by infusing isotonic solutions. Under these conditions norepinephrine, dopamine and phenylepinephrine given in doses to achieve MAP of 75 mmHg were without selective effects on regional blood flow. A benefical effect of norepinephrine on splanchnic oxygenation in septic patients was shown in a study by Marik et al. [60] who compared norepinephrine and dopamine given as vasopressors. Patients who were treated with norepinephrine had an increase in gastric mucosal pH (pHi) whereas dopamine led to a decrease in pHi.

We measured the splanchnic blood flow in 10 patients with septic shock by the green dye dilution technique. Changing the catecholamine treatment from a combination of dobutamine with norepinephrine to norepinephrine alone led to a parallel decrease in splanchnic perfusion and cardiac output. The relationship between splanchnic perfusion and cardiac output remained unchanged. Furthermore, the splanchnic VO_2 remained unchanged (Table 3). Due to the decrease in splanchnic DO_2, hepatic venous O_2 extraction increased. Therefore, in situations where there is a further decrease in splanchnic DO_2, there is an increased risk that splanchnic VO_2 becomes supply dependent with norepinephrine treatment alone.

In conclusion it should be pointed out that treatment with vasopressors is often indispensable in the therapeutical management of septic shock. Provided that the DO_2 is in a supranormal range, treatment with norepinephrine alone is without negative tissue oxygenation effects. Animal studies have shown that the negative effect of norepinephrine on splanchnic perfusion is only seen in nonseptic conditions.

Epinephrine

Epinephrine is advocated in the treatment of septic shock [61–63] because it leads to a beta receptor mediated increase in cardiac output and an alpha receptor mediated increase in perfusion pressure. Low doses of epinephrine have predominantly beta mimetic effects and only in higher doses do the alpha mimetic effects become predominant [64]. Bollaert et al. [61] investigated the effects of epinephrine in doses between 0.5 and 1.0 µg/kg/min in 13 patients with septic

Table 3. Effects of changing catecholamine treatment from a combination of dobutamine with norepinephrine to norepinephrine alone

	dobutamine/ norepinephrine	norepinephrine alone	
DO_2 (ml/min/m²)	796 ±151	598 ±113	*
VO_2 (ml/min/m²)	159 ± 27	152 ± 26	n.s.
CI (l/min/m²)	6.0± 1.2	4.3± 0.8	*
DO_2hep (ml/min/m²)	210 ±108	171 ± 88	*
VO_2hep (ml/min/m²)	77 ± 41	72 ± 21	n.s.
HBF (l/min/m²)	1.6± 0.8	1.1± 0.6	*
DO_2/DO_2hep	4.3± 1.4	4.1± 1.7	n.s.
VO_2/VO_2hep	4.9± 2.5	4.8± 1.3	n.s.
CI/HBF	4.3± 1.4	4.1± 1.7	n.s.
SvO_2 (%)	76 ± 4	71 ± 6	*
$ShvO_2$ (%)	58 ± 13	49 ± 15	*

DO_2: oxygen delivery; VO_2: oxygen consumption; CI: cardiac index; DO_2hep: splanchnic oxygen delivery; VO_2hep: splanchnic oxygen consumption; HBF: hepatic blood flow; SvO_2: mixed venous O_2 saturation; $ShvO_2$: hepatic venous O_2 saturation; * statistically significant; n.s.: not significant

shock that could not stabilized by 15 µg/kg/min dopamine. Epinephrine increased MAP, systemic vascular resistance and cardiac output in these patients. Furthermore the DO_2 and VO_2 increased. Elevated arterial lactate levels were interpreteted as a metabolic effect due to epinephrine. Moran et al. [65] reported an increase in DO_2 from 481 to 531 ml/min/m² and an increase in VO_2 from 165 to 193 ml/min/m² with an epinephrine infusion in doses up to 18 µg/min in patients with septic shock. According to the dose dependent effects of epinephrine both a reduction [66–68] and an improvement [69] of splanchnic perfusion is reported in animal studies. Little is known about the effects of epinephrine on splanchnic and renal perfusion in septic shock states.

In our own investigations, changing the catecholamine treatment from a combination of dobutamine and norepinephrine to epinephrine alone decreased the $ShvO_2$ but did not change the SvO_2, so the difference between the two catecholamine regimens was significantly increased [70]. Dahn et al. [71] reported a parallel decrease in $ShvO_2$ and SvO_2 under hypoxia. In contrast, in 33 patients undergoing liver surgery the $ShvO_2$ decreased and the SvO_2 did not change after skin incision [72]. The authors explained this discrepancy as being a selective decrease in splanchnic perfusion mediated by endogeneous catecholamines liberated following skin incision. The selective decrease in $ShvO_2$ seems to be a marker for deterioration in splanchnic oxygenation. We measured splanchnic perfusion, DO_2 and VO_2 in 8 patients with septic shock treated with a combination of dobutamine and norepinephrine. After a change of treatment to epinephrine alone, titrated to achieve the same MAP as before, the DO_2 and VO_2 were unchanged, but epinephrine decreased the splanchnic perfusion in the presence of an unchanged cardiac output (Table 4). The decreased splanchnic DO_2 lead to a decreased

Table 4. Effects of changing catecholamine treatment from a combination of dobutamine with norepinephrine to epinephrine alone

	dobutamine/ norepinephrine		norepinephrine alone		
DO_2 (ml/min/m^2)	819	±120	822	±249	n.s.
VO_2 (ml/min/m^2)	145	± 27	152	± 45	n.s.
CI (l/min/m^2)	5.9 ±	0.9	5.9 ±	1.7	n.s.
DO_2hep (ml/min/m^2)	380	±170	222	± 92	*
VO_2hep (ml/min/m^2)	107	± 59	78	± 39	*
HBF (l/min/m^2)	2.8 ±	1.4	1.6 ±	0.6	*
Fractional HBF (%)	47	± 19	29	± 14	*
Lac arterial (mmol/L)	1.6 ±	0.8	2.9 ±	1.5	*
Lac mixed venous (mmol/L)	1.6 ±	0.8	3.0 ±	1.6	*
Lac hepatic venous (mmol/L)	1.3 ±	0.8	2.4 ±	1.5	*
Gastric mucosal pH	7.27±	0.08	7.19±	0.05	*

DO$_2$: oxygen delivery; *VO$_2$:* oxygen consumption; *CI:* cardiac index; *DO$_2$hep:* splanchnic oxygen delivery; *VO$_2$hep:* splanchnic oxygen consumption; *HBF:* hepatic blood flow; *Lac:* lactate; * statistically significant; *n.s.:* not significant

splanchnic VO$_2$. These extreme changes in splanchnic oxygenation were not detected by whole body DO$_2$ and VO$_2$, underlying the importance of measuring DO$_2$ and VO$_2$ in specific regions. Furthermore, an increase in lactate levels and a decrease in pHi indicates tissue hypoxia in the splanchnic region [73].

Due to the lack of more information regarding epinephrine in the treatment of septic shock a conclusion is not yet possible. Our preliminary results have demonstrated a decrease in splanchnic perfusion and oxygenation accompanied by signs of severe tissue hypoxia. If further investigations also demonstrate these negative effects, the use of epinephrine in patients with septic shock will not be recommended.

Dopamine

Dopamine has effects on alpha, beta and dopaminergic receptors. The dopaminergic receptors can be divided into presynaptic (DA1) and postsynaptic (DA2) receptors. Stimulation of DA1 receptors causes renal and splanchnic vasodilation. Stimulation of DA2 receptors blocks norepinephrine output from sympathetic nerves [74].

Dopaminergic receptors are found in renal, mesenteric and hepatic vessels [74]. The effects of dopamine are dose dependent. In doses up to 3 µg/kg/min, dopamine selectively stimulates the dopaminergic receptors. In doses up to 5 µg/kg/min there is stimulation of beta receptors and in doses greater than 5 µg/kg/min the alpha receptors are also stimulated.

Vincent and Preiser [75] advocated dopamine as the drug of choice in the primary management of decreased MAP in patients in septic shock. It is the opinion of other authors that the alpha mimetic effects of dopamine are a disadvantage because a previously disturbed microcirculation could be further compromised [26, 27]. In 437 critical care patients Shoemaker et al. more frequently induced an increase in DO_2 and VO_2 with dobutamine than with dopamine [42]. In brain dead patients treatment with dopamine to elevate MAP to within a normal range caused a lower mitochondrial redox state in liver cells as compared to patients with a lower MAP who were not treated with dopamine [76]. This effect of dopamine can be interpreted as a hypoxia mediated organ failure.

Dopamine in low doses is often recommended as an additional drug for the improvement of renal function and splanchnic perfusion [77, 78]. In non septic patients Duke et al. [79] showed that low dose dopamine increased urine output without changing creatinine clearance, whereas low dose dobutamine did not change urine output but increased creatinine clearance. Nevertheless, it is not yet proven that treatment with low dose dopamine is beneficial to patients in septic shock.

In animals and healthy humans an increase in the inulin clearance, renal plasma flow, and sodium excretion has been shown after dopamine infusion [74]. Mousdale et al. [32] demonstrated that dopamine in doses of 2.5, 5.0 and 10.0 µg/kg/min induced a significantly higher renal plasma flow than dobutamine in a similar dosage and dopexamine in doses of 1.0, 2.0 and 4.0 µg/kg/min in healthy humans. The effects of dopamine on renal function in patients with septic shock is not completely understood. It is not known if dopamine influences the incidence of renal failue in septic shock patients.

Dopamine improved a decreased hepatic blood flow in dogs ventilated with positive end-expiratory pressure [80]. In septic rats dopamine induced a selective improvement of hepatic blood flow [81]. An increase in hepatic blood flow does not guarantee improved splanchnic oxygenation because a redistribution of blood flow in the splanchnic area may lead to a deterioration in tissue oxygenation. Giraud et al. [39] infused dogs with dopamine and were able to measure an increase in blood flow in the superior mesenteric artery and in the muscularis of the gut with a decreased blood flow to the gut mucosa accompanied by a decrease in splanchnic VO_2. The improvement of global blood flow measured in a major artery seems to be accompanied by a deterioration of blood flow and oxygenation in other tissues such as the gut mucosa. Pawlik et al. [82] demonstrated that intraarterial infusion of dopamine 1 µg/kg/min in dogs caused splanchnic vasoconstriction with reduction of blood flow and splanchnic VO_2. In the same investigation epinephrine also led to a reduction in splanchnic blood flow but did not influence the splanchnic VO_2. Therefore the authors suggested that dopamine is a drug with deleterious side effects on splanchnic oxygenation. In contrast to these findings Kullmann et al. [83] showed an increased blood flow to the intestinal organs and an improved perfusion of the mucosa and submucosa in rabbits measured by microsphere technique. Leier [31] reported in congestive heart failure patients that 3 µg/kg/min dopamine significantly increased renal blood flow and did not change splanchnic blood flow. In non septic pigs Roytblat et al. [84] measured a dose independent increase in splanchnic DO_2 and a dose dependent increase in splanchnic VO_2 after dopamine infusion. Since higher doses of dopamine increased splanchnic VO_2 to a greater extent than splanchnic DO_2 the authors conclude that dopamine did not improve splanchnic oxygenation and explained the increased splanchnic VO_2 as a calorigenic effect of dopamine [85–87].

In 11 patients with septic shock treated with norepinephrine we added dopamine in a dosage of 2.8 to 3.0 µg/kg/min. In the patients who had a fractional splanchnic flow in a normal range, low dose dopamine increased splanchnic perfusion, whereas in patients with an elevated fractional splanchnic flow before treatment we measured no further increase or even a decrease in splanchnic flow [88]. This finding suggests that the effect of dopamine depends on the individual splanchnic flow, which could vary from normal to markedly elevated in septic patients.

To summarize, whether management with a higher dose of dopamine alone compared to the combination of dobutamine and norepinephrine is of advantage in the treatment of septic shock has not yet proven. The improvement of renal function is an argument for the use of low dose dopamine although under the conditions of septic shock there are only few and nonequivocal studies. Animal studies reported deleterious effects of dopamine on splanchnic oxygenation. One study demonstrated an increased splanchnic VO_2 after dopamine infusion, but it remained unclear if the increased VO_2 was the result of improved oxygenation or only the calorigenic effect of dopamine.

Dopexamine

The relatively new catecholamine dopexamine has predominantly $beta_2$ and dopaminergic receptor activity. Many animal and human studies have described the usefulness of dopexamine in heart failure [89–92]. Tan et al. [93] demonstrated a direct inotropic effect of dopexamine in patients with low-output cardiac failure.

To date, only a few studies have examined the effects of dopexamine in patients with septic shock. Colardyn et al. [94] reported an increase in cardiac index and heart rate and a decrease in systemic vascular resistance. Unfortunately, data regarding the DO_2 and VO_2 were not mentioned. Cain and Curtis [95] did not note a difference in mesenteric venous blood flow in a group of septic dogs treated with dopexamine and a control group without catecholamine treatment. The gut of the dopexamine treated animals produced less lactate and the authors concluded that dopexamine caused gut mucosa to be preferentially perfused. Biro et al. [96] measured a relatively higher skeletal muscle and gastric blood flow in non septic dogs with dopexamine in comparison to dobutamine. In dogs in hemorrhagic shock Lokhandwala and Jandhyala [97] demonstrated an increase in splanchnic perfusion to 40–50% from baseline after blood retransfusion, whereas splanchnic perfusion increased to 80–90% of baseline if dopexamine was added to the transfusion. Uusaro et al. [98] reported an increase in whole body DO_2 and splanchnic DO_2 to similar extent after dopexamine infusion in cardiac surgery patients. They did not seen a special effect on splanchnic perfusion by dopexamine infusion, as indicated by an unchanged fractional splanchnic perfusion. Smithies et al. [99] reported an increase in pHi in 10 septic patients treated with dopexamine to a maximum dose of 6.0 µg/kg/min. A benefical effect on outcome in 54 high risk patients was reported from Boyd et al. [100], who treated patients perioperatively with dopexamine to achieve an DO_2 greater than 600 ml/min/m². Whether the reduced mortality in the study from Boyd was really an effect of the dopexamine treatment is the purpose of an ongoing multicenter trial.

In our studies the addition of 4.0 µg/kg/min dopexamine did not influence the difference between SvO_2 and $ShvO_2$. This finding is consistent with Leier [31] who reported in patients with heart failure that an increase in cardiac output accompanied an increase in splanchnic perfusion.

To date, little is known concerning the effects of dopexamine on renal blood flow in patients with septic shock. Dopexamine increased urine output in both healthy subjects and patients with heart failure [101]. In comparison to dopamine, dopexamine caused no further increase in urine output in patients undergoing hepatic surgery [102]. Stephan et al. [103] demonstrated a more profound decrease in renal vascular resistance under dopamine than under dopexamine in patients with cardiac surgery. The increase in renal blood flow was proportional to the increase in cardiac output. The authors therefore concluded that a selective dopaminergic effect of dopexamine was not proven. Magrini et al. [104] reported an increase in renal blood flow to a higher extent than an increased cardiac output in patients with hypertension. Mousdale et al. [32] demonstrated that dopamine in doses of 2.5, 5.0, and 10.0 µg/kg/min increased renal plasma flow more than dopexamine in doses of 1.0, 2.0, and 4.0 µg/kg/min.

In conclusion, some investigators recommend dopexamine to improve splanchnic oxygenation and renal function. Further studies are required to prove the usefulness of dopexamine in the treatment of septic shock patients and to compare the effects with those of low dose dopamine.

Conclusions

Only a few, conflicting studies have looked at the effects of the various catecholamines on regional blood flow. Therefore a clear recommendation for a specific catecholamine regimen in septic shock is impossible. Furthermore, it is unknown whether the choice of a specific catecholamine in the treatment of septic shock influences the patient's outcome. It is suggested that an increase in DO_2 within a supranormal range is associated with an improved patient outcome [34, 105, 106].

A fundamentel step in the treatment of septic shock is adequate volume replacement. We have demonstrated that volume treatment alone can improve pHi [107]. Figure 1 demonstrates the change in whole body DO_2 and VO_2 and splanchnic DO_2 and VO_2 in a patient in septic shock after the infusion of 1800 ml colloid, which increased the pulmonary capillary wedge pressure from 12 mmHg to 17 mmHg. The increase in whole body and splanchnic VO_2 emphasized the importance of adequate volume substitution.

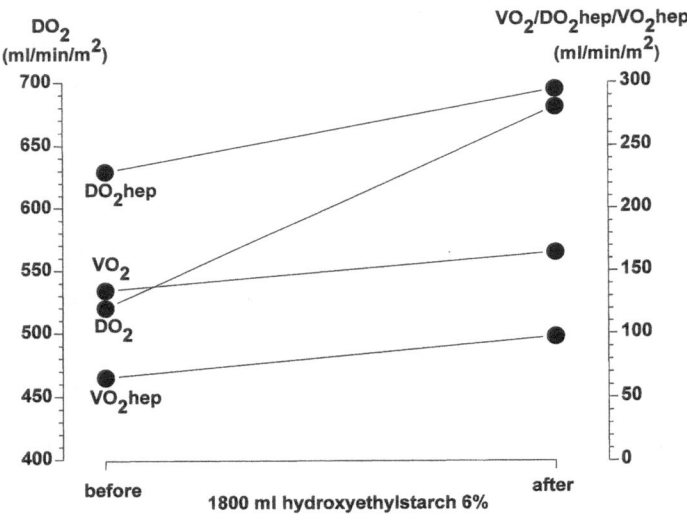

Fig. 1. Effects of volume management with 1800 ml Hydroxyethylstarch on oxygen delivery (DO_2), oxygen consumption (VO_2), splanchnic oxygen delivery (DO_2hep) and splanchnic oxygen consumption (VO_2hep)

In most patients, the use of vasopressors is indispensable because adequate hemodynamic perfusion pressure is not achieved with volume alone. The negative effects of vasopressors on splanchnic perfusion are known from studies carried out under non septic conditions. Norepinephrine and dopamine in doses of 10 µg/kg/min in septic animals are without negative effects on splanchnic perfusion. Preliminary results show a decrease in splanchnic oxygenation in patients with septic shock treated with epinephrine.

Catecholamines with beta mimetic effects are often used to increase DO_2. The question as to whether dobutamine or dopamine should be used first in treatment of septic shock cannot be yet answered.

Whether treatment with low dose dopamine or dopexamine actually improves renal function and splanchnic oxygenation is the purpose of ongoing studies.

References

1. Fiddian-Green RG (1991) Role of gut in shock and resuscitation. In: Stoutenbeck CP, van Saene HKF (eds) Infection and the anesthetist, Vol 5 (1). Bailliere Tindall/WB Saunders Company, London, pp 75–99
2. Schumacker P, Cain S (1987) The concept of a critical oxygen delivery. Intensive Care Med 13:223–229
3. Sibbald WJ, Bersten A, Rutledge FS (1989) The role of tissue hypoxia in multiple organ failure. In: Reinhart K, Eyrich K (eds) Clinical aspects of oxygen transport and tissue oxygenation. Springer, Berlin Heidelberg New York 1989, pp 102–114

4. Gilbert EM, Haupt MT, Mandanas RY, Huaringa AJ, Carlson RW (1986) The effect of fluid loading, blood transfusion, and catecholamine infusion on oxygen delivery and consumption in patients with sepsis. Am Respir Dis Rev 134:873–878
5. Kaufman BS, Rackow EC, Falk JL (1984) The Relationship Between Oxygen Delivery and Consumption during Fluid Resuscitation of Hypovolemic and Septic Shock. Chest 85,3: 337–340
6. Parker MM, Parillo JF (1983) Septic shock. Hemodynamics and pathogenesis. JAMA 250: 3324–3327
7. Fry DE, Pearlstein L, Fulton RL (1980) Multiple-system organ failure: the role of uncontrolled infection. Arch Surg 115:136–140
8. Lucas CE (1976) The renal response to acute injury and sepsis. Surg Clin North Am 56: 953–975
9. Tran DD, Groeneveld ABJ, Van der Meulen J, et al (1990) Age, chronic disease, sepsis, organ system failure, and mortality in a medical intensive care unit. Crit Care Med 18:474–479
10. Deitch EA, Berg R, Specian R (1987) Endotoxin promotes the translocation of bacteria from the gut. Arch Surg 122:185–190
11. Marshall JC, Christou NV, Horn R, et al (1988) The microbiology of multiple organ failure: the proximal GI tract as an occult reservoir of pathogens. Arch Surg 123:309–315
12. Meakins JL, Marshall JC (1989) The gut as the 'motor of multiple system organ failure. In: Marston A, Bulkley GB, Fiddian Green RG, et al (eds) Splanchnic Ischemia and Multiple Organ Failure. CV Mosby, St Louis, pp 339–348
13. Nelson DP, Samsel RW, Wood LD, Schumacker PT (1988) Pathologic supply dependence of systemic and intestinal O_2 uptake during endotoxemia. J Appl Physiol 64:2410–2419
14. Dahn MS, Lange P, Lobdell K, Hans B, Jacobs LA, Mitchel RA (1989) Hepatic blood flow and splanchnic oxygen consumption measurements in clinical sepsis. Surgery 107:295–301
15. Dahn MS, Lange P, Lobdell K, Hans B, Jacobs LA, Mitchell RA (1987) Splanchnic and total body oxygen consumption differences in septic and injured patients. Surgery 101:69–80
16. Lang CH, Bagby GJ, Ferguson JL, Spitzer JJ (1984) Cardiac output and redistribution of organ blood flow in hypermetabolic sepsis. Am J Physiol 246 R:331–337
17. Wang P, Ba ZF, Chaudry IH (1991) Hepatic extraction of indocyanine green is depressed early in sepsis despite increased hepatic blood flow and cardiac output. Arch Surg 126: 219–224
18. Fong Y, Marano MA, Moldawer LL, et al (1990) The acute splanchnic and peripheral tissue metabolic response to endotoxin in humans. J Clin Invest 85:1896–1904
19. Johnson GA, McNamara JJ (1981) Organ ischemia after hemorrhagic shock. Surg Forum 32:24–26
20. Leevy CM, George W, Lesko W, et al (1961) Observations on hepatic oxygen metabolism in man. JAMA 178:565–567
21. Brown RS, Carey JS, Mohr PA, Monson DO, Shoemaker WC (1966) Comparative evaluation of sympathomimetic amines in clinical shock. Circulation 34:260–271
22. Sibbald WJ, Calvin JE, et al (1983) Concepts in the pharmacologic and nonpharmacologic support of cardiovascular function in critically ill surgical patients. Surg Clin North Am 63:456–465
23. Dhainaut JF, Edwards JD, Grootendorst AF, et al (1990) Practical aspects of oxygen transport: conclusions and recommendations of the Round Table Conference. Int Care Med 16: 179–180
24. Reinhart K, Hannemann L, Kuss B (1990) Optimal levels of O_2 delivery in the critically ill. Int Care Med 16:149–154
25. Shoemaker WC, Appel PL, Kram HB, Bishop M, Abraham E (1993) Hemodynamic and oxygen transport monitoring to titrate therapy in septic shock. New Horizons 1:145–159
26. Shoemaker WC, Appel PL, Kram HB, Duarte D, Harrier D, Ocampo HA (1989) Comparison of hemodynamic and oxygen transport effects of dopamine and dobutamine in critically ill surgical patients. Chest 96:120–126
27. Vincent JL, Van der Linden P, Domb M, Blecic S, Azimi G, Bernard A (1987) Dopamine compared with dobutamine in experimental septic shock: Relevance to fluid administration. Anesth Analg 66:565–571

28. Vincent JL, Roman A, Kahn RJ (1990) Dobutamine administration in septic shock: Addition to a standard protocol. Crit Care Med 18:689-693
29. Silverman HJ, Tuma P (1992) Gastric tonometry in patients with sepsis. Effects of dobutamine infusions and packed red blood cell transfusions. Chest 102:184-188
30. Schneider AJ, Groeneveld ABJ, Teule GJJ, Nauta J, Heidendal GAK, Thijs LG (1987) Volume expansion, dobutamine and noradrenaline for treatment of right ventrikular dysfunction in porcine septic shock: A combined invasive and radionuclide study. Circ Shock 23: 93-106
31. Leier CV (1988) Regional blood flow responses to vasodilators and inotropes in congestive heart failure. Am J Cardiol 62:86E-93E
32. Mousdale S, Clyburn PA, Mackie AM, Groves ND, Rosen M (1988) Comparison of the effects of dopamine, dobutamine, and dopexamine upon renal blood flow: a study in normal healthy volunteers. Br J Clin Pharmac 25:555-560
33. Hayes MA, Timmins AC, Yau EHS, Palazzo M, Hinds CJ, Watson D (1994) Elevation of systemic oxygen delivery in the treatment of critically ill patients. N Engl J Med 330: 1717-1722
34. Shoemaker WC, Appel PL, Kram HB, Waxman K, Lee TS (1988) Prospective trial of supranormal values of survivors as therapeutic goals in high risk surgical patients. Chest 94: 1176-1186
35. Bland RD, Shoemaker WC, Abraham E, Cobo JC (1995) Hemodynamic and oxygen transport patterns in surviving and nonsurviving postoperative patients. Crit Care Med 13: 85-90
36. Shoemaker WC, Appel PL, Kram HB, Waxman K, Lee TS (1988) Prospective trial of supranormal values of survivors as therapeutic goals in high risk surgical patients. Chest 94: 1176-1186
37. Gutierrez G, Clark C, Brown SD, Price K, Ortiz L, Nelson C (1994) Effect of dobutamine on oxygen consumption and gastric mucosal pH in septic patients. Am J Respir Crit Care Med 150:324-329
38. Granger DN, Richardson PDI, Kvietys PR, Mortillaro NA (1980) Intestinal blood flow. Gastroenterology 78:837-863
39. Giraud GD, MacCannell KL (1984) Decreased nutrient blood flow during dopamine- and epinephrine-induced intestinal vasodilatation. J Pharm Exp Ther 230:214-220
40. Reilly FD, McCuskey RS, v Cilento E (1981) Hepatic microvascular regulatory mechanisms. I. Adrenergic mechanisms. Microvasc Res 21:103-116
41. Mills LC, Moyer JH, Handley CA (1960) Effects of various sympathicomimetic drugs on renal hemodynamics in normotensive and hypotensive dogs. Am J Physiol 198:1279
42. Shoemaker WC, Appel PL, Kram HB (1991) Oxygen transport measurements to evaluate tissue perfusion and titrate therapy: Dobutamine and dopamine effects. Crit Care Med 19: 672-688
43. Melchior JC, Pinaud M, Blanloeil Y, Bourreli B, Potel G, Souron R (1987) Hemodynamic effects of continious norepinephrine infusion in dog with and without hyperkinetic endotoxic shock. Crit Care Med 15:687-691
44. Bakker J, Vincent JL (1993) Effects of norepinephrine and dobutamine on oxygen transport and consumption in a dog model of endotoxic shock. Crit Care Med 21:425-432
45. Schreuder WO, Schneider AJ, Groeneveld ABJ, Thijs LG (1989) Effect of dopamine vs norepinephrine on hemodynamics in septic shock. Emphasis on right ventricular performance. Chest 95:1282-1288
46. Meadows D, Edwards JD, Wilkins RG, Nightingale P (1988) Reversal of intractable septic shock with norepinephrine therapy. Crit Care Med 16:663-666
47. Specht M, Meier-Hellmann A, Hannemann L, Spies C, Wirbelauer Ch, Heil Th, Reinhart K (1993) Effects of dobutamine vs norepinephrine therapy on oxygen supply and oxygen consumption in septic patients. Crit Care Med 21:S276
48. Desjars P, Pinaud M, Potel G, Tasseau F, Touze MD (1987) A reappraisal of norepinephrine in human septic shock. Crit Care Med 15:134-137
49. Hesselvik JF, Brodin B (1989) Low dose norepinephrine in patients with septic shock and oliguria: Effects on afterload, urine flow, and oxygen transport. Crit Care Med 17:179-180

50. Martin C, Eon B, Saux P, Aknin P, Gouin F (1990) Renal effects of norepinephrine used to treat septic shock patients. Crit Care Med 18:282–285
51. Redl-Wenzl EM, Armbruster C, Edelmann G, Fischl E, Kolacny M, Wechsler-Fördös A, Sporn P (1993) The effects of norepinephrine on hemodynamics and renal function in severe septic shock states. Intensive Care Med 19:151–154
52. Fukuoka T, Nishimura M, Imanaka H, Taenaka N, Yoshiya I, Takezawa J (1989) Effects of norepinephrine on renal function in septic patients with normal and elevated lactate levels. Crit Care Med 17:1104–1107
53. Bersten AD, Hersch M, Cheung H, Rutledge FS, Sibbald WJ (1992) The effect of various sympathomimetics on the regional circulations in hyperdynamic sepsis. Surgery 112:549–561
54. Baker CH, Wilmoth FR (1984) Microvascular responses to E. Coli endotoxin with altered adrenergic activity. Circ Shock 12:165–176
55. Gray GA, Furman BL, Parratt JR (1990) Endotoxin-induced impairment of vascular reactivity in the pithed rat: Role of arachidonic acid metabolites. Circ Shock 31:395–406
56. Hollenberg SM, Cunnion RE, Parrillo JE (1992) Effect of septic serum on vascular smooth muscle: In vitro studies using rat aortic rings. Crit Care Med 20:993–998
57. Kato T, Hayashi K, Takamizawa K (1988) Response of femoral arteries to norepinephrine following endotoxicosis. Circ Shock 26:383–390
58. Seaman KL, Greenway CV (1984) Loss of hepatic venous responsiveness after endotoxin in anesthetized cats. Am J Physiol 246:H658–H663
59. Breslow MJ, Miller CF, Parker SD, Walman AT, Traystman RJ (1987) Effect of vasopressors on organ blood flow during endotoxin shock in pigs. Am J Physiol 252:H291–H300
60. Marik PE, Mohedin M (1994) The contrasting effects of dopamine and norepinephrine on systemic and splanchnic oxygen utilization in hyperdynamic sepsis. JAMA 272:1354–1357
61. Bollaert PE, Bauer Ph, Audibert G, Lambert H, Larcan A (1990) Effects of epinephrine on hemodynamics and oxygen metabolism in dopamine-resistant septic shock. Chest 98:949–953
62. Lipman J, Roux A, Kraus P (1991) Vasoconstrictor Effects of Adrenaline in Human Septic Shock. Anaesth Intens Care 19:61–65
63. Mackenzie SJ, Kapadia F, Nimmo GR, Armstrong IR, Grant IS (1991) Adrenaline in treatment of septic shock: effects on hemodynamics and oxygen transport. Intensive Care Med 17:36–39
64. Innes IR, Nickerson M (1975) Norepinephrine, epinephrine and the sympathomimetic amines. In: Goodman LD, Gilman A (eds) The Pharmalogical Basis of Therapeutics. MacMillan, New York, pp 483–504
65. Moran JL, O'Fathartaigh MS, Peisach AR, Chapman MJ, Leppard Ph (1993) Epinephrine as an inotropic agent in septic shock: A dose-profile analysis. Crit Care Med 21:70–77
66. Haddy FJ, Chou CC, Scott JB, et al (1967) Intestinal vascular responses to naturally occurring vasoactive substances. Gastroenterology 52:444–451
67. Haddy FJ, Molnar JI, Borden CW, et al (1962) Comparison of direct effects of angiotensin, and other vasoactive agents on small and large blood vessels in several vascular beds. Circulation 25:239–246
68. Pawlik W, Shepherd AP, Jacobson ED (1975) Effects of vasoactive agents on intestinal oxygen consumption and blood flow in dogs. J Clin Invest 56:484–490
69. Greenway CV, Lawson A (1966) The effects of adrenaline and noradrenaline on venous return and regional blood flow in the anesthetized cat with special reference to intestinal blood flow. J Physiol (Lond) 187:579–595
70. Meier-Hellmann A, Hannemann L, Specht M, Schaffartzik W, Spies C, Reinhart K (1994) The relationship between mixed venous and hepatic venous O_2 saturation in patients with septic shock. In: Oxygen transport to tissues XV. Vaupel P (ed) Adv Exp Med Biol 345:701–707
71. Dahn MS, Lange P, Jacobs LA (1988) Central mixed and splanchnic venous oxygen saturation monitoring. Int Care Med 14:373–378
72. Kainuma M, Fujiwara Y, Kimura N, Shitaokoshi A, Nakashima K, Shimado Y (1991) Monitoring hepatic venous hemoglobin oxygen saturation in patients undergoing liver surgery. Anesthesiology 74:49–52

73. Meier-Hellmann A, Reinhart K, Bredle DL, et al (in press) Epinephrine impairs splanchnic perfusion in septic shock. Crit Care Med
74. Goldberg LI (1972) Cardiovascular and renal actions of dopamine. Potential clinical applications. Pharmacol Rev 24:1–29
75. Vincent JL, Preiser JC (1993) Inotropic agents. New Horizons 1:137–144
76. Nakatani T, Ishikawa Y, et al (1991) Hepatic mitochondrial redox state in hypotensive brain-dead patients and an effect of dopamine administration. Int Care Med 17:103–107
77. Lundberg J, Lundberg D, Norgren L, Ribbe E, Thörne J, Werner O (1990) Intestinal Hemodynamics during Laparotomy: Effects of Thoracic Epidural Anesthesia and Dopamine in Humans. Anesth Analg 71:9–15
78. Winsö O, Biber B, Martner J (1985) Does Dopamine Suppress Stress-Induced Intestinal and Renal Vasoconstriction? Acta Anaesthesiol Scand 29:508–514
79. Duke GJ, Briedis JH, Weaver RA (1994) Renal support in critically ill patients: Low dose dopamine or low dose dobutamine. Crit Care Med 22:1919–1925
80. Johnson DJ, Johannigman JA, Branson RD, Davis K, Hurst JM (1991) The Effect of Low Dose Dopamine on Gut Hemodynamics during PEEP Ventilation for Acute Lung Injury. J Surg Research 50:344–349
81. Townsend MC, Schirmer WJ, Schirmer JM, Fry DE (1987) Low-dose dopamine improves effective hepatic blood flow in murine peritonitis. Circ Shock 21:149–153
82. Pawlik W, Shepherd AP, Mailman D, Shanbour LL, Jacobson ED (1976) Effects of dopamine and epinephrine on intestinal blood flow and oxygen uptake. In: Grote J, Reneau D, Thews G (eds) Oxygen transport to the tissue – II. Plenum Press, New York London, pp 511–516
83. Kullmann R, Breull WR, Reinsberg J, Wassermann K, Konopatzki A (1983) Dopamine produces vasodilation in specific regions and layers of the rabbit gastrointestinal tract. Life Sciences 32:2115–2122
84. Roytblat L, Gelman S, Bradley EL, Henderson T, Parks D (1990) Dopamine and hepatic oxygen supply-demand relationship. Can J Physiol Pharmacol 1165–1169
85. Jackson LK, Key BM, Cain SM (1982) Total and hindlimb O_2 uptake and blood flow in hypoxic dogs given dopamine. Crit Care Med 10:327–331
86. Regan CJ, Duckworth R, Fairhurst JA, Maycock PF, Frayn KN, Campbell IT (1990) Metabolic effects of low-dose dopamine infusion in normal volunters. Clin Science 79:605–611
87. Ruttimann Y, Chidero R, et al (1989) Effects of dopamine on total oxygen consumption and oxygen delivery in healthy men. Am J Physiol 257:E541–546
88. Meier-Hellmann A, Reinhart K, Bredle DL, Specht M, Spies C, Hannemann L, Heiss-Dunlop W (1996) The effects of low-dose dopamine on splanchnic perfusion and oxygen uptake in patients with septic shock. Intensive Care Med (in press)
89. Baumann G, Gutting M, Pfafferott C, Ningel K, Klein G (1988) Comparison of acute haemodynamic effects of dopexamine hydrochloride, dobutamine and sodium nitroprusside in chronic heart failure. Eur Heart J 9:503–512
90. De Marco T, Kwasman M, Au D, Chatterjee K (1988) Dopexamine Hydrochloride in chronic congestive heart failure with improved cardiac performance without increased metabolic cost. Am J Cardiol 62:57C–62C
91. Parratt JR, Wainwright CL, Fagbemi O (1988) Effect of dopexamine hydrochloride in the early stages of experimental myocardial infarction and comparison with dopamine and dobutamine. Am J Cardiol 62:18C–23C
92. Svenson G, Strandberg LE, Lindvall B, Erhardt L (1988) Haemodynamic response to dopexamine hydrochloride in postinfarction heart failure: lack of tolerance after continuous infusion. Br Heart J 60:489–496
93. Tan LB, Littler A, Murray RG (1987) Beneficial haemodynamic effects of intravenous dopexamine in patients with low-output heart failue. J Cardiovasc Pharmacol 10:280–286
94. Colardyn FC, Vandenbogaerde JF, Vogelaers DP, Verbeke JH (1989) Use of dopexamine hydrochloride in patients with septic shock. Crit Care Med 17:999–1003
95. Cain SM, Curtis SE (1991) Systemic and regional oxygen uptake and delivery and lactate flux in endotoxic dogs infused with dopexamine. Crit Care Med 19:1552–1560

96. Biro GP, Douglas JR, Keon WJ, Taichman GC (1988) Changes in regional blood flow distribution induced by infusions of dopexamine hydrochloride or dobutamine in anesthetized dogs. Am J Cardiol 62:30C–36C
97. Lokhandwala MF, Jandhyala BS (1992) Effects of dopaminergic agonists on organ blood flow and function. Clin Int Care 3 (1) (Suppl):12–16
98. Uusaro A, Ruokonen E, Takala J (1995) Gastric mucosal pH does not reflect changes in splanchnic blood flow after cardiac surgery. Br J Anaesth 74:149–154
99. Smithies M, Yee TH, Jackson L, Beale R, Bihari D (1994) Protecting the gut and the liver in the critically ill: Effects of dopexamine. Crit Care Med 22:789–795
100. Boyd O, Grounds RM, Bennett ED (1993) A randomized clinical trial of the effect of deliberate perioperative increase of oxygen delivery on mortality in high-risk surgical patients. JAMA 270:2699–2707
101. Baumann G, Felix SB, Filcek SAL (1990) Usefulness of dopexamine hydrochloride versus dobutamine in chronic congestive heart failure and effects on hemodynamics and urine output. Am J Cardiol 65:748–754
102. Gray PA, Bodenham AR, Park GR (1991) A comparison of dopexamine and dopamine to prevent renal impairment in patients undergoing orthotopic liver transplantation. Anaesthesia 46:638–641
103. Stephan H, Sonntag H, Henning H, Yoshimine K (1990) Cardiovascular and renal haemodynamic effects of dopexamine: comparison with dopamine. Brit J Anaesth 65:380–387
104. Magrini F, Foulds RA, Roberts N, Macchi G, Mondadori C, Zanchetti A (1988) Renal hemodynamic effects of dopexamine hydrochloride. Am J Cardiol 62:53C–56C
105. Shoemaker WC, Appel PL, Kram HB (1988) Tissue oxygen debt as a determinant of lethal and nonlethal postoperative organ failure. Crit Care Med 16:117–120
106. Tuchschmidt J, Fried J, Swinney R, et al (1989) Early hemodynamic correlations of survival in patients with septic shock. Crit Care Med 17:719–723
107. Hannemann L, Meier-Hellmann A, Specht M, Spies C, Reinhart K (1993) O_2-Angebot, O_2-Verbrauch und Mucosa pH-Wert des Magens. Anaesthesist 42:11–14

Extracorporeal Support

A. Pesenti and M. Bombino

Extracorporeal organ substitution can temporaneously support a failing organ, allowing to buy time for recovery or if recovery is not achievable can be used as a bridge to transplantation.

While extracorporeal substitution of renal function became a technology at hand of any critical care physician, cardiovascular and respiratory support are implemented only in specialized centers.

We will briefly review the rationale, indications and the techniques currently available focusing mainly on respiratory extracorporeal support.

A Historical Overview

Extracorporeal support technology has evolved over the last forty years Gibbon successfully performed the first open-heart surgical procedure in 1953 using total circulatory support by an extracorporeal pump oxygenation system [1]. During the following years this technology, named cardiopulmonary bypass (CPB), gained widespread acceptance and became a routine procedure for open-heart surgery.

Three methods of oxygenating blood have been used over the years [2]. The first, bubble oxygenation, stems from Brown-Sequard's observation that blood could be oxygenated if vigorously whipped with air: oxygen is bubbled through the blood, bubbles are then filtered out and the oxygenated blood is pumped back into the patient. A different method is applied in film oxygenators: a thin layer of blood is spread on a surface and exposed to oxygen. In both methods the occurrence of hemolysis due to the direct contact between the blood and the gaseous phases was the major time-limiting factor. The introduction of heparin in clinical practice and the pioneer observation of Kolff [3] that "blue blood turns red" through dialysis membranes opened the era of extracorporeal membrane oxygenation (ECMO), in which a synthetic semipermeable membrane acts as blood/gas interface for exchange of oxygen and carbon dioxide.

During the late '50s and '60s the ECMO investigation focused on the development of several "membrane oxygenators" looking for the best surface and design in terms of gas exchange and biocompatibility [4, 5]. The separation of the blood and gaseous phases by the oxygenator membrane decreased the blood components damage allowing longer perfusion times. Soon the application of extracorporeal support was extended to the long term assistance of patients with acute respiratory failure. ECMO was first applied to newborns with idiopathic respiratory failure; but the high incidence of intracranial bleeding was initially a major problem [6, 7]. Perfusions were then tried in adults and in 1971 Hill reported the first long-term ECMO survivors [8].

Indications for Extracorporeal Cardiac Assist

Beside the widespread use of CPB in the operating theatre, other clinical indications for temporary and even permanent cardiac assist have become evident. First, some patients cannot be weaned from cardiopulmonary bypass after open-heart surgery and require prolonged mechanical assist [9]. Cardiogenic shock following acute myocardial infarction carries a high mortality rate; some of these patients will benefit from combined aggressive pharmacological therapy and short-term cardiopulmonary support, in others the implementation of an extracorporeal assist will make safer invasive maneuvers such as cardiac catheterization and subsequent coronary artery surgery [10]. Acute overwhelming cardiac failure due to myocardial infarction or myocarditis is another indication for the temporary use of an assist device as a bridge to transplant [11]. The need for long term or permanent circulatory support devices is increasing. In 1985 the National Heart, Lung and Blood Institute (NIH), reported 17 000 to 35 000 candidates for heart transplant per year in the United States [12]; donor hearts availability is far less. Many patients die waiting a donor heart, possibly some of them would benefit from long term cardiac assist [13].

The different indications briefly outlined require different amount of extracorporeal assist. Therefore extracorporeal cardiac support ranges from short-term to permanent, partial or total assist device.

Intraaortic balloon pump (IABP) is an example of short term partial cardiovascular assist providing a cardiac output supplementation of 20–30% by counterpulsation. On the other end implementation of a veno-arterial bypass with a pump, either roller or centrifugal, accomplishes total temporaneous support of the circulation providing 5–6 liters of extracorporeal blood flow. Implantable ventricle assist devices (VAD) and total artificial hearts (TAH) are the other available techniques used for total cardiac assist as bridges to transplantation [13].

Rationale and Indications of Respiratory Extracorporeal Support

The idea of lung rest while buying time for lung to heal was one of the dreams of the extracorporeal perfusion teams as early as 1972 [14]. In the last years scientific evidences were gathered that mechanical ventilation, which is a life-saving maneuver in acute respiratory failure, can lead per se to pulmonary damage.

Adult respiratory distress syndrome (ARDS) is the term introduced by Asbaugh in 1967 to describe an acute form of respiratory failure characterized by severe hypoxemia, bilateral pulmonary infiltrates and decreased lung compliance [15]. Different insults can determine the initial diffuse lung injury, manifested as an increased permeability leading to interstitial edema and lung consolidation. A subsequent evolution towards a non homogeneous pattern is described in autoptic and radiographic studies. Different kinds of lesions, such as fibrosis, alveolar and/or interstitial edema, vascular occlusions, focal (secondary) sepsis, occur in the same lung [16]. CT scan morphologic studies suggest the presence of "normal" areas interspersed with well defined lung densities (collapse or consolidation), mainly localized in the dependent lung fields [17, 18]. The dependent collapsed regions are excluded from gas exchange and therefore are responsible for the refractory hypoxemia due to right to left shunt [19]. Some poorly aerated lung regions can indeed be recruited to gas exchange if an adequate opening-pressure is provided.

The size of the relatively normal part of ARDS lung, roughly estimated by the total static lung compliance (TSLC) measurement [20], can be compared to a "baby lung" [18]. This "baby lung" takes the entire burden of ventilation to accomplish the metabolic needs of an adult body.

Impairment of gas exchange in ARDS almost always requires intubation and mechanical ventilation.

Ventilators were introduced in clinical practice to substitute respiration in the setting of neuromuscular impairment. These machines mainly pump air in and out the lungs providing CO_2 removal; control of inspired oxygen concentration (FiO_2) and manipulation of mean airway pressure are byproducts which act as aids to oxygenation.

An "ideal" artificial support should avoid further damage to organ structure. Both FiO_2 and airway pressures, the means to increase oxygenation through a ventilator, demonstrated major adverse effects on lung structure. In fact, even normal lungs exposed to high FiO_2 showed pathological lesions similar to those seen in ARDS [21–23] and experimental models of lung damage have been created utilizing high inspiratory volumes and pressures [24–26].

The deleterious effects of volume, pressure and FiO_2 will be even enhanced on an already damaged lung structure. This iatrogenic damage is known under the name of barotrauma, or volotrauma [27–30]. Tidal volume is mainly directed toward the more compliant but relatively small residual healthy areas ("baby lung"), causing local hyperventilation, known to adversely affect lung function and structure [31,32], and overdistention. Stretching of the "baby lung" is reflected by the upper inflection point on the TSLC curve [33]. New mechanical ventilation strategies have been recently proposed to titrate tidal ventilation to the size of the "baby lung". Low-tidal volume pressure-limited ventilation leading to permissive hypercapnia is now widely applied in severe ARDS [34]; it reduces but it does not completely abolish the volotrauma to the residual healthy lung.

Mechanical ventilation with positive airway pressure is a life saving supportive maneuver in most ARDS cases, but gas exchange is maintained through overdistension, stretching and ripping of the residual healthy portions of the ARDS lungs. The appropriate artificial organ for respiratory insufficiency is indeed an ideal membrane lung, capable of substituting the gas exchange function of the natural lungs without major side effects.

ECLS Technique

Whichever organ need substitution, extracorporeal support connotes the implementation of an extracorporeal perfusion through cannulae introduced into veins or arteries. Exposure of blood to artificial surfaces requires some kind of anticoagulation to prevent clot formation; anticoagulation, mainly achieved with heparin, carries the risk of bleeding.

Current techniques are fully described elsewhere [35].

Different acronyms have been used in the literature to outline some aspects of the extracorporeal techniques (Extracorporeal Membrane Oxygenation, ECMO; Extracorporeal CO_2 removal, $ECCO_2R$; Extracorporeal Lung Assist, ECLA). We need to stress that a comprehensive description of a extracorporeal circulation and pulmonary support comprises:

1. The vascular access used, veno-arterial (V-A) or veno-venous (V-V). In V-A bypasses the artificial lung works in parallel with the natural lung, the amount of blood directed to the artificial lung will not perfuse the natural lung. In V-V bypasses the artificial lung is placed in series with the natural one, all the cardiac output perfuses the natural lung. V-A bypasses provide also circulation assist.
2. The amount of extracorporeal blood flow (ECBF) as a proportion of cardiac output (CO). The greater the ECBF/CO ratio (high-flow bypass), the greater is the contribution of the extracorporeal system to the oxygenation.
3. The ventilatory management of the patient's lung.

When extracorporeal support of gas exchange was introduced in clinical practice the ventilatory management of the natural lung didn't achieve "lung rest". During the ECMO trial funded by the NIH [36], the main goals were to maximize oxygenation through the extracorporeal system and to decrease the pulmonary hypertension, therefore a high flow veno-arterial bypass (ECBF of approximately 60–80% of the cardiac output) was preferred. A reduction of FiO_2 was achieved, but patient's lung ventilation was slightly modified from pre bypass setting [37]. 90 patients were enrolled into the ECMO study: 48 were randomized to conventional mechanical ventilation and 4 of them survived (8%); 42 were randomized to receive ECMO plus mechanical ventilation and 4 patients survived (10%) [38].

The different approach proposed by Kolobow and Gattinoni focused to achieve "lung rest" by low frequency ventilation and apneic oxygenation, extracorporeal support was required to completely remove the CO_2 produced, therefore a low-flow veno-venous bypass needed to be implemented [39–42]. A scheme of the $ECCO_2R$ system is depicted in Fig. 1.

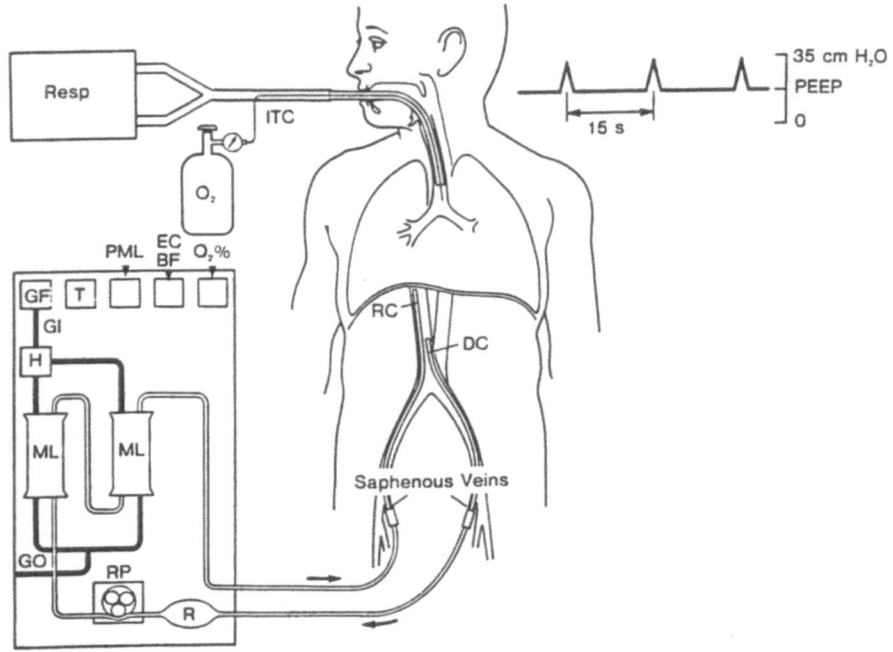

Fig. 1. ECCO$_2$R system.
DC: blood drainage catheter; *ECBF:* extracorporeal blood flow; *GF:* gas flowmeters; *GI:* gas inlet; *GO:* gas outlet; *H:* humidifier; *ITC:* intratracheal catheter; *ML:* membrane lung; *O$_2$%:* venous drainage blood oxygen monitor; *PML:* membrane lung pressure, in–out; *R:* venous reservoir; *RC:* blood return catheter; *Resp:* respirator; *RP:* roller pump; *PEEP:* positive end expiratory pressure; *T:* ambient temperature control. (From [47])

Clinical Results

The reported European experience with extracorporeal support for ARDS in the last 25 years account to 615 patients with 327 survivors. Similar results are reported in the adult population in U.S. and in Japan [43].

Starting from 1980 we supported 104 ARDS patients. During the years the entry criteria for extracorporeal support have been evolving. New supportive means to enhance gas exchange in ARDS patients, nitric oxide, permissive hypercapnia etc., lead to a decrease need for extracorporeal support. In the meantime we introduced some technical innovations to reduce the risk of bleeding and to simplify the technique [44–46]. The evolution of our experience is exemplified in Fig. 2.

Our current population differs from the previous one mainly for the ventilatory parameters before institution of extracorporeal support (Fig. 3). Higher PaCO$_2$ values are not only the result of the introduction of permissive hypercapnia to avoid volotrauma pre bypass, but reflect a profound derangement of lung compliance and in gas exchange.

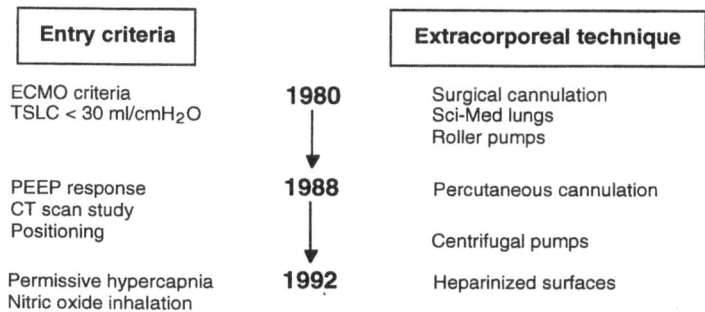

Entry criteria		Extracorporeal technique
ECMO criteria TSLC < 30 ml/cmH₂O	**1980**	Surgical cannulation Sci-Med lungs Roller pumps
PEEP response CT scan study Positioning	**1988**	Percutaneous cannulation Centrifugal pumps
Permissive hypercapnia Nitric oxide inhalation	**1992**	Heparinized surfaces

Fig. 2. Evolution of entry criteria and extracorporeal technique

All the centers performing extracorporeal support in ARDS report the need for high extracorporeal blood flow to support oxygenation during perfusions which may last weeks with a completely lost natural lung function (shunt fraction approximately 100%).

We also observed an increase in bypass length over the last years affecting both survivors and non survivors (Fig. 4). When we first reported our clinical results we divided the population in "responders" and "non responder" to the bypass [47]. "Responders" showed a brisk improvement in oxygenation over few days, all the survivors were "responders". Starting from 1989 however we observed some survivors showing improvement of their oxygenation and lung mechanics after some weeks of bypass.

Complications and Cause of Death

We had few technical complications on over 32000 hours of bypass. Bartlett pointed out that a skilled team need to be prepared and maintained through

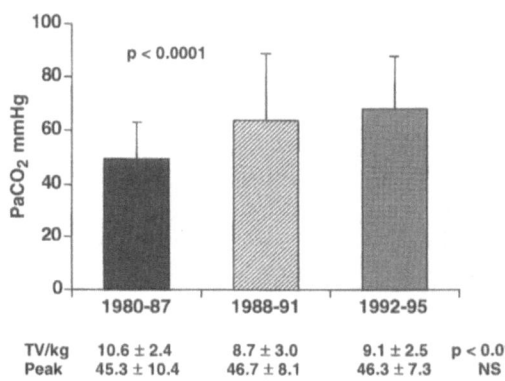

Fig. 3. Ventilatory parameters before bypass

		1980-87	1988-91	1992-95	
	TV/kg	10.6 ± 2.4	8.7 ± 3.0	9.1 ± 2.5	p < 0.01
	Peak	45.3 ± 10.4	46.7 ± 8.1	46.3 ± 7.3	NS

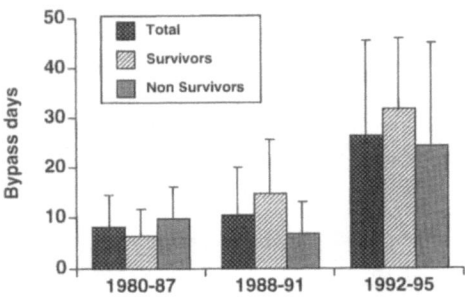

ANOVA F = 25.21 p < 0.0001   Fig. 4. Bypass length

experience gathered in the laboratory first and in clinical practice year after year [43].

The longer bypass length and the occurrence of haemolysis with heparinized centrifugal pumps (mean duration approximately 5–7 days) lead to frequent changes of extracorporeal circuits components in the same patient. If the patient is hemodynamically unstable or is almost completely dependent on extracorporeal support for oxygenation, we are used to modify the circuit inserting a second drainage line in parallel with is own pump and artificial lung, assuring in this way a continuous support also during the changes of circuit components [48]. In other centers a second parallel circuit is implemented from the beginning [49].

Bleeding complications have been always reported as the major side effect, sometimes life-threatening, of the necessary heparinization. We observed a significant drop in transfusions requirements with the introduction of percutaneous cannulation first and with heparinized circuits thereafter [50] (Table 1).

The need for a major surgical procedure (thoracotomy, laparotomy, etc.) during bypass carries high risk of life-threatening bleeding. We performed surgery in 24 patients (23%), out of whom 6 (25%) eventually survived. Also during surgery the use of heparinized surfaces, with the possibility to temporaneously stop heparin infusion lead to a decrease in transfusions need.

A life-threatening complication, intracranial hemorrhage (ICH) increased in incidence over the years. Risk factors identified in the 14 patients who developed

Table 1. Transfusions requirements (packed red blood cells ml/kg/day)

	Total	Surgery	NO Surgery
1980–1987 surgical cannulation	17.3 ± 14.1 (n = 52)	31.6 ± 21.4 (n = 11)	13.5 ± 8.2 (n = 41)
1988–1991 percutaneous cannulation	9.4 ± 10.2 (n = 23)	20.2 ± 18.2 (n = 5)	6.4 ± 3.5 (n = 18)
1992–1995 heparinized circuits	7.4 ± 5.4 (n = 22)	11.1 ± 6.2 (n = 8)	5.3 ± 3.6 (n = 14)

ANOVA F = 13.83; p < 0.0001

ICH were a $PaCO_2$ higher than 75 mmHg, DIC and a positive head CT scan before bypass it looks like the sickest patients are the most prone to develop ICH when exposed to systemic heparinization.

The major cause of death in our population is multiple organ failure and secondary sepsis. In our experience patients requiring two organ substitution (extracorporeal respiratory support and continuous hemofiltration or secondary implementation of V-A bypass for cardiac assist) have a very low survival rate.

Conclusions

While extracorporeal support technology keeps evolving indications for extracorporeal life support are changing. The rationale for extracorporeal substitution of lung function in ARDS stems from the increased evidence that mechanical ventilators do harm the natural lung. In spite of the implementation of new supportive techniques (permissive hypercapnia, nitric oxide, almitrine) some patients still require extracorporeal support as a salvage technique. New applications of ECLS techniques, for examples in cardiopulmonary resuscitation, are in an early phase of development [51].

The role of extracorporeal gas exchange is already established in the neonatal population. The neonatal results arise from the comprehension of factors affecting survival and complications that lead to close entry criteria [52, 53].

The rationale of extracorporeal support as a mean to substitute the alveolar-capillary function allowing a non-harmful treatment of the diseased lung is well established also for the pediatric and adult population. We still need to learn more about ARDS to establish the correct place of extracorporeal gas exchange in its supportive treatment. In the meantime the efforts of the groups implementing ECLS techniques will hopefully provide new devices and materials that will expand the application of the principle.

References

1. Gibbon JH Jr (1954) Application of a mechanical heart and lung apparatus to cardiac surgery. Minnesota Medicine 37:171–180
2. Livesey SA, Lennox SC (1992) Historical aspects. In: Kay PH (ed) Techniques in extracorporeal circulation. 3rd edition. Butterworth-Heinemann, Oxford, England, pp 1–7
3. Kolff WJ, Berk HT Jr (1944) Artificial kidney: a dialyzer with a great area. Acta Med Scand 117:121
4. Clowes GHA Jr, Hopkins AL, Neville WE (1956) An artificial lung dependent upon diffusion of oxygen and carbon dioxide through plastic membranes. J Thoracic Surg 32 (5):630–637
5. Kolobow T, Bowman RL (1963) Construction and evaluation of an alveolar membrane artificial heart lung. Trans Am Soc Artif Intern Organs 9:238–243
6. Dorson W Jr, Baker E, Cohen ML, Mayer B, Molthan M, Trum D, Elgas R (1969) A perfusion system for infants. Trans Am Soc Artif Intern Organs 15:155–160
7. White JJ, Andrews HG, Risemberg H, Mazur D, Haller JA Jr (1971) Prolonged respiratory support in newborn infants with a membrane oxygenator. Surgery 70:288–296
8. Hill JB, O'Brian TG, Murray JJ, Dontigny L, Bramson ML, Osborn JJ, Gerbode F (1972) Prolonged extracorporeal oxygenation for acute post-traumatic respiratory failure (shock-lung syndrome). Use of the Bramson membrane lung. N Engl J Med 286:629–634

9. Pae WE Jr (1987) Temporary ventricular support. Current indications and results. Trans Am Soc Artif Intern Organs 33:4–7
10. Smalling RW, Sweeny M, Lachterman B, Hess MJ, Morris R, Anderson HV, Heibig J, Li G, Willerson JT, Frazier OH, Warnpler RK (1994) Transvalvular left ventricular assistance in cardiogenic shock secondary to acute myocardial infarction. JACC 23:637–644
11. Chiu RCJ, Riebman JB (1991) Mechanical left ventricular assist progress and new horizons. J Invest Surg 4:111–123
12. The Working Group on Mechanical Circulatory Support of the National Heart, Lung, and Blood Institute (1985) Artificial heart and assist devices: directions, needs, costs, societal, and ethical issues. US Dept of Health and Human Services, Public Health Service. Publication No NIW 85-2723. Washington, DC
13. Hill DJ (1989) Bridging to cardiac transplantation. Ann Thorac Surg 47:167–171
14. Zapol WM, Kitz RJ (1972) Buying time with the artificial lungs. New Engl J Med 286, 12:657–658
15. Ashbaugh DG, Bigelow DB, Petty TL, Levine B (1967) Acute respiratory distress in adults. Lancet 2:319–323
16. Zapol WM, Qvist J, Trelstad RL, Lemaire F (1992) Pathophysiological pathways of the adult respiratory distress syndrome. In: Tinker J, Zapol WM (eds) Care of the critically ill. 2nd Edition. Springer-Verlag, London, pp 435–455
17. Maunder RJ, Shuman WP, McHugh JW, Marglin SI, Butler J (1986) Preservation of normal lung regions in the adult respiratory distress syndrome. Analysis by computed tomography. JAMA 255:2463–2465
18. Gattinoni L, Pesenti A (1987) ARDS: the non-homogeneous lung; facts and hypothesis. Intensive and Crit Care Digest 6:1–3
19. Gattinoni L, Pesenti A, Bombino M, Baglioni S, Rivolta M, Rossi F, Rossi GP, Fumagalli R, Marcolin R, Mascheroni D, Torresin A (1988) Relationship between lung computed tomographic densities, gas exchange, and PEEP in acute respiratory failure. Anesthesiology 69:824–832
20. Gattinoni L, Pesenti A, Avalli L, Rossi F, Bombino M (1987) Pressure/volume curve of total respiratory system in acute respiratory failure. Computed tomographic scan study. Am Rev Respir Dis 136:730–736
21. Nash G, Blennerhasset JB, Pontoppidan H (1967) Pulmonary lesions associated with oxygen therapy and artificial ventilation. N Engl J Med 276:368–374
22. Deneke SM, Fanbourg BL (1982) Oxygen toxicity of the lung: an update. Br J Anaesth 54:737–749
23. Bryan CL, Jenkinson SG (1988) Oxigen toxicity. Clinics in Chest Medicine 9:141–152
24. Kolobow T, Moretti MP, Fumagalli R, Mascheroni D, Prato P, Chen V, Joris M (1987) Severe impairment in lung function induced by high peak airway pressure during mechanical ventilation. Am Rev Respir Dis 135:312–315
25. Kolobow T (1988) Acute respiratory failure. On how to injure healthy lungs (and prevent sick lungs from recovery). Trans Am Soc Artif Intern Organs 34:31–34
26. Dreyfuss D, Soler P, Basset G, Saumon G (1988) High inflation pressure pulmonary edema. Respective effects of high airway pressure, high tidal volume and positive end-expiratory pressure. Am Rev Respir Dis 137:1159–1164
27. Baeza OR, Wagner RB, Lowery BD, Gott VL (1975) Pulmonary hyperinflation. A form of barotrauma during mechanical ventilation. J Thorac Cardiovasc Surg 70:790–805
28. Churg A, Golden J, Fligiel S, Hogg JC (1983) Bronchopulmonary dysplasia in the adult. Am Rev Respir Dis 127:117–120
29. Slavin G, Nunn JF, Crow J, Doré CJ (1982) Bronchiolectasis – a complication of artificial ventilation. Brit Med J 285:931–934
30. Haake R, Schlichtig R, Ulstad DR, Henschen RR (1987) Barotrauma. Pathophysiology, risk factors, and prevention. Chest 91:608–613
31. Mascheroni D, Kolobow T, Fumagalli R, Moretti MP, Chen V, Buckhold D (1988) Acute respiratory failure following pharmacologically induced hyperventilation: an experimental animal study. Intensive Care Med 15:8–14

32. Kolobow T, Spragg R, Pierce J (1981) Massive pulmonary infarction during total cardiopulmonary bypass in unanesthetized spontaneously breathing lambs. Int J Artif Organs 4: 76–81

33. Roupie E, Dambrosio M, Servillo G, Mentec H, El Atrous S, Beydon L, Brun-Buisson C, Lemaire F, Brochard L (1995) Titration of tidal volume and induced hypercapnia in acute respiratory distress syndrome. Am J Respir Crit Care Med 152:121–128

34. Hickling KG, Henderson SJ, Jackson R (1990) Low mortality associated with low volume pressure limited ventilation with permissive hypercapnia in severe adult respiratory distress syndrome. Intensive Care Med 16:372–377

35. Gattinoni L, Pesenti A, Bombino M (1995) Artificial lung in acute respiratory failure. In "The thorax" 2nd edition, edited by C. Roussos, Marcel Dekker, Inc., New York, Part C Chapter 85:2521–2539

36. Protocol for extracorporel support for respiratory insufficiency, collaborative program (1974) National Heart, Lung and Blood Institute, Division of Lung Diseases. Bethesda, Maryland, May

37. National Heart Lung and Blood Institute, Division of Lung Diseases (1979) Extracorporeal support for respiratory insufficiency: A collaborative study in response to RFP-NHLI-73-20. National Heart Lung and Blood Institute, Bethesda, MD, pp 1–390

38. Zapol WM, Snider MT, Hill JD, Fallat RJ, Bartlett RH, Edmunds LH, Morris AH, Bagniewski A, Miller RG Jr (1979) Extracorporeal membrane oxygenation in severe acute respiratory failure. A randomized prospective study. JAMA 242:2193–2196

39. Gattinoni L, Pesenti A, Kolobow T, Damia G (1983) A new look at therapy of the adult respiratory distress syndrome: motionless lung. Int Anesthesiol Clin 21:97–117

40. Kolobow T, Gattinoni L, Tomlison TA, Pierce JE (1977) Control of breathing using an extracorporeal membrane lung. Anesthesiology 46:138–141

41. Kolobow T, Gattinoni L, Tomlison T, Pierce JE (1978) An alternative to breathing. J Thorac Cardiovasc Surg 75:261–266

42. Gattinoni L, Kolobow T, Tomlison T, Iapichino G, Samaja M, White D, Pierce J (1978) Low-frequency positive pressure ventilation with extracorporeal carbon dioxide removal (LFPPV-ECCO$_2$R): an experimental study. Anesth Analg 57:470–477

43. Bartlett RH, DeLosh T, Tracey T (1995) Extracorporeal life support (ECLS) for adult respiratory failure: the North American experience. Int J Artif Organs 18:620–623

44. Pesenti A, Rossi GP, Pelosi P, Brazzi L, Gattinoni L (1990) Percutaneous extracorporeal CO$_2$ removal in a patient with bullous emphysema with recurrent bilateral pneumothoraces and respiratory failure. Anesthesiology 72:571–573

45. Bindslev L, Eklund J, Norlander O, Swedenborg J, Olsson P, Nilsson E, Larm O, Gouda I, Malmberg A, Scholander E (1987) Treatment of acute respiratory failure by extracorporeal carbon dioxide elimination performed with a surface heparinized artificial lung. Anesthesiology 67:117–120

46. Musch G, Verweij M, Bombino M, Banfi G, Fumagalli R, Pesenti A (1996) Small pore size microporous membrane oxygenator reduces plasma leakage during prolonged extracorporeal circulation: a case report. Int J Artif Organs 19:177–180

47. Gattinoni L, Pesenti A, Mascheroni D, Marcolin R, Fumagalli R, Rossi F, Iapichino G, Romagnoli G, Uziel L, Agostoni A, Kolobow T, Damia G (1986) Low Frequency positive-pressure ventilation with extracorporeal CO$_2$ removal in severe acute respiratory failure. JAMA 256: 881–886

48. Verweij M, Bombino M, Mush G, Benini A, Marcolin R, Pesenti A (1996) Cardiopulmonary resuscitation (CPR) during substitution of deteriorated circuit elements in patients treated with long term ECCO$_2$R. 5th European Congress of Extracorporeal Life Support, June 26–29, Stockholm, Sweden, P 18, p 86

49. Borg UR, Reynolds HN, Habashi NM (1996) ECLA, ECMO, ECCO$_2$R: is your system safe? Part I: ECLA circuit. 5th European Congress of Extracorporeal Life Support, June 26–29, Stockholm, Sweden, 27a, p 58

50. Gattinoni L, Pesenti A, Bombino M, Pelosi P, Brazzi L (1993) Role of extracorporeal circulation in adult respiratory distress syndrome management. New Horizons 1:603–612

51. Hill J (1995) Adult emergency cardiopulmonary support systems. In: "ECMO – Extracorporeal cardiopulmonary support in critical care". Zwischenberger JB, Bartlett RH (eds) Extracorporeal Life Support Organization, Chapter 28:491–510
52. Bartlett RH, Roloff DW, Cornell RG, Andrews AF, Dillon PW, Zwischenberger JP (1985) Extracorporeal circulation in neonatal respiratory failure. A prospective randomized study. Pediatrics 76:479–487
53. Rosenberg EM, Seguin JH (1995) Selection criteria for use of ECLS in neonates. In: "ECMO – Extracorporeal cardiopulmonary support in critical care". Zwischenberger JB, Bartlett RH (eds) Extracorporeal Life Support Organization, Chapter 15:261–271

Subject Index

Springer-Verlag
and the Environment

We at Springer-Verlag firmly believe that an international science publisher has a special obligation to the environment, and our corporate policies consistently reflect this conviction.

We also expect our business partners – paper mills, printers, packaging manufacturers, etc. – to commit themselves to using environmentally friendly materials and production processes.

The paper in this book is made from low- or no-chlorine pulp and is acid free, in conformance with international standards for paper permanency.